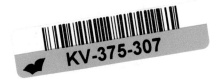

DERMATOLOGY: CLINICAL & BASIC SCIENCE SERIES

SENSITIVE SKIN SYNDROME

DERMATOLOGY: CLINICAL & BASIC SCIENCE SERIES

Series Editor Howard I. Maibach, M.D.

Published Titles:

Bioengineering of the Skin: Cutaneous Blood Flow and Erythema
Enzo Berardesca, Peter Elsner, and Howard I. Maibach

Bioengineering of the Skin: Methods and Instrumentation
Enzo Berardesca, Peter Elsner, Klaus P. Wilhelm, and Howard I. Maibach

Bioengineering of the Skin: Skin Biomechanics
Peter Elsner, Enzo Berardesca, Klaus-P. Wilhelm, and Howard I. Maibach

Bioengineering of the Skin: Skin Surface, Imaging, and Analysis
Klaus P. Wilhelm, Peter Elsner, Enzo Berardesca, and Howard I. Maibach

Bioengineering of the Skin: Water and the Stratum Corneum, Second Edition
Joachim W. Fluhr, Peter Elsner, Enzo Berardesca, and Howard I. Maibach

Contact Urticaria Syndrome
Smita Amin, Arto Lahti, and Howard I. Maibach

Cutaneous T-Cell Lymphoma: Mycosis Fungoides and Sezary Syndrome
Herschel S. Zackheim and Howard I. Maibach

Dermatologic Botany
Javier Avalos and Howard I. Maibach

Dermatologic Research Techniques
Howard I. Maibach

Dry Skin and Moisturizers: Chemistry and Function, Second Edition
Marie Lodén and Howard I. Maibach

The Epidermis in Wound Healing
David T. Rovee and Howard I. Maibach

Hand Eczema, Second Edition
Torkil Menné and Howard I. Maibach

Human Papillomavirus Infections in Dermatovenereology
Gerd Gross and Geo von Krogh

The Irritant Contact Dermatitis Syndrome
Pieter van der Valk, Pieter Coenrads, and Howard I. Maibach

Latex Intolerance: Basic Science, Epidemiology, and Clinical Management
Mahbub M. V. Chowdhry and Howard I. Maibach

Nickel and the Skin: Absorption, Immunology, Epidemiology, and Metallurgy
Jurij J. Hostýneck and Howard I. Maibach

Pesticide Dermatoses
Homero Penagos, Michael O'Malley, and Howard I. Maibach

Protective Gloves for Occupational Use, Second Edition
Anders Boman, Tuula Estlander, Jan E. Wahlberg, and Howard I. Maibach

Sensitive Skin Syndrome
Enzo Berardesca, Joachim W. Fluhr, and Howard I. Maibach

Skin Cancer: Mechanisms and Human Relevance
Hasan Mukhtar

Skin Reactions to Drugs
Kirsti Kauppinen, Kristiina Alanko, Matti Hannuksela, and Howard I. Maibach

DERMATOLOGY: CLINICAL & BASIC SCIENCE SERIES

SENSITIVE SKIN SYNDROME

Edited by

Enzo Berardesca
San Gallicano Dermatological Institute
Rome, Italy

Joachim W. Fluhr
Friedrich-Schiller University
Jena, Germany

Howard I. Maibach
University of California
San Francisco, California, U.S.A.

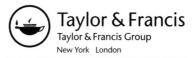

Taylor & Francis
Taylor & Francis Group
New York   London

Taylor & Francis is an imprint of the
Taylor & Francis Group, an informa business

Published in 2006 by
Taylor & Francis Group
270 Madison Avenue
New York, NY 10016

© 2006 by Taylor & Francis Group, LLC

No claim to original U.S. Government works
Printed in the United States of America on acid-free paper
10 9 8 7 6 5 4 3 2 1

International Standard Book Number-10: 0-8493-3058-0 (Hardcover)
International Standard Book Number-13: 978-0-8493-3058-2 (Hardcover)

This book contains information obtained from authentic and highly regarded sources. Reprinted material is quoted with permission, and sources are indicated. A wide variety of references are listed. Reasonable efforts have been made to publish reliable data and information, but the author and the publisher cannot assume responsibility for the validity of all materials or for the consequences of their use.

Library of Congress Cataloging-in-Publication Data

Catalog record is available from the Library of Congress

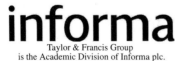

Taylor & Francis Group
is the Academic Division of Informa plc.

Visit the Taylor & Francis Web site at
http://www.taylorandfrancis.com

Preface

Sensitive skin is becoming a common clinical condition that dermatologists should be prepared to recognize, understand, and treat.

Subjects experiencing this condition report exaggerated reactions when their skin is in contact with cosmetics, soaps, and other substances, and they often report worsening after exposure to dry and cold climates. Sensitive skin and subjective irritation are widespread in western countries, but still far from being completely defined and understood. The development in these recent years of cosmetic sciences and in particular of cosmetic dermatology has provided solutions and answers to many needs of the dermatological patient with cosmetic problems; nevertheless, the management of sensitive skin is still a difficult task where the rate of patient dissatisfaction is tremendously high.

We hope with this book to give a deep overview on the main physiological basis of skin reactivity as well as on the many mechanisms which may generate this condition that to our understanding should be referred to as "sensitive skin syndrome."

Enzo Berardesca
Joachim W. Fluhr
Howard I. Maibach

Contents

Contributors

David A. Basketter   Safety and Environmental Assurance Centre, Unilever Colworth, Bedford, U.K.

Enzo Berardesca   San Gallicano Dermatological Institute, Rome, Italy

A. Bonfigli   Institute of Skin and Product Evaluation, Milan, Italy

Maria Breternitz   Department of Dermatology and Allergology, Friedrich-Schiller University, Jena, Germany

Manuela Carrera   San Gallicano Dermatological Institute, Rome, Italy

Carole Collard   Department of Dermatopathology, University Hospital Sart Tilman, Liège, Belgium

Sylvie Consoli   Cabinet Médical, Paris, France

Karen J. Cooper   Safety and Environmental Assurance Centre, Unilever Colworth, Bedford, U.K.

R. D'Agostino   Institute of Skin and Product Evaluation, Milan, Italy

F. Distante   Institute of Skin and Product Evaluation, Milan, Italy

Zoe Diana Draelos   Department of Dermatology, Wake Forest University School of Medicine, Winston-Salem, North Carolina, and Dermatology Consulting Services, High Point, North Carolina, U.S.A.

Patricia G. Engasser   Department of Dermatology, University of California, San Francisco, California, U.S.A.

Joachim W. Fluhr   Department of Dermatology and Allergology, Friedrich-Schiller University, Jena, Germany

Marina Goldovsky   Department of Dermatology, University of California, San Francisco, California, U.S.A.

Kathryn L. Hatch   Department of Agricultural and Biosystems Engineering, College of Agriculture and Life Sciences, University of Arizona, Tucson, Arizona, U.S.A.

Swen Malte John   Department of Dermatology, Environmental Medicine, Health Theory, University of Osnabrueck, Osnabrueck, Germany

Giovanni Leone   Phototherapy Unit, San Gallicano Dermatologic Institute, IRCCS, Rome, Italy

Harald Löffler   Department of Dermatology, Philipp University of Marburg, Marburg, Germany

Howard I. Maibach   Department of Dermatology, University of California, San Francisco, California, U.S.A.

Marie C. Marriott   Safety and Environmental Assurance Centre, Unilever Colworth, Bedford, U.K.

Nicolas Martin   Département Santé Publique, Laboratoires Pierre Fabre, Boulogne, France

Francis McGlone   Department of Neurological Sciences, Liverpool University, Liverpool, U.K.

Laurent Misery   CHU Morvan, Service de Dermatologie, Brest, France

Eric Myon   Département Santé Publique, Laboratoires Pierre Fabre, Boulogne, France

Thérèse Nocera   Laboratoires Avène, Avène, France

Alessia Pacifico   Phototherapy Unit, San Gallicano Dermatologic Institute, IRCCS, Rome, Italy

Manisha J. Patel   Department of Dermatology, Wake Forest University Health Sciences Center, Winston-Salem, North Carolina, U.S.A.

Marc Paye   Colgate-Palmolive R&D, Milmort, Belgium

Lisa Peters   Safety and Environmental Assurance Centre, Unilever Colworth, Bedford, U.K.

Gérald E. Piérard   Department of Dermatopathology, University Hospital Sart Tilman, Liège, Belgium

Claudine Piérard-Franchimont   Department of Dermatopathology, University Hospital Sart Tilman, Liège, Belgium

David Reilly   Life Sciences Group, Unilever Research & Development, Colworth, U.K.

L. Rigano   Institute of Skin and Product Evaluation, Milan, Italy

Michael K. Robinson   Procter & Gamble Company, Cincinnati, Ohio, U.S.A.

Martin Schmelz   Department of Anesthesiology and Intensive Care Medicine, Faculty of Clinical Medicine Mannheim, University of Heidelberg, Mannheim, Germany

Päivikki Susitaival   Department of Dermatology, North Karelia Central Hospital, Joensuu, Finland

Charles Taieb   Département Santé Publique, Laboratoires Pierre Fabre, Boulogne, France

Emmanuelle Xhauflaire-Uhoda   Department of Dermatopathology, University Hospital Sart Tilman, Liège, Belgium

Gil Yosipovitch   Department of Dermatology, Neurobiology, and Anatomy, Wake Forest University Health Sciences Center, Winston-Salem, North Carolina, U.S.A.

1

What Is Sensitive Skin?

Enzo Berardesca
San Gallicano Dermatological Institute, Rome, Italy

Joachim W. Fluhr
*Department of Dermatology and Allergology, Friedrich-Schiller University,
Jena, Germany*

Howard I. Maibach
*Department of Dermatology, University of California, San Francisco,
California, U.S.A.*

Sensitive skin is a condition of subjective cutaneous hyperreactivity to environmental factors. Subjects experiencing this condition report exaggerated reactions when their skin is in contact with cosmetics, soaps, and sunscreens, and they often report worsening after exposure to dry and cold climates.

Although no sign of irritation is commonly detected, itching, burning, stinging, and a tight sensation are constantly present. Generally, substances that are not commonly considered irritants are involved in this abnormal response. They include many ingredients of cosmetics such as dimethyl sulfoxide, benzoyl peroxide preparations, salicylic acid, propylene glycol, amyldimethylaminobenzoic acid, and 2-ethoxyethyl methoxycinnamate (1).

Sensitive skin and subjective irritation are widespread but still far from being completely defined and understood.

Burckhardt (2) hypothesized a correlation between sensitive skin and constitutional anomalies and/or other triggering factors such as occupational skin diseases or chronic exposure to irritants. On the other hand, Bjornberg (3) supported that no constitutional factors play a role in the pathogenesis of sensitive skin, although the presence of dermatitis demonstrates a general increase in skin reactivity to primary irritants lasting months.

Actually, sensitive skin is considered a category identified as being hypersensitive to stimuli—an increased permeability of the stratum corneum and acceleration of the nerve response in skin are considered to be involved (4). Hyperreactors may have a thinner stratum corneum with a reduced corneocyte area, causing higher transcutaneous penetration of water-soluble chemicals (5). Frosch and Kligman (6), by testing different irritants, showed a 14% incidence of sensitive skin in the normal population likely correlated to a thin permeable stratum corneum, which makes these subjects more susceptible to chemical irritation.

Moreover, the declined barrier function in sensitive skin has already been reported as the result of an imbalance of intercellular lipid of stratum corneum (7). Although impaired barrier function is easily understood as a mechanism of sensitive skin, other factors are also possible—implications such as changes in the nerve system and/or the structure of the epidermis. In a recent study (4), detailed characteristics of sensitive skin have been investigated using non-invasive methods. Sensitive skin has been classified into three different types on the basis of their physiological parameters. Type I has been defined as the low-barrier function group. Type II has been defined as the inflammation group with normal barrier function and inflammatory changes. Type III has been specified as the pseudo-healthy group in terms of normal barrier function and no inflammatory changes. In all types, a high content of nerve growth factor has been observed in the stratum corneum, relative to that of non-sensitive skin. Both in Types II and III, the sensitivity to electrical stimuli was high. As these data suggest, the hypersensitive reaction of sensitive skin is closely related to nerve fibers innervating the epidermis.

EPIDEMIOLOGY

Many epidemiologic studies have been carried out to assess whether or not a correlation with sex, age, skin type, or race could be found (8). Contradictory findings have been reported. Some authors (8–10) documented a higher reactivity to irritants mostly in females; some others noted that male subjects were directionally or significantly more reactive than female (11). Other experimental studies did not confirm this observation. Bjornberg (12), using six different irritants by patch test application, found no sex-related differences. Moreover, Lammintausta et al. (13), studying the response to open and patch test application of sodium lauryl sulfate (SLS), found mild interindividual variations in transepidermal water loss (TEWL) and dielectric water content values, but no sex-related differences in the reaction pattern.

In 1982, Frosch and Wissing (14), using dimethylsulfoxide, demonstrated a correlation between the minimal erythema dose (MED) and the response to irritants—the higher the inflammation, the lower the MED. Subsequently, a correlation between skin reactivity and skin type was reported—higher reactions were detected in subjects with skin Type I (15). However, in a total of 110 subjects covering all six skin types, the SLS dose–response generated by applying the substance under four-hour occlusion demonstrated that there was no significant difference between the groups. Even for Type VI skin, the dose–response curve fell within the general pattern (16). In fact, conflicting findings have been reported on the incidence of allergic contact dermatitis in different races (17–20). Although there is a clinical consensus that Blacks are less reactive and Asians are more reactive than Caucasians, the data supporting this hypothesis rarely reach statistical significance (21). Conflicting data have also been found on subjective (sensory) irritation. Frosch and Kligman (22) reported that most common "stingers" were light-complexioned persons of Celtic ancestry who sunburned easily and tanned poorly. Grove et al. (23) found no skin type propensity to stinging. He noted that increased stinging was related mainly to the person's history of sensitivity to soaps, cosmetics, and drugs. Arakami et al. (20) instead found no significant differences after SLS testing, but significant subjective sensory differences between Japanese and German women. So they concluded that Japanese women may complain about stronger sensations, reflecting a different cultural behavior rather than measurable differences in skin physiology; however, a faster penetration of SLS in Japanese cannot be excluded.

Moreover, skin reactivity is enhanced in eczema (24). Studies performed on animal models demonstrated that strong irritant reactions in guinea pigs significantly reduced the threshold of skin irritation (25). In contrast, hyporeactive states may be induced by skin treatment. Subclinical dermatitis, after repeated cutaneous irritation by open application, may induce skin hyporeactivity (26). This can also be one of the mechanisms of false-negative patch test.

Skin reactivity seems also to change depending on age, although contradictory findings are reported in the literature. For example, Nilzen and Voss Lagerlund (27) reported higher reactivity patch test reactions to soaps and detergents in the elderly, whereas Bettley and Donoghue (28) reported a lower reactivity in the same group. Coenraads et al. (29) demonstrated a higher skin reactivity to croton oil in the older patient group, but no differences by testing thimochinone or croton aldehyde. In 1993, Grove (30), by testing croton oil, cationic and anionic surfactants, weak acids, and solvents, reported a lower susceptibility in older subjects in terms of less severe skin reactions. Recently, Robinson (8) confirmed this lower reactivity; in fact, in his study, the oldest age cluster of subjects (56–74 years of age) was directionally or significantly less reactive than the younger age clusters. Moreover, Wohrl et al. (11) noted that although the rate of positive reactions to nickel and thimerosal decreased with age, fragrance mix and metallic mercury reactions stayed at the same level throughout all ages. The overall sensitization rate was highest in children less than 10 years old and decreased steadily, to be lowest among patients more than 70 years.

Patients over 70 years of age seem to have a reduced inflammatory response either to chemical irritants or to irritation induced by ultraviolet (UV) light (31). The ultraviolet B (UVB)-induced irritation, increased in both TEWL and DNA synthesis, was significantly diminished, with decreased epidermal hyperplasia evident in intrinsically aged versus young mouse epidermis (32).

In contrast, following skin irritation, increased TEWL values were recorded in the older subjects compared with the young. This finding could be related to a deficient "early warning detection system" in the elderly. Moreover, the skin of women in menopause becomes more sensitive to various environmental threats. It has been reported that the skin gets more sensitive in women at the beginning of menopause. This can be due to the fact that at this stage the skin becomes thinner, with a decrease of its function as a barrier that leads to a higher percutaneous absorption (33).

CLINICAL PARAMETERS

Sensitive skin can be defined in both subjective and objective terms. Subjective perceptions of sensitive skin are derived from patient observations regarding stinging, burning, pruritus, and tightness, following various environmental stimuli. Because of the lack of clinical signs, the phenomenon of sensitive skin is difficult to document. Attempts to identify clinical parameters in subjects with subjective irritation indicate that these individuals tend to have a less hydrated, less supple, more erythematous, and more teleangiectatic skin, compared with the normal population. In particular, significant differences were found for erythema and hydration/dryness (34).

CONCLUSIONS

Sensitive skin represents a widespread condition of susceptibility to exogenous factors. To find an effective approach to improve sensitive skin, it is important to know the detailed mechanism of sensitive skin. The reason why some subjects react with subjective symptoms such as itching, burning, stinging, prickling, or tingling is unclear. An increased permeability of the stratum corneum and acceleration of the nerve response in skin are considered to be involved (4). Approximately 40% of the population consider themselves to possess the characteristics of sensitive skin, and 50% of these patients with sensitive skin demonstrate these uncomfortable symptoms without accompanying visible signs of inflammation (35). Non-invasive evaluation of sensitive skin may successfully predict individual susceptibility to cosmetic-related adverse reaction. All the efforts in this direction appear undoubtedly important to improve tolerance to the majority of cosmetic products. Moreover, if sensitive skin involves several different causes, skin treatment must be selected to fit each mechanism. An appropriate approach to improve the sensitivity of skin should be taken considering the different mechanisms of skin sensitivity among various skin types.

REFERENCES

1. Amin S, Engasser PG, Maibach HI. Side-effects and social aspects of cosmetology. In: Baran R, Maibach HI, eds. Textbook of Cosmetic Dermatology. London: Martin Dunitz, 1993:205.
2. Burckhardt W. Praktische und theoretische bedeutung der alkalineutralisation und alkaliresistenzproben. Arch Klin Exp Derm 1964; 219:600.
3. Bjornberg A. Skin reactions to primary irritants in patients with hand eczema. Thesis, Isaccsons, Goteborg, 1968.
4. Yokota T et al. Classification of sensitive skin and development of a treatment system appropriate for each group. IFSCC Magazine 2003; 6:303.
5. Berardesca E et al. In vivo transcutaneous penetration of nicotinates and sensitive skin. Contact Dermatitis 1991; 25:35.
6. Frosch PJ, Kligman AM. A method for appraising the stinging capacity of topically applied substances. J Cosmet Sci 1977; 28:197.
7. Ohta M, Hikima R, Ogawa T. Physiological characteristics of sensitive skin classified by stinging test. J Cosmet Sci Soc Jpn 2000; 23:163.
8. Robinson MK. Population differences in acute skin irritation responses. Contact Dermatitis 2002; 46:86.
9. Agrup G. Hand eczema and other hand dermatoses in South Sweden. Academic Dissertation. Acta Derm Venereol 1969; 49(suppl 161).
10. Fregert S. Occupational dermatitis in 10 years material. Contact Dermatitis 1975; 1(96):107.
11. Wohrl S, Hemmer W, Focke M, et al. Patch testing in children, adults, and the elderly: influence of age and sex on sensitization patterns. Pediatr Dermatol 2003; 20:119.
12. Bjornberg A. Skin reactions to primary irritants in men and women. Acta Derm Venereol 1975; 55:191.
13. Lammintausta K, Maibach HI, Wilson D. Irritant reactivity in males and females. Contact Dermatitis 1987; 17:276.
14. Frosch P, Wissing C. Cutaneous sensitivity to ultraviolet light and chemical irritants. Arch Derm Res 1982; 272:269.
15. Lammintausta K, Maibach HI, Wilson D. Susceptibility to cumulative and acute irritant dermatitis: an experimental approach in human volunteers. Contact Dermatitis 1988; 19:84.
16. McFadden JP, Wakelin SH, Basketter DA. Acute irritation thresholds in subjects with type I skin. Contact Dermatitis 1998; 38:147.
17. Berardesca E, Maibach H. Ethnic skin: overview of structure and function. J Am Acad Dermatol 2003; 48:S139.
18. Berardesca E, Maibach HI. Contact dermatitis in blacks. Dermatol Clin 1998; 6:363.
19. Robinson MK. Racial differences in acute and cumulative skin irritation responses between Caucasian and Asian populations. Contact Dermatitis 2000; 42:134.
20. Arakami J et al. Differences of skin irritation between Japanese and European women. Br J Dermatol 2002; 146:1052.
21. Modjtahedi SP, Maibach HI. Ethnicity as a possible endogenous factor in irritant contact dermatitis: comparing the irritant response among Caucasian, Blacks and Asians. Contact Dermatitis 2002; 47:272.
22. Frosch P, Kligman AM. A method for appraising the stinging capacity of topically applied substances. J Soc Cosmet Chem 1981; 28:197.

23. Grove GL, Soschin DM, Kligman AM. Adverse subjective reactions to topical agents. In: Drill VA, Lazar P, eds. Cutaneous Toxicology. New York: Raven Press, 1984:200–210.

24. Bettley FR. Non-specific irritant reactions in eczematous subjects. Br J Dermatol 1964; 76:116.

25. Roper SS, Jones EH. An animal model for altering the irritability threshold of normal skin. Contact Dermatitis 1985; 13:91.

26. Lammintausta K, Maibach HI, Wilson D. Human cutaneous irritation: induced hyporeactivity. Contact Dermatitis 1987; 17:193.

27. Nilzen A, Voss Lagerlund K. Epicutaneous tests with detergents and a number of other common allergens. Dermatologica 1962; 124:42.

28. Bettley FR, Donoghue E. The irritant effect of soap upon the normal skin. Br J Dermatol 1960; 72:67.

29. Coenraads PJ, Bleumink E, Nofer JP. Susceptibility to primary irritants: age dependence. Contact Dermatitis 1975; 1:377.

30. Grove GL. Age-associated changes in integumental reactivity. In: Léveque JL, Agache PG, eds. Aging Skin: Properties and Functional Changes. New York: Marcel Dekker, 1993:189.

31. Haratake A et al. Intrinsically aged epidermis displays diminished UVB-induced alterations in barrier function associated with decreased proliferation. J Invest Dermatol 1997; 108:319.

32. Gilchrest BA, Stoff JS, Soter NA. Chronologic aging alters the response to ultraviolet-induced inflammation in human skin. J Invest Dermatol 1982; 79:11.

33. Paquet F et al. Sensitive skin at menopause; dew point and electrometric properties of the stratum corneum. Maturitas 1998; 28:221.

34. Seidenari S, Francomano M, Mantovani L. Baseline biophysical parameters in subjects with sensitive skin. Contact Dermatitis 1998; 38:311.

35. Simion FA, Rau AH. Sensitive skin. Cosmet Toiletries 1994; 109:43.

2

The Somatosensory System

Francis McGlone

Department of Neurological Sciences, Liverpool University, Liverpool, U.K.

David Reilly

Life Sciences Group, Unilever Research & Development, Colworth, U.K.

SOMATOSENSATION

The primary sensory modality subserving the body senses is collectively described as the somatosensory system, and comprises all those peripheral afferent nerve fibers and specialized receptors subserving proprioceptive (joint, muscle) and cutaneous sensitivity. The former processes information about limb position and muscle forces which the central nervous system (CNS) uses to monitor and control limb movements and, via elegant feedback and feedforward mechanisms, ensures that a planned action or movement is executed fluently. This chapter will focus on sensory inputs arising from the skin surface—cutaneous sensibility—and describe the neurobiological processes that enable the skin to be "sensitive." Skin sensations are multimodal and are classically described as subserving the three submodalities of touch, temperature, and pain. We will also consider the growing evidence for a fourth submodality, present only in hairy skin, that is preferentially activated by slowly moving, low force, mechanical stimuli.

This brief introduction to somatosensation will start with the discriminative touch system. The component that is relayed via the spinal cord includes the entire body from the neck down; information from the face is relayed by cranial nerves, but both parts of this system share a common central organization. Sensation enters the periphery via sensory axons that have their cell bodies sitting just outside the spinal cord in the dorsal root ganglia, with one ganglion for each spinal nerve root. Neurons are the building blocks of the nervous system and somatosensory neurons are unique in that, unlike most neurons, the electrical signal does not pass through the cell body but the cell body sits off to one side, without dendrites, the signal passing directly from the distal axon process to the proximal process which enters the dorsal half of the spinal cord, and immediately turns up the spinal cord forming a white matter column, the dorsal columns, which relay information to the first brain relay nucleus in the medulla. These axons are called the primary afferents because they are the same axons that carry the signal into the spinal cord. Sensory input from the face does not enter the spinal cord, but instead enters the brainstem via the trigeminal nerve (one of the cranial nerves). Just as with inputs from the body, there are three modalities of touch, temperature, and pain with each modality having different receptors traveling along different tracts projecting to different targets in the brainstem. Once the pathways synapse in the brainstem, they join the pathways from the body on their way up to the thalamus and higher cortical structures. Sensory information arising from the skin is represented in the brain in the primary and secondary somatosensory cortices, where the contralateral body surfaces are mapped in each hemisphere. In line with other sensory modalities, information is then fed forward to higher-order neural systems controlling perception, recognition, attention, and emotion, as well as systems that integrate this information with other sensory modalities, such as vision, to enable the brain to maximize the information it receives from the senses about conditions in the external world.

THE PERIPHERAL NERVOUS SYSTEM

The skin is the most extensive and versatile organ of the body and in a fully grown adult it covers a surface area approaching 2 m^2. This surface, despite the comment made by a famous, now deceased, U.K. comedian, Spike Milligan: "Oh wonderful stuff is skin, It's the stuff that keeps you in!" is far more than just a passive barrier. Apart from its role in the etiology of "sensitive skin," the topic of this book, skin contains in excess of 2 million sweat glands and 5 million hairs that may be either fine vellous types covering all surfaces, apart from the soles of the feet and the palms of the hands (glabrous skin), or over 100,000 of the coarser type found on the scalp. Evidence is also emerging that non-glabrous skin contains a system of nerves that code specifically for the pleasant properties of touch. It consists of an outer, waterproof, stratified squamous epithelium of ectodermal origin—the epidermis—plus an inner, thicker, supporting layer of connective tissue of mesodermal origin—the dermis. The thickness of this layer, and thereby its susceptibility to irritation, varies from 0.5 mm over the eyelid to >5.0 mm over the palm and sole of the foot.

Touch

Most primate research into skin-sensory processing has focused on the glabrous surface of the hand, in particular, the digits, and a description of this somatic site will provide a good general understanding of somatosensation (1–6). Of the three "classical" submodalities of the somatosensory system, discriminative touch subserves the perception of pressure, vibration, and texture and relies upon four different receptors in the digit skin—(1) Meissner's corpuscles, (2) Pacinian corpuscles, (3) Merkel's discs, and (4) Ruffini endings—collectively known as low-threshold mechanoreceptors (LTMs), a class of cutaneous receptors that are specialized to transduce mechanical forces impinging the skin into nerve impulses (Fig. 1). The first two are classified as fast adapting (FA) as they only respond to the initial and final contacts of a mechanical stimulus on the skin, and the second two are classified as slowly adapting (SA) as they continue firing during a constant mechanical stimulus. A further classification relates to the LTMs' receptive field (RF), that is, the surface area of skin to which they are sensitive. The RF is determined by the LTMs' anatomical location within the skin with those near the surface at the dermal/epidermal boundary, Meissner's corpuscles and Merkel's discs, having small RFs, and those lying deeper within the dermis, Pacinian corpuscles and Ruffini endings, having large RFs (Fig. 1).

Psychophysical procedures have been traditionally employed to study the sense of touch and, as in hearing research where the sensory receptor is another type of specialized mechanoreceptor, different frequencies of vibration are used to quantify the response properties of this sensory system. Von Bekesy (7) was the first to use vibratory stimuli as an extension of his research interests in audition. In a typical experiment, participants are asked to respond with a simple button-press when they can just detect the presence of a vibration presented to a digit within one of the two time periods. This two-alternative forced choice paradigm provides a threshold-tuning curve, the slopes of which provide information about a particular class of LTMs' response properties. As can be seen from Figure 2, a U-shaped function is generated, with increasingly lower detection thresholds being measured as vibrotactile frequency increases to a "peak" at around 300 Hz, at which point the curve begins to increase again as sensitivity decreases.

By carefully controlling the spatial configuration of the vibrating probe (i.e., its diameter and the gap between it and a static surround), the vibratory frequency, amplitude, stimulus duration, the skin surface temperature, and the use of various masking techniques, Bolanowski et al. (8) proposed that there are four distinct psychophysical channels mediating tactile perception in the glabrous skin of the hand. This model proposes that each psychophysically determined channel is represented by one of the four anatomical end organs and nerve fiber subtypes with frequencies in the 40 to 500 Hz range providing a sense of vibration, transmitted by Pacinian corpuscles (PC channel or FAI), Meissner corpuscles being responsible for the sense of "flutter" in the 2 to 40 Hz range

(A)

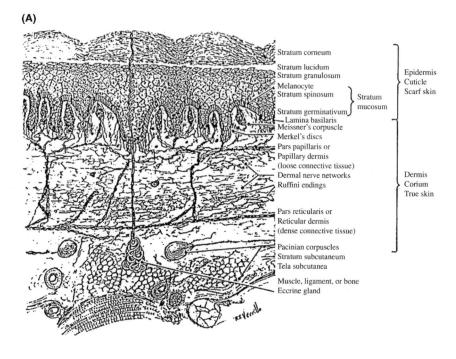

(B)

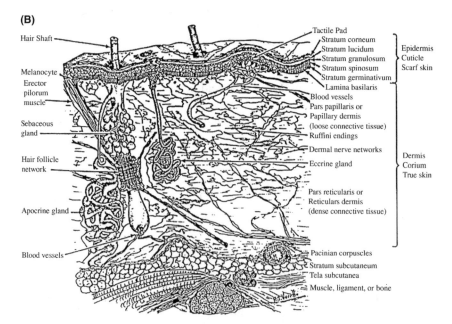

Figure 1   A cross-sectional perspective of glabrous (**A**) and hairy (**B**) skin.

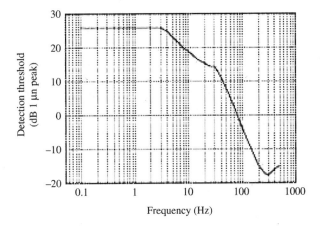

Figure 2 Absolute detection thresholds for sinusoidal stimuli (from Ref. 8) where it can be seen that as vibration frequency increases, detection thresholds decrease (note—log axes).

(NPI channel or FAII), the sense of "pressure" being mediated by Merkel's discs in the 0.4 to 2.0 Hz range (NPIII or SAI), and Ruffini end organs producing a "buzzing" sensation in the 100 to 500 Hz range (NPII or SAII). Neurophysiological studies have by and large supported this model, but there is still some way to go to link the anatomy with perception (refer to Table 1 for a summary of the properties of these LTMs).

There have been relatively few studies of tactile sensitivity on hairy skin, the cat being the animal of choice for most of these studies. Mechanoreceptive afferents (A-β fibers) have been described that are analogous to those found in

Table 1 Main Characteristics of Primary Sensory Afferents Innervating Human Skin

Class	Modality	Axonal diameter (μm)	CV (m/sec)
Myelinated			
A-α	Proprioceptors from muscles and tendons	20	120
A-β	LTMs	10	80
A-δ	Cold, noxious, thermal	2.5	12
Unmyelinated			
C-Pain	Noxious, heat, thermal	1	<1
C-Tactile	Light stroking, gentle touch	1	<1
C-Autonomic	Autonomic, sweat glands, vasculature	1	<1

Abbreviations: CV, conduction velocity; LTM, low-threshold mechanoreceptor.

human glabrous skin (FAI, FAII, SAI, and SAII) and Essick and Edin (9) have described sensory fibers with these properties in human facial skin. The relationship between these sensory fibers and tactile perception is still uncertain and this is exemplified by the response properties of SAI afferents. Harrington and Merzenich (10) have found that these afferents are responsive to levels of stimulation that are below perceptual thresholds and Jarvilehto et al. (11) describe high levels of activity in human hairy skin SAIs that are not perceivable, in contrast to the responses of this class of afferent in glabrous skin where SAI nerve activity is directly correlated with a sense of pressure.

Sensory axons are classified according to their degree of myelination, the fatty sheath that surrounds the nerve fiber. The degree of myelination determines the speed with which the axon can conduct nerve impulses and hence the conduction velocity (CV) of the nerves. The largest and fastest axons are called A-α and include some of the proprioceptive neurons, such as the muscle stretch receptors. The second largest group, called A-β, includes all the discriminative touch receptors being described here. Pain and temperature include the third and fourth groups, A-δ and C fibers, and will be dealt with in "Temperature" (Table 1).

Electrophysiological studies by Vallbo and Johansson (12), on single peripheral nerve fibers innervating the human hand, have provided a generally accepted model of touch that relates the four anatomically defined types of cutaneous or subcutaneous sense organs to their neural response patterns. The technique they employed and developed is called microneurography and involves inserting a fine tungsten microelectrode, of tip diameter <5 μm, through the skin of the wrist and into the underlying median nerve which innervates the thumb and first two digits. A sensitive biological amplifier records and amplifies the spike discharges conveyed by the axons and feeds these to a loudspeaker to enable the experimenter to hear the spike activity and "home-in" on a single unit. Skilled manual micromanipulation of the electrode, coupled with stroking across the hand to stimulate LTMs, results first in a population response being recorded, that is, neural activity in a nerve fascicle containing hundreds of peripheral axons until finally, sometimes after many hours, a single axon is isolated. At this stage, the RF of the single unit is mapped with a Von-Frey hair and the unit subtype (i.e., FA or SA) identified. Once this stage is completed, a small pulsed current of a few microamperes (typically <10 μA) is delivered to the nerve that provides a final, perceptual confirmation of the unit subtype. If, for example, an RA unit has been isolated, microstimulation is perceived as a "flutter" or "vibration," depending on the frequency of the electrical pulses, and is perceptually localized to the previously mapped RF. Figure 3 depicts the relationships between RF, adaptation rate, and unit type from studies carried out on the human hand (13).

Temperature

The cutaneous somatosensory system detects changes in ambient temperature over an impressive range, initiated when thermal stimuli that differ from a

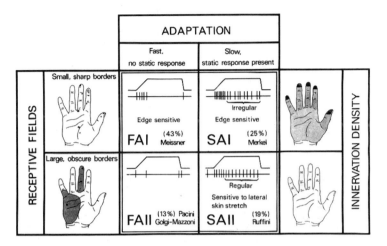

Figure 3 The four types of LTMs in human glabrous skin are depicted. The four panels in the center show the nerve-firing responses to a ramp-and-hold indentation and in % the frequency of occurrence and putative morphological correlate. The black dots in the left panel show the RFs of Type I (top) and Type II (bottom) afferents. The right panel shows the average density of Type I (top) and Type II (bottom) afferents with darker area depicting higher densities [after Westling, 1986 (13)]. *Abbreviations*: LTM, low-threshold mechanoreceptor; RF, receptive field.

homeostatic set-point excite temperature-specific sensory nerves in the skin, and relays this information to the spinal cord and brain. It is important to recognize that these nerves code for temperature change, not absolute temperature, as a thermometer does. The system does not have specialized receptor end organs such as those found with LTMs, but uses free nerve endings throughout the skin to sense changes in temperature. Within the innocuous thermal-sensing range, there are two populations of thermosensory fibers, one that responds to warmth (warm receptors) and one that responds to cold (cold receptors), and include fibers from the A-δ and C range. Specific cutaneous cold and warm receptors have been defined as slowly conducting units that exhibit a steady-state discharge at constant skin temperature and a dynamic response to temperature changes (14,15). Cold- and warm-specific receptors can be distinguished from nociceptors that respond to noxious low and high temperatures (<20 and $>45°C$) (16,17) and also from thermosensitive mechanoreceptors (14,18). Konietzny (18) recorded from 13 cold-specific units in humans employing the microneurography technique and measured CVs which were in the C-fiber range ($0.43–2.04$ m s^{-1}). Serra et al. (19) reported a number of spontaneously active fibers employing microneurography, which were sensitive to small temperature changes and that were described as cold-specific units, but all had CVs in the C-fiber range ($0.43–1.27$ m s^{-1}). Standard medical textbooks describe the cutaneous cold sense in man as being mediated by myelinated A-fibers with CVs in the range 12 to 30 m s^{-1} (20), but recent work from Campero et al. (21) concludes that either human cold-specific afferent fibers are incompletely myelinated "BC" fibers, described by Duclaux et al. (22) as having electrophysiological and morphological properties of C-fibers in their distal part and B fibers in their proximal part, or else there are C as well as A cold fibers, with the C-fiber group contributing little to sensation. An example of a feature of these units can be seen in Figure 4 where it can be seen that the resting discharge at room temperature (21°C) is characterized by a low-frequency discharge (~1 Hz) and that this steady-state activity is suppressed by sudden warming of the RF and increased by cooling the RF (Fig. 4).

The free nerve endings for cold- or warm-sensitive nerve fibers are located just beneath the skin surface. The terminals of an individual temperature-sensitive fiber do not branch profusely or widely. Rather, the endings of each fiber form a small, discretely sensitive point, which is separate from the sensitive points of neighboring fibers. The total area of skin occupied by the receptor endings of a single temperature-sensitive nerve fiber is relatively small (~1 mm in diameter) with the density of these thermo-sensitive points varying in different body regions. For example, there are up to 15 to 25 cold points per cm^2 in the lips, three to five cold points per cm^2 in the finger, and less than one cold point per cm^2 in some broad areas of the trunk. There are 3- to 10-times

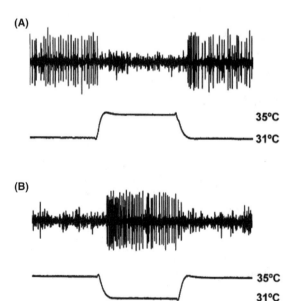

Figure 4 Resting discharge of a C cold fiber at room temperature. (**A**) The resting discharge is suppressed by warming of the RF from 31 to 35°C. (**B**) From a holding temperature of 35°C, at which the unit is silent, activity is initiated by cooling the RF to 31°C (time bar: 5 sec). *Abbreviation*: RF, receptive field. *Source*: From Ref. 21.

as many cold-sensitive points as warm-sensitive points in most areas of the body. It is well established from physiological and psychological testing that warm- and cold-sensitive nerve fibers are distinctively different from one another in both structure and function.

Pain

Here we consider a system of peripheral sensory nerves that innervate all cutaneous structures and whose sole purpose is to protect the skin against potential or actual damage. These primary afferents include A-δ and C-fibers which respond selectively and linearly to the levels of thermal, mechanical, and chemical intensity/strength that are tissue-threatening, that is, have the potential to damage the skin. This initial encoding mechanism is termed nociception and describes the sensory process detecting any overt, or impending, tissue damage. The term "pain," on the other hand, describes the perception of irritation, stinging, burning, soreness, or painful sensations arising from the skin. It is important to recognize, especially when we are investigating an area such as "sensitive skin," that the perception of pain depends not only on nociceptor inputs, but also on other processes and pathways giving information about, for example, emotional or contextual components. Pain is, therefore, described in terms of an "experience" rather than just a simple sensation. There are again submodalities within the nociceptive system which at the peripheral anatomical level are evident with respect to the degree of myelination of the nerve fibers (A-δ and C) subserving nociception (Table 2). A-δ fibers are thin (1–5 μm), poorly myelinated axons of mechanical nociceptors, thermal receptors, and mechanoreceptors with axon potential CVs average 12 m/sec, and C-fibers are very thin (<1 μm) slowly conducting axons (<1 m/sec). Mechanical nociceptors are in

Table 2 Major Findings in Bolanowski et al. (8) and Previous Work Done by These Researchers at the Institute for Sensory Research at Syracuse University (79–82)

Channel	Pacinian	NPI	NPII	NPIII
Frequency response (Hz)	40–80	3–100	15–400	<0.3 to >100
Threshold (at 1 μm)	<−20 dB at 300 Hz	28 dB at 3 Hz	10 dB at 300 Hz	28 dB at 3 Hz
Sensation	Vibration	Flutter	Not known	Pressure
Temporal summation	Yes	No	Yes	No
Spatial summation	Yes	No	Not known	No
Receptor type	FAI Pacinian corpuscle	FAII Meissner's corpuscle	SAII Ruffini end organ	SAI Merkel's disc

the A-δ range and possess RFs distributed as 5 to 20 small sensitive spots over an area approximately 2 to 3 mm in diameter. In many cases, activation of these spots depends upon stimuli intense enough to produce tissue damage, such as a pin-prick. A-δ units with a short latency response to intense thermal stimulation in the range 40 to 50°C have been described as well as other units excited by heat after a long latency—usually with thresholds in excess of 50°C.

Over 50% of the unmyelinated axons (C-fibers) of a peripheral nerve respond not only to intense mechanical stimulation, but also to heat and noxious chemicals, and are therefore classified as polymodal nociceptors (23) or C-mechano-heat (CMH) nociceptors (24). A subgroup of polymodal nociceptors has been reported to respond to extreme cold; however, many of these units develop an excitatory response to cooling after prior exposure to noxious heat. A small number of C-fibers have mechanical thresholds in the nociceptor range with no response to heat, whereas others have been found that respond preferentially to noxious heating. RFs consist of single zones with distinct borders and in this respect they differ from A-δ nociceptors that have multipoint fields. Innervation densities are high and responses have been reported to a number of irritant chemicals such as dilute acids, histamine, bradykinin, and capsaicin. Employing microneurography, Schmidt et al. (25) described not only CMH-responsive units, but also a novel class of C nociceptors responding only to mechanical stimuli (CM), units responding only to heating (CH), and units that were insensitive to mechanical and heating stimuli and also to sympathetic provocation tests (CMiCHi). Of relevance here is that some CM, CH, and CMiCHi units were sensitized to thermal and/or mechanical stimuli after topical application of skin irritants such as mustard oil or capsaicin; these units then acquired responsiveness to stimuli to which they were previously unresponsive. Recruitment of these "silent nociceptors" implies spatial summation to the nociceptive afferent barrage at central levels and may, therefore, contribute to primary hyperalgesia after chemical irritation and to secondary hyperalgesia as a consequence of central sensitization (detailed subsequently).

Nociceptors do not show the kinds of adaptation response found with rapidly adapting LTMs (i.e., they fire continuously to tissue damage), but pain sensation may come and go and pain may be felt in the absence of any nociceptor discharge. They rely on chemical mediators around the nerve ending which are released from nerve terminals and skin cells in response to tissue damage. Koltenzenburg et al. (26) have shown that nerve growth factor (NGF) is an important mediator in painful inflammatory skin states, with levels increasing in inflamed tissue. Following carrageenan inflammation of rodent skin, a marked increase in the proportion of nociceptors which displayed ongoing activity was observed, and this was reflected in a significant increase in the average ongoing discharge activity. Spontaneously active C-fibers were sensitized to heat and displayed a more than twofold increase in their discharge to a standard noxious heat stimulus. Furthermore, the number of nociceptors responding to the algesic mediator bradykinin increased significantly from 28% to 58%.

In contrast, the mechanical threshold of nociceptive afferents did not change during inflammation. When the NGF-neutralizing molecule trkA-IgG was co-administered with carrageenan at the onset of the inflammation, primary afferent nociceptors did not sensitize and displayed essentially normal response properties, although the inflammation as evidenced by tissue edema developed normally, demonstrating that NGF is a crucial component for the sensitization of primary afferent nociceptors associated with tissue inflammation.

The axon terminals of nociceptive axons possess no specialized end organ structure and for that reason are referred to as free nerve endings. This absence of any encapsulation renders them sensitive to chemical agents, both intrinsic and extrinsic, and inflammatory mediators released at a site of injury can initiate or modulate activity in surrounding nociceptors over an area of several millimeters leading to two kinds of sensory responses termed hyperalgesia—the phenomenon of increased sensitivity of damaged areas to painful stimuli; primary hyperalgesia occurs within the damaged area and secondary hyperalgesia occurs in undamaged tissues surrounding this area.

One further sensation mediated by afferent C-fibers is that of itch and this is dealt with in detail in Part I of this book (Schmelz).

Pleasure

It is generally accepted that human tactile sensibility is solely mediated by LTMs with fast-conducting large myelinated afferents (as described earlier). However, in recent years a growing body of evidence has been accumulating, from anatomical, psychophysical, electrophysiological, and neuroimaging studies, that a further submodality of afferent slowly conducting unmyelinated C-fibers exists in human hairy skin that are neither nociceptive nor pruritic, but that respond preferentially to low force, slowly moving mechanical stimuli traversing across their RFs. These nerve fibers have been classified as C- tactile afferents (CT-afferents) and were first described by Nordin in 1990 (27) in the face, and previously by Johansson et al. (28) in the same region, employing the technique of microneurography. Evidence of a more general distribution of CT-afferents have subsequently been found in the arm and the leg, but never in glabrous skin sites such as the palms of the hands or the soles of the feet (29). It is well known that mechanoreceptive innervation of the skin of many mammals is subserved by A- and C-afferents (23,30,31), but until the observations of Nordin and Vallbo, C-mechanoreceptive afferents in human skin appeared to be lacking entirely.

The functional role of CT-afferents is not fully known (32), but their neurophysiological response properties, fiber class, and slow CVs preclude their role in any rapid mechanical discriminative or cognitive tasks, and point to a more limbic function, particularly the emotional aspects of tactile perception (33,34). However, the central neural identification of low-threshold C mechanoreceptors, responding specifically to light touch, and the assignment of a functional role in human skin have only recently been achieved. In a study on a unique patient lacking large myelinated A-β fibers, it was discovered that activation of CT-afferents produced a faint sensation of pleasant touch, and functional neuroimaging showed activation in the insular cortex, but no activation in the primary sensory cortex identifying CT-afferents as a system for limbic touch that might underlie emotional, hormonal, and affiliative responses to skin-to-skin contacts between individuals engaged in grooming and bonding behaviors—pleasant touch (35,36). If pain is elicited via sensory C- and A-δ-fibers, then it is reasonable to speculate that the same system may be alternatively modulated to deliver a sensation of pleasure. One hypothesis is that pleasant touch stimulates opioid and cannabinoid receptors on these peripheral nerve fibers (both opioids and cannabinoids also have anti-nociceptive and anti-inflammatory activities) and that this signal is decoded in areas of the brain such as the insular cortex, which is associated with pleasure. Further evidence of the representation of pleasant touch in the brain has been provided by Francis et al. (37), where it was shown that discriminative and affective aspects of touch are processed in different brain areas. Activation of the primary somatosensory cortex was found in the physical aspects of stimulation, whereas the orbitofrontal cortex (an area of the frontal lobes involved in emotion) was activated by pleasant aspects. This area has also been shown to represent painful as well as pleasant touch, demonstrating the relevance of this brain region for representing the emotional dimensions of skin sensitivity—the positive and the negative (38).

Work is in progress to identify this class of C-fibers anatomically and histologically, and a study employing the pan-neuronal marker PGP9.5 and confocal laser microscopy has identified a population of free nerve endings located solely within the epidermis that may represent the putative anatomical substrate for this submodality (39).

Sympathetic Nerves

Although this chapter deals with sensory aspects of skin innervation, it is important to briefly review the role of a class of efferent (motor) nerves that innervate various skin structures: (a) blood vessels, (b) cutaneous glands, and (c) unstriated muscle in the skin, for example, the erectors of the hairs. In sensitive skin conditions and some painful neuropathic states, sympathetic nerves play a role in exacerbating inflammation and irritation. The efferent sympathetic fibers that leave the CNS in connection with certain cranial and spinal nerves and end in sympathetic ganglia are known as preganglionic fibers. From these ganglia, postganglionic fibers arise and conduct nerve impulses to the different organs in the skin such as the vasoconstrictor fibers to the blood vessels, the pilomotor fibers to the hairs, and the motor fibers to the sweat glands. Most of the postganglionic neurons utilize the organic chemical noradrenalin as their neurotransmitter, which is released at the effector synapse where the neuron ends. Noradrenalin and adrenaline stimulate two types of adrenergic receptors, namely α and β

receptors. Adrenaline stimulates both α and β receptors almost equally, whereas noradrenalin acts more pronouncedly on the α receptors. Stimulation of the two different types can produce different results; for example, stimulation of the α receptors on capillaries causes vasoconstriction, whereas stimulation of the β receptors causes vasodilation. Most of the postganglionic neurons are adrenergic; however, those which serve the sweat glands are cholinergic in their action except those on the palms of the hands, which are adrenergic.

In some cases, the sympathetic nervous system has been purported to play an important role in sustaining pain in recent theories, suggesting that pain receptors in the affected part of the body become responsive to a family of nervous system messengers known as catecholamines. Animal studies indicate that noradrenalin, released from sympathetic nerves, acquires the capacity to activate pain pathways after tissue or nerve injury. Complex regional pain syndrome is a chronic pain condition that is believed to be the result of dysfunction in the central or peripheral nervous systems. Typical features include dramatic changes in the color and temperature of the skin over the affected limb or body part, accompanied by intense burning pain, skin sensitivity, sweating, and swelling.

Receptors and Channels

Signaling of stimuli such as heat, pain, or chemical challenge acting on nociceptors is controlled peripherally via a complex regulation of activity in a series of ion channels. A candidate receptor for chemosensory agents such as capsaicin and menthol eluded scientific characterization until 1997 and 2002, respectively (40,41). Recent developments in molecular cloning of receptor types (e.g., the vanilloid receptor and associated thermoTRP channels—a subset of transient receptor potential [TRP] ion channels) combined with electrophysiological and receptor–ligand characterization have shed new light on the understanding of how noxious stimuli are encoded at the cellular level (42). The vanilloid receptor subtype 1 (VR1, also referred to as trpV1) is a classical cation channel and is expressed in cutaneous sensory nerve fibers, mast cells, and epithelial cells of appendage structures (43). Interestingly, activity for temperature (heat and cold), pain, and chemesthetic activity can all be explained in terms of the plasticity of a family of thermoTRP cation channels (44). Development of transgenic mouse models lacking expression of the VR1 gene shows that phenotypic characteristics in VR1 null $(-/-)$ mice support a functional role for VR1 in sensory transduction of nociceptive stimuli, although it was apparent that another unidentified receptor could partially compensate for the loss of VR1 function (45,46).

As an understanding of the process involved in sensing temperature and chemical stimulation of nociceptors has evolved, it has become apparent that there are additional non-TRP proteins and receptors which also play a role in nociception, for example, the acid-sensing ion channels and the P2×3 Adenosine tri-phosphate (ATP) receptor (47,48).

Opioids

The pain relief produced by opiates, such as morphine, derived from the opium poppy (*Papaver somniferum*), has been used and studied extensively for more than 5000 years. In addition to narcotic effects caused by activities within the CNS, opioids are also known for their antinociceptive and anti-inflammatory effects in the periphery. Coggeshall et al. (49) used light microscopic techniques to demonstrate the presence of μ- and δ-opioid receptors on ummyelinated afferents in human skin. In more recent years, Stander et al. (50) have shown a co-localization of μ-opioid receptor isoform 1A (MOR 1A) and calcitonin gene-related peptide in sensory fibers, suggesting a functional relationship for opiate agonists in terms of anti-inflammatory and anti-nociceptive activities. Opiates also cause vasodilatation of skin, although this does not appear to account for a reduction in pain via a local warming mechanism, that is, the analgesic effect is clearly MOR-mediated (51). The activity of opiates in the periphery does appear to be dependent on the extent of inflammation and local tissue damage and this may account for many of the discrepancies reported by various authors (52–54).

A range of cell types, including neurons, keratinocytes, and immune cells, produce endogenous opioids. There are three families of peptides identified to date, each arising from alternate processing of the gene products for pro-opiomelanocortin (POMC), pro-encephalin, and pro-dynorphin. In skin, the opioid, β-endorphin, is produced by post-translational cleavage of the POMC gene and acts both on MOR on nerves and keratinocytes (55). The expression of MOR on keratinocytes and involvement in the pathogenesis of clinical skin disease such as psoriasis suggest an additional role for opiates as immunoregulatory molecules in skin (56).

Cannabinoids

Cannabis (*Cannabis sativa* L.), like the opiates, has long been used for its narcotic effects. The recent discovery of specific cannabinoid receptors and endogenous ligands, produced in the periphery, has led to a new therapeutic potential as an analgesic and anti-inflammatory molecule (57,58). To date, two G-protein-coupled cannabinoid receptors, referred to as CB1 and CB2, have been identified in both the central and peripheral nervous systems (59,60). Differential localization using in situ hybridization and immunohistochemistry has shown the presence of CB receptors on both nociceptive and non-nociceptive afferents, in addition to staining on non-neuronal tissues, for example, keratinocytes and leukocytes (61,62).

Several studies have shown that both classical agonists, such as HU210, and endogenous cannabinoid (endocannabinoids) agonists, such as anandamide, have anti-inflammatory and anti-nociceptive benefits (63,64). The lipid metabolic pathways leading to production of endocannabinoids, their interactions with receptors, deactivation, and clearance pathways have been reviewed by Piomelli (65).

An interesting development in the understanding of the role of endocannabinoids in skin has been the observation that they can also activate VR1. Anandamide has been shown to activate VR1 (66,67) and this may explain the ability of anandamide to act as a vasodilator, although there is still some controversy over levels required to activate VR1 and its physiological relevance.

THE CENTRAL PROJECTIONS

The submodalities of skin-sensory receptors and nerves that convey information to the brain about mechanical, thermal, and painful stimulation of the skin are grouped into three different pathways in the spinal cord and project to different target areas in the brain. They differ in their receptors, pathways, and targets, and also in the level of decussation (crossing over) within the CNS. Most sensory systems en route to the cerebral cortex decussate at some point, as projections are mapped contralaterally. The discriminative touch system crosses in the medulla, where the spinal cord joins the brain; the pain system crosses at the point of entry into the spinal cord.

Spinal Cord

All the primary sensory neurons described earlier have their cell bodies situated outside the spinal cord in the dorsal root ganglion, there being one ganglion for every spinal nerve. Sensory neurons have a unique property in that, unlike most neurons, the nerve signal does not pass through the cell body but, as the cell body sits off to one side, the signal passes directly from the distal axon process to the proximal process which enters the dorsal half of the spinal cord.

Tactile primary afferents, or first-order neurons, immediately turn up the spinal cord toward the brain, ascending in the dorsal white matter and forming the dorsal columns. In a cross-section of the spinal cord at cervical levels, two separate tracts can be seen—the midline tracts comprise the gracile fasciculus conveying information from the lower half of the body (legs and trunk) and the outer tracts comprise the cuneate fasciculus conveying information from the upper half of the body (arms and trunk). At the medulla, situated at the top of spinal cord, the primary tactile afferents make their first synapse with second-order neurons where fibers from each tract synapse in a nucleus of the same name—the gracile fasciculus axons synapse in the gracile nucleus and the cuneate axons synapse in the cuneate nucleus. The neurons receiving the synapse provide the secondary afferents and cross immediately to form a new tract on the contralateral side of the brainstem—the medial lemniscus—which ascends through the brainstem to the next relay station in the midbrain, the thalamus.

As with the tactile system, pain, and thermal afferents, primary afferents synapse ipsilaterally and then the secondary afferents cross, but the crossings occur at different levels. Pain and temperature afferents enter the dorsal horn of the spinal and synapse within one or two segments, forming Lissauer's tract as they do so. The dorsal horn is a radially laminar structure; the thin outermost layer is called the posterior marginalis layer, the second layer is the substantia gelatinosa, and the layer deeper to that is the nucleus proprius. The two types of pain fibers, C and A-δ, enter different layers of the dorsal horn. A-δ fibers enter the posterior marginalis and the nucleus proprius, and synapse on a second set of neurons. These are the secondary afferents which will relay the signal to the thalamus. The secondary afferents from both layers cross to the opposite side of the spinal cord and ascend in the spinothalamic tract. The C-fibers enter the substantia gelatinosa and synapse, but they do not synapse on secondary afferents. Instead, they synapse on interneurons—neurons which do not project out of the immediate area but relay the signal to the secondary afferents in either the posterior marginalis or the nucleus proprius. The spinothalamic tract ascends the entire length of the cord and the entire brainstem, and by the time it reaches the midbrain appears to be continuous with the medial lemniscus. These tracts enter the thalamus together.

It is important to note that although the bulk of afferent input adheres to the plan outlined earlier, there is degree mixing that goes on between the tracts. Some light touch information, for example, travels in the spinothalamic tract with the result that damage to the dorsal columns does not completely remove touch and pressure sensation. Some proprioception also travels in the dorsal columns and follows the medial lemniscus all the way to the cortex, so there is conscious awareness of body position and movement. The pain and temperature system also has multiple targets in the brainstem and other areas.

We have concentrated on somatosensory inputs from the body thus far, but as facial skin is often the source of sensitive reactions to topical applications, its peripheral and central anatomy/neurophysiology will be briefly summarized here. The trigeminal nerve innervates all facial skin structures (including the oral mucosa) and, just as with the spinal afferents, these neurons have their cell bodies outside of the CNS in the trigeminal ganglion with their proximal processes entering the brainstem. Just as in the spinal cord, the three modalities of touch, temperature, and pain have different receptors in the facial skin, travel along different tracts, and have different targets in the brainstem—the trigeminal nucleus, a relatively large structure that extends from the midbrain to the medulla.

The large-diameter (A-β) fibers enter directly into the main sensory nucleus of the trigeminal and, as with the somatosensory neurons of the body, synapse and then decussate, the secondary afferents joining the medial lemniscus as it projects to the thalamus. The small-diameter fibers conveying pain and temperature enter midbrain with the main Vth cranial nerve, but then descend down the brainstem to the caudal medulla where they synapse and cross. These descending axons form a tract, the spinal tract of V, and synapse in the spinal nucleus of V, so called because it reaches as far down as the upper cervical spinal cord. The spinal nucleus of V comprises three regions along its length: the subnucleus oralis, the subnucleus interpolaris, and the subnucleus caudalis. The secondary afferents from the subnucleus caudalis cross to the opposite side and join the spinothalamic tract where the somatosensory information from the face joins that from the body, entering the thalamus in a separate nucleus, the ventroposterior medial nucleus (VPM).

Brain

The third-order thalamocortical afferents (from thalamus to cortex) travel up through the internal capsule to reach the primary somatosensory cortex, located in the post-central gyrus, a fold of cortex just posterior to the central sulcus (Fig. 5A).

The thalamocortical afferents convey all the signals, whether from ventro posterio lateral (VPL) or ventro posterio medial (VPM), to primary somatosensory cortex where the sensory information from all body surfaces is mapped in a somatotopic (body-mapped) manner (68,69), with the legs represented medially, at the top of the head, and the face represented laterally (Fig. 5B). Within the cortex, there are thought to be nine separate areas primarily subserving somatosensation: primary somatosensory cortex, SI, comprised four subregions (2, 1, 3a, and 3b), secondary somatosensory cortex, SII, located along the superior bank of the lateral sulcus (70–74), the insular cortex (75), and the posterior parietal cortex, areas 5 and 7b (Fig. 6).

As with studies of the peripheral nervous system, outlined in "The Peripheral Nervous System," the technique of microneurography has again been employed, in this case to study the relationship between skin-sensory nerves and their central projections, as evidenced by the use of concurrent functional magnetic resonance imaging (fMRI). Microstimulation of individual LTM afferents, projecting to RFs on the digit, produces robust, focal, and orderly (somatotopic) hemodynamic blood oxygen level dependent (BOLD) responses in both primary and secondary somatosensory cortices (76), in accordance with the findings of Penfield and Boldrey (77). It is expected that this technique will permit the study of many different topics in somatosensory neurophysiology, such as sampling from FA and SA mechanoreceptors and C-fibers with neighboring or overlapping RFs on the skin, and quantifying their spatial and temporal profiles in response to electrical chemical and/or mechanical stimulation of the skin areas they innervate, as well as perceptual responses to microstimulation.

Finally, the forward projections from these primary somatosensory areas to limbic and prefrontal structures have been studied with fMRI to understand the

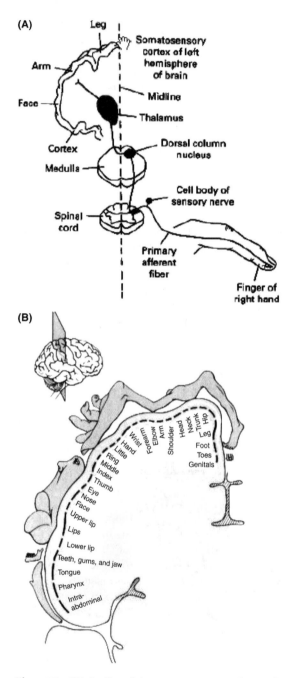

Figure 5   (**A**) Outline of the somatosensory pathways from the digit tip to primary somatosensory cortex, via the dorsal column nuclei and the thalamus. (**B**) Penfield's somatosensory homunculus. Note the relative overrepresentation of the hands and lips, and the relative underrepresentation of the trunk and arms.

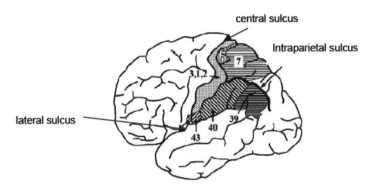

Figure 6 Cortical areas subserving somatosensation. SI is located in the posterior bank of the central sulcus and the posterior gyrus and comprises areas 2, 1, 3a, and 3b; secondary somatosensory cortex is located in the upper bank of the lateral sulcus with two further somatosensory regions in the posterior parietal cortex, areas 5 and 7b. *Abbreviation*: SI, primary somatosensory cortex.

effective representations of skin stimulation for both pain and pleasure (37,78) and it is hoped that studies of this nature will help us to better understand the emotional aspects of both negative ("sensitive" skin) and positive (pleasant touch) skin sensations.

REFERENCES

1. Johansson RS. Receptive field sensitivity profile of mechanosensitive units innervating the glabrous skin of the human hand. Brain Res 1976; 219:13–27.
2. Darian-Smith I. The sense of touch: performance and peripheral neural processes. In: Brookhart JM, Mountcastle VB, eds. Handbook of Physiology. Section 1: The Nervous System. Vol. 3. UK: OUP, 1984.
3. Gescheider GA, Bolanowski SJ, Verrillo RT. Sensory, cognitive and response factors in the judgement of sensory magnitude. In: Algom D, ed. Psychophysical Approaches to Cognition. Amsterdam: Elsevier, 1992:575–621.
4. Greenspan JD, Lamotte RH. Cutaneous mechanoreceptors of the hand: experimental studies and their implications for clinical testing of tactile sensation. J Hand Ther 1993; 6:75–82.
5. Vallbo AB, Hagbarth K, Torebjork E & Wallin BG. Somatosensory, proprioceptive and sympathetic activity in human peripheral nerves. Physiol Rev 1979; 59:919–957.
6. Willis WD, Coggeshall RE. Sensory Mechanisms of the Spinal Cord. 2nd ed. New York: Plenum Press, 1991.
7. von Bekesy G. Uber die Vibrationsempfindung [On the vibration sense]. Akustische Zeitschrift 1939; 4:315–334.
8. Bolanowski SJ, Gescheider GA, Verrillo RT, Checkosky CM. Four channels mediate the mechanical aspects of touch. J Acoustic Soc Am 1988; 84:1680–1694.

9. Essick GK, Edin BB. Receptor encoding of moving tactile stimuli in humans. II. The mean response of individual low-threshold mechanoreceptors to motion across the receptive field. J Neurosci 1995; 15:848–864.

10. Harrington T, Merzenich M. Neural coding in the sense of touch: human sensations of skin indentation compared with responses of slowly adapting mechanoreceptive afferents innervating the hairy skin of monkeys. Exp Brain Res 1970; 10:251–264.

11. Jarvilehto T, Hamalainen H, Laurinen P. Characteristics of single mechanoreceptive fibres innervating hairy skin of the human hand. Exp Brain Res 1976; 25:45–61.

12. Vallbo AB, Johansson RS. The tactile sensory innervation of the glabrous skin of the human hand. In: Gordon G, ed. Active Touch. New York: Pergamon, 1978:29–54.

13. Westling GK. Sensori-motor mechanisms during precision grip in man. Umea University Medical Dissertations. New Series 171, Umea, Sweden, 1986.

14. Hensel H, Boman KKA. Afferent impulses in cutaneous sensory nerves in human subjects. J Neurophysiol 1960; 23:564–578.

15. Hensel H. Cutaneous thermoreceptors. In: IGGO, A. ed. Somatosensory System. Berlin: Springer, 1973:79–110.

16. Torebjörk, Hallin. A new method for classification of C-unit activity in intact human skin nerves. In: Bonica JJ, Albe-Fessard D, eds. Advances in Pain Research and Therapy. New York: Raven Press, 1976:29–34.

17. Campero M, Serra J, Ochoa JL. C-polymodal nociceptors activated by noxious low temperature in human skin. J Physiol 1966; 497:565–572.

18. Konietzny F. Peripheral neural correlates of temperature sensations in man. Hum Neurobiol 1984; 3:21–32.

19. Serra J, Campero M, Ochoa JL, Bostock H. Activity-dependent slowing of conduction differentiates functional subtypes of C fibres innervating human skin. J Physiol 1999; 515:799–811.

20. Darian-Smith I, ed. Thermal sensibility. In: Handbook of Physiology, Section 1, The Nervous System, Vol. 3, Sensory Processes, Part 2. Bethesda, MD, USA: American Physiological Society, 1984:879–913.

21. Campero M, Serra J, Bostock H, Ochoa JL. Slowly conducting afferents activated by innocuous low temperature in human skin. J Physiol 2001; 535(3):855–865.

22. Duclaux R, Mei N, Ranieri F. Conduction velocity along afferent vagal dendrites: a new type of fibre. J Physiol 1976; 260:487–495.

23. Bessou M, Perl ER. Response of cutaneous sensory units with unmyelinated fibres to noxious stimuli. J Neurophysiol 1969; 32:1025–1043.

24. Campbell JN, Raja SN, Cohen RH, Manning DC, Khan AA, Meyer RA. Peripheral neural mechanisms of nociception. In: Wall PD, Melzack R, eds. Textbook of Pain. New York: Churchill Livingstone, 1989:22–45.

25. Schmidt R, Schmelz M, Forster C, Ringkamp M, Torebjork E, Handwerker H. Novel classes of responsive and unresponsive C nociceptors in humans skin. J Neurosci 1995; 15(1):333–341.

26. Koltenzenburg M, Bennett DL, Shelton DL, McMahon SB. Neutralization of endogenous NGF prevents the sensitization of nociceptors supplying inflamed skin. Eur J Neurosci 1999; 11(5):1698–1704.

27. Nordin M. Low threshold mechanoreceptive and nociceptive units with unmyelinated (C) fibres in the human supraorbital nerve. J Physiol 1990; 426:229–240.

28. Johansson RS, Trulsson M, Olsson KA, Westberg KG. Mechanoreceptor activity from the human face and oral mucosa. Exp Brain Res 1988; 72:204–208.

29. Vallbo AB, Hagbarth K-E, Torebjork HE, Wallin BG. Somatosensory, proprioceptive, and sympathetic activity in human peripheral nerves. Physiological Reviews 1979; 59:919–957.

30. Zotermann Y. Touch, pain and tickling: an electrophysiological investigation on cutaneous sensory nerves. J Physiol 1939; 95:1–28.

31. Iggo A, Korhuber HHA. A quantitative study of C-mechanoreceptors in the hairy skin of the cat. J Physiol 1977; 271:549–565.

32. MacKenzie RA, Burke D, Skuse NF, Lethlean AK. Fibre function and perception during cutaneous nerve block. J Neurol Neurosurg Phychiatry 1975; 38:865–873.

33. Vallbo AB, Olausson H, Wessberg J, Norsell U. A system of unmyelinated afferents for innocuous mechanoreception in the human skin. Brain Res 1993; 628:301–304.

34. Essick G, James A, McGlone FP. Psychophysical assessment of the affective components of non-painful touch. Neuroreport 1999; 10:2083–2087.

35. Olausson H, Lamarre Y, Backlund H, Morin C, Wallin BG, Starck S, Strigo K, Worsley K, Vallbo AB, Bushnell MC. Unmyelinated tactile afferents signal touch and project to the insular cortex. Nat Neurosci 2002; 5:900–904.

36. Wessberg J, Olausson H, Fernstormm KW, Vallbo AB. Receptive field properties of unmyelinated tactile afferents in the human skin. J Neurophysiol 2003; 89:1567–1575.

37. Francis ST, Rolls ET, Bowtell R, McGlone F, O'Doherty JO, Browning A, Clare S, Smith E. The representation of pleasant touch in the brain and its relationship with taste and olfactory areas. Neuroreport 1999; 10:453–459.

38. Rolls ET, O'Doherty JO, Kringelbach ML, Francis S, Bowtell R, McGlone F. Representations of pleasant and painful touch in the human orbitofrontal cortices. Cerebral Cortex 2003; 13:308–317.

39. Reilly DM, Ferdinando D, Johnston C, Shaw C, Buchanan KD, Green M. The epidermal nerve fibre network: characterization of nerve fibres in human skin by confocal microscopy and assessment of racial variations. Br J Dermatol 1997; 137:163–170.

40. Caterina MJ, Schumaker MJ, Tominaga M, Rosen TA, Levin JD, Julius D. The capsaicin receptor: a heat-activated ion channel in the pain pathway. Nature 1997; 389:816–824.

41. McKemy DD, Neuhausser WM, Julius D. Identification of a cold receptor reveals a general role for TRP channels in thermosensation. Nature 2002; 416:52–58.

42. Patapoutian A, Peier AM, Story GM, Viswanath V. ThermoTRP channels and beyond: mechanisms of temperature sensation. Nat Rev Neurosci 2003; 4:529–538.

43. Stander S, Moormann C, Schumacher M, Buddenkotte J, Artuc M, Shpacovitch V, Brzoska T, Lippert U, Henz BM, Luger TA, Metze D, Steinhoff M. Expression of vanilloid receptor subtype 1 in cutaneous sensory nerve fibres, mast cells, and epithelial cells of appendage structures. Exp Dermatol 2004; 13:129–139.

44. Montell C, Birnaumer L, Flockerzi V. The TRP channels, a remarkably functional family. Cell 2002; 108:595–598.

45. Caterina MJ, Leffer A, Malmberg AB, Martin WJ, Trafton J, Petersen-Zeitz M, Koltzenburg M, Basbaum Ai, Julius D. Impaired nociception and pain sensation in mice lacking the capsaicin receptor. Science 2000; 288:306–313.

46. Davis JB, Gray J, Gunthorpe MJ, Hatcher JP, Davey PT, Overend P, Harries MH, Latcham J, Clapham C, Atkinson K, et al. Vanilloid receptor-1 is essential for inflammatory thermal hyperalgesia. Nature 2000; 405:183–187.

47. Askwith CC, Benson CJ, Welsh MJ, Snyder PM. DEG/EnaC ion channels involved in sensory transduction are modulated by cold temperature. PNAS USA 2001; 98:6459–6463.
48. Souslova V, Cesare P, Ding Y, Akopian AN, Stanfa L, Suzuki R, Carpenter K, Dickenson A, Boyce S, Hill R, Oosthuizen DN, Smith AJH, Kidd EJ, Wood JN. Warm-coding deficits and aberrant inflammatory pain in mice lacking P2X3 receptors. Nature 2000; 407:1015–1017.
49. Coggeshall RE, Zhou S, Carlton SM. Opioid receptors on peripheral sensory axons. Brain Res 1997; 764:126–132.
50. Stander S, Gunzer M, Metze D, Luger T, Steinhoff M. Localization of μ-opioid receptor 1A on sensory nerve fibres in human skin. Regulatory Peptides 2002; 110:75–83.
51. Holland RL, Harkin NE, Coleshaw RK, Jones DA, Peck AW, Telekes A. Dipipanone and nifedipine in cold induced pain: analgesia not due to skin warming. Br J Clin Pharmacol 1987; 24:823–826.
52. Yuge O, Matsumoto M, Kitahata LM, Collins JG, Senami M. Direct opioid application to peripheral nerves does not alter compound action potentials. Anesth Analg 1985; 64:667–671.
53. Frank GB, Sudha TS. Effects of encephalin, applied intracellularly, on action potentials in vertebrate A and C nerve fibre axons. Neuropharmacology 1987; 26:61–66.
54. Antoijevic I, Mousa SA, Schafer M, Stein C. Perineural defect and peripheral opioid analgesia during inflammation. J Neurosci 1995; 15:165–172.
55. Bigliardi PL, Bigliardi-Qi M, Buechner S, Ruffi T. Expression of μ-opiate receptor in human epidermis and keratinocytes. J Invest Dermatol 1998; 111:297–301.
56. Bigliardi-Qi M, Bigliardi PL, Eberle AN, Buechner S, Ruffi T. β-Endorphin stimulates cytokeratin 16 expression and downregulates μ-opiate receptor expression in human epidermis. J Invest Dermatol 1998; 114:527–532.
57. Dvorak M, Watkinson A, McGlone F, Rukweid R. Histamine-induced responses are attenuated by a cannabinoid receptor agonist in human skin. Inflamm Res 2003; 52:238–245.
58. Johanek LM, Simone DA. Activation of peripheral cannabinoid receptors attenuates cutaneous hyperalgesia produced by a heat injury. Pain 2004; 109:432–442.
59. Matsuda LA. Molecular aspects of cannabinoid receptors. Crit Rev Neurobiol 1997; 11:143–166.
60. Munro S, Thomas KL, Abu-Shaar M. Molecular characterization of a peripheral receptor for cannabinoids. Nature 1993; 365:61–65.
61. Price TJ, Helesic G, Parghi D, Hargreaves KM, Flores CM. The neuronal distribution of cannabinoid receptor type 1 in the trigeminal ganglion of the rat. Neuroscience 2003; 120:155–162.
62. Galiegue S, Mary S, Marchand J, Dussossoy D, Carriere D, Carayon P, Bouaboula M, Shire D, Le Fur G, Casellas P. Expression of central and peripheral cannabinoid receptors in human immune tissues and leukocytes subpopulations. Eur J Biochem 1995; 232:54–61.
63. Rukweid R, Watkinson A, McGlone F, Dvorak M. Cannabinoid agonists attenuate capsaicin-induced responses in human skin. Pain 2003; 102:283–288.
64. Walker JM, Huang SM, Strangman NM, Tsou K, Sanudo-Pena MN. Pain modulation by release of the endogenous cannabinoid anandamide. PNAS 1999; 96:12198–12203.

65. Piomelli D. The molecular logic of endocannabinoid signalling. Nat Rev Neurosci 2003; 4:873–884.

66. DiMarzo V, Bisogno T, Melck D, Ross R, Brochic H, Stevenson L, Pertwee R, DePetrocellis L. Interactions between synthetic vanilloids and the endogenous cannabinoid system. FEBS Lett 1998; 436:449–454.

67. DiMarzo V, Bisogno T, Petrocellis L. Anandamide: some like it hot. Trends Pharmacol Sci 2001; 22:346–349.

68. Penfield R, Rasmussen T. The Cerebral Cortex of Man. New York: Macmillan, 1952.

69. Maldjian JA, Gotschalk A, Patel RS, Detre JA, Alsop DC. The sensory somatotopic map of the human hand demonstrated at 4 T. Neuroimage 1999; 10:55–62.

70. Woolsey C. Second somatic receiving areas in the cerebral cortex of the cat, dog and monkey. Fed Proc 2 1946; 55–56.

71. Maeda K, Kakigi R, Hoshiyama M, Koyama S. Topography of the secondary somatosensory cortex in humans: a magentoencephalographic study. Neuroreport 1999; 10:301–306.

72. Coghill RC, Talbot JD, Evans AC, Meyer E, Gjedde A, Bushnell MC, Duncan GH. Distributed processing of pain and vibration by the human brain. J Neurosci 1994; 14:4095–4108.

73. Francis ST, Kelly EF, Bowtell R, Dunseath WJ, Folger SE, McGlone FP. FMRI of the responses to vibratory stimulation of digit tips. Neuroimage 2000; 11:188–202.

74. McGlone FP, Kelly EF, Trulsson M, Francis ST, Westling G, Bowtel R. Functional neuroimaging studies of human somatosensory cortex. Behav Brain Res 2002; 135:147–158.

75. Schneider RJ, Friedman DP, Mishkin M. A modality-specific somatosensory area within the insula of the rhesus monkey. Brain Res 1993; 621:116–120.

76. Trulsson M, Francis ST, Kelly EF, Westling G, Bowtell R, McGlone FP. Cortical responses to single mechanoreceptive afferent microstimulation revealed with fMRI. Neuroimage 2001; 13:613–622.

77. Penfield R, Boldrey E. Somatic motor and sensory representation in the cerebral cortex of man as studied by electrical stimulation. Brain 1937; 60:389–443.

78. Rolls E, O'Doherty J, Kringelbach M, Francis S, Bowtell R, McGlone F. Representation of pleasant and painful touch in the human orbitofrontal cortex. Cerebral Cortex 2003; 10(3):284–294,

79. Gescheider GA, O'Malley MJ, Verrillo RT. Vibrotactile forward masking: evidence for channel independence. J Acoustic Soc Am 1983; 74:474–485.

80. Gescheider GA, Sklar BF, Van Doren CL, Verrillo RT. Vibrotactile forward masking: psychophysical evidence for a triplex theory of cutaneous mechanoreception. Sensory Process 1985; 1:187–203.

81. Gescheider GA, Verrillo RT, Van Doren CL. Prediction of vibrotactile masking functions. J Acoustic Soc Am 1982; 72:1421–1426.

82. Verrillo RT. Effect of contactor area on the vibrotactile threshold. J Acoustic Soc Am 1963; 35:1962–1966.

3

Neurophysiology of Itch

Martin Schmelz

*Department of Anesthesiology and Intensive Care Medicine, Faculty of Clinical
Medicine Mannheim, University of Heidelberg, Mannheim, Germany*

NEUROPHYSIOLOGY OF ITCH

Common complaints of patients with sensitive skin include sensory phenomena, especially pain and itch. Itch (lat. pruritus) is a peculiar modality in the realm of somatic sensations. Obviously, it serves nociceptive functions, but it is clearly distinct from pain as a sensation and also with respect to inducing stimuli. It is restricted to the skin and some adjoining mucosae. For the neurophysiologist, the most striking difference applies to the connected reflex apparatus; whereas painful stimuli applied to the skin—in particular, at the extremities—provoke withdrawal reflexes, itching stimuli provoke very characteristic scratching reflexes. One might also describe scratching as a reflex pattern that is used in situations in which the noxious stimulus has already invaded the skin. In this situation, withdrawal would be useless; instead, attending to the injured site by scratching and a close inspection appear to be more adequate. On the other hand, pathological pruritus raises a major therapeutic problem in a number of diseases. In some cases, itching may be so severe that it heavily impedes the quality of life of the patient.

SPECIALIZED "ITCH NEURONS"

The neurophysiological basis for the itch sensation was unclear for decades. Several competing theories coexisted, until finally in 1997, itch-selective neurons were found in humans, which could explain the histamine-induced itch sensation (1).

Primary Afferent Neurons

C-fibers, responding to histamine application in parallel to the itch ratings of subjects, have been discovered among the group on mechano-insensitive C-afferents (1), suggesting that there is a specific pathway for itch (Fig. 1). In contrast, the most common type of C-fibers, mechano-heat nociceptors (CMH or polymodal nociceptors), are either insensitive to histamine or only weakly activated by it (2,3). This fiber type cannot account for the prolonged itch induced by the intradermal application of histamine.

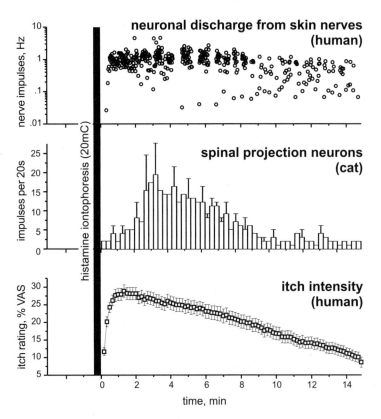

Figure 1 The *upper panel* shows instantaneous discharge frequency of a primary afferent mechano- and heat-insensitive C-fiber (CMiHi) in the superficial peroneal nerve, following histamine iontophoresis (20 mC; marked as the *black bar* in the diagram). The unit was not spontaneously active before histamine application. The *middle panel* depicts the response of a dorsal horn neuron in the cat, following the application of histamine in the skin receptive field. The *lower panel* shows average itch magnitude ratings of a group of 21 healthy volunteers after an identical histamine stimulus. Ratings at 10-second intervals on a visual analog scale with the endpoints "no itch–unbearable itch." *Bars*: standard error of means. *Source*: From Refs. 1,6.

The histamine-sensitive "itch" fibers or pruriceptors are characterized by a particular low conduction velocity, large innervation territories, mechanical unresponsiveness, and high transcutaneous electrical thresholds (1,4,5).

Spinal Neurons

The concept of dedicated pruriceptive neurons has now been complemented and extended by recordings from the cat spinal cord. A specialized class of dorsal horn neurons projecting to the thalamus has been demonstrated that responds strongly to histamine administered to the skin by iontophoresis (6). The time course of these responses was similar to that of itch in humans and matched the responses of the peripheral C-itch fibers (Fig. 1). These units were also unresponsive to mechanical stimulation and differed from the histamine-insensitive nociceptive units in lamina I of the spinal cord. In addition, their axons had a lower conduction velocity and anatomically distinct projections to the thalamus. Thus, the combination of dedicated peripheral and central neurons with a unique response pattern to pruritugenic mediators and anatomically distinct projections to the thalamus provides the basis for a specialized neuronal pathway for itch.

PRURITIC MEDIATORS

Histamine

Histamine has been a widely used pruritogen in experimental settings. It has been shown that most experimental itch stimuli act indirectly via release of histamine from cutaneous mast cells. This activity is mediated by H_1 receptors and is of major relevance for some chronic itch conditions such as urticaria, in which pruritus is responsive to H_1-antihistamines. Upon activation by histamine, prurituceptors release vasodilatory neuropeptides such as substance P (SP) and calcitonin gene-related peptide. These neuropeptides are released not only from the stimulated terminals, but also from the axon collaterals, which are excited by an axon reflex, thereby inducing erythema around the application site. In turn, when exogenous SP is injected intradermally in high concentrations, it degranulates mast cells and consequently provokes an itch sensation (7). However, under physiological conditions, the concentrations of endogenous neuropeptides released by activation of nociceptors are too low to degranulate mast cells (8,9).

Neuropeptides

Neuropeptides, especially SP, have been implicated in the mechanism of itch (10–12). Although it has been suggested that the direct excitatory effects of SP can explain itch in humans (13), experimental evidence for histamine-independent

SP-induced itch in humans (14) has been denied by most studies (15–20). Similarly, SP does not excite skin nociceptors (21).

At high concentrations, SP degranulates mast cells, but not via specific binding to SP receptors (NKI) (22,23). However, even at high concentrations of up to 10^{-5} M, SP does not evoke any sensation or axon reflex, even though protein extravasation and vasodilation can be elicited at a concentration of 10^{-8} M, without any detectable histamine release (16). In contrast to rodents, physiological concentrations of endogenously released SP are obviously too low to provoke mast cell degranulation (17,16) or even protein extravasation in human skin (9). Thus, it can be concluded that SP-induced vasodilation and wheal formation are mast cell independent.

Although there is probably no direct role for SP as peripheral pain or itch mediators in human, this does not exclude a major role of released neuropeptides in inflammation. Trophic and immunomodulatory effects of neuropeptides have been observed at concentrations of about 10^{-11} M (24–26), which might reflect their important role under physiological conditions. In addition, in disease, the concentrations of neuropeptides in the skin might well be increased and hence, neuropeptides may play a major role in pathophysiological mechanisms, for example, in patients with chronic pain (27).

Opioids

Intradermally injected opioids can activate mast cells by a non-receptor-mediated mechanism (23,28). Weak opioids, such as codeine, have been used as a positive control in skin prick tests. The consecutive release of histamine and mast cell tryptase can be specifically monitored by measuring tryptase concentration with dermal microdialysis following intraprobe delivery (29). In contrast to morphine, the highly potent μ-opioid agonist, fentanyl, does not provoke any mast cell degranulation, even if applied at concentrations having μ-agonistic effects exceeding those of morphine. Thus, one can conclude that morphine-induced mast cell degranulation is not mediated by μ-opioid receptors (28). As high local concentrations of opioids are required to degranulate mast cells, systemic administration of opioids in therapeutic doses does not cause pruritus by non-receptor-mediated mast cell degranulation, but probably by central mechanisms.

Proteinases

Although previous research has mainly focused on histamine as the main pruritic mediator in patients with itch, microdialysis has also provided evidence for mast-cell-derived histamine-independent mediators, which may also induce itch. In atopic subjects, mast cell degranulation by compound 48/80 provokes itch, which is not suppressed by H_1-antihistamines (30). It has been postulated that mast-cell-derived tryptase is a possible candidate for this effect, as it specifically activates proteinase-activated receptors (PAR-2). Although proteinases, such as papain, have been identified as histamine-independent mediators of itch decades ago (31,32), they received little attention until recently. In contrast, the identification of specific PAR-2 in the membrane of afferent nerve fibers (33) has prompted several successful investigations of the role of PAR-2 in the pain pathway (34,35). Meanwhile, there is convincing evidence for the involvement of PAR-2 in activation and sensitization of both somatic (36) and visceral afferent nerve fibers (37–39).

Apart from its involvement in pain pathways, recent studies of PAR-2 knockout mice indicate also a role of PAR-2 in itchy skin diseases, including atopic dermatitis (40). Recent microdialysis data suggest that the concentrations of tryptase is elevated in patients with atopic dermatitis, as would be expected from the increased numbers of tryptase-positive mast cells in this condition (41). Activation of PAR-2 may induce itch in patients with atopic dermatitis (42). In this context, it is noteworthy that proteinase activity can also be found in common allergens, such as house dust mites. However, it is unknown whether this activity contributes only to enhanced allergic potency (43) or whether it might also directly excite PAR-2 on sensory nerves (35).

Moreover, PAR-2 activation increases the release of interleukin (IL)-6 and granulocyte/macrophage colony-stimulating factor (44), which has been found elevated in keratinocytes of Alzheimer's disease (AD) patients (45). The importance of PAR-2 signaling for the induction of dermatitis has recently been shown by a markedly decreased contact dermatitis in PAR-2 knockout mice (40). As PAR-2 is expressed by various inflammatory cells, including mast cells (46) and T-cells (47), one may speculate that PAR-2 is critically involved in both neurogenic and non-neurogenic inflammations of human skin.

Interleukins

Supernatants of mitogen-stimulated leukocytes, which were pruritic in atopics but not in controls, contained larger amounts of IL-2 and IL-6 (48). However, no correlation of IL-6 content with itch intensity was found in atopics (49). IL-6 and IL-6 receptors are expressed in nerve and Schwann cells (50) and IL-6-like immunoreactivity was increased in nerve fibers of patients with positive epicutaneous patch tests and prurigo nodularis (51), which might indicate a role of IL-6 in the pathophysiology of some types of itch. However, intradermal injections of IL-2 did not induce considerable itch sensations in AD patients (52) or controls (53). Only upon IV injection, it caused some pruritus in cancer patients (54). Thus, the exact role of IL for the induction of pruritus remains to be established.

Prostanoids

There are only a few examples of mediators that can induce histamine-independent pruritus. As mentioned earlier, prostaglandins were found to enhance histamine-induced itch in the skin (55) and also to act directly as pruritugens (56,57).

SENSITIZATION FOR ITCH

Interaction of Pain and Itch

Itch Modulation by Painful and Non-painful Stimuli

It is a common experience that the itch sensation can be reduced by the pain caused by scratching. The inhibition of itch by painful stimuli has been experimentally demonstrated by the use of various painful thermal, mechanical, and chemical stimuli. Recently, electrical stimulation via an array of pointed electrodes ("cutaneous field stimulation") has also been successfully used to inhibit histamine-induced itch for several hours in an area around a stimulated site, 20 cm in diameter. The large area of inhibition suggests a central mode of action (58). Consistent with these results, itch is suppressed inside the secondary zone of capsaicin-induced mechanical hyperalgesia (59). This central effect of nociceptor excitation by capsaicin should clearly be distinguished from the neurotoxic effect of higher concentrations of capsaicin, which destroy most C-fiber terminals, including fibers that mediate itch (60,61). The latter mechanism, therefore, also abolishes pruritus locally, until the nerve terminals have regenerated.

Not only is itch inhibited by enhanced input of pain stimuli, but vice versa: inhibition of pain processing may reduce its inhibitory effect, and thus, enhance itch (62). This phenomenon is particularly relevant to spinally administered μ-opioid receptor agonists (Fig. 2), which are widely used in the treatment of pain and typically may cause pruritus.

Central inhibition of itch can also be achieved by cold stimulation (63) in agreement with the observation that histamine-induced activation of nociceptors is temperature-dependent (64). Cooling of a histamine-treated skin site reduces the activity of the primary afferents and decreases the area of "itchy skin" or "hyperknesis" around the source of the pruritus (65). Conversely, warming the

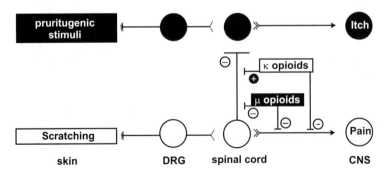

Figure 2 Simplified schematic view of central interaction between pain and itch under physiological conditions. Although having a similar inhibitory effect on the pain processing, μ- and κ-opioids differentially modify the spinal itch processing. *Abbreviations*: DRG, dorsal root ganglion; CNS, central nervous system.

skin would lead to an exacerbation of itch. However, as soon as the heating becomes painful, central inhibition of pruritus will counteract this effect.

Sensitization for Itch

Peripheral Sensitization for Itch

Increased intradermal nerve fiber density has been found in patients with chronic pruritus (66,67). In addition, increased epidermal levels of neurotrophin 4 (NT_4) have been found in patients with atopic dermatitis (68) and massively increased serum levels of nerve growth factor (NGF) and SP have been found to correlate with the severity of the disease in such patients (69). Increased fiber density and higher local NGF concentrations were also found in patients with contact dermatitis (70). It is known that NGF and NT_4 can sensitize nociceptors (71,72). These similarities between localized painful and pruritic lesions might suggest that on a peripheral level, similar mechanisms of nociceptor sprouting and sensitization exist. It has not been possible to morphologically differentiate nociceptors from pruriceptors. There is no way yet to test for a specific sprouting of pruriceptors that would spare the nociceptors. Apart from this obvious lack of knowledge, it is very unlikely that peripheral mechanisms alone account for the obvious differences between patients with localized chronic itch and pain.

Central Sensitization for Itch

There is remarkable similarity between the phenomena associated with central sensitization to pain and itch. Activity in chemo-nociceptors not only leads to acute pain, but also can sensitize second-order neurons in the dorsal horn, thereby leading to increased sensitivity to pain (hyperalgesia). In itch-processing, similar phenomena have been described: touch- or brush-evoked pruritus around an itching site has been termed "itchy skin" (73,74). It requires ongoing activity in primary afferents and is most probably elicited by low-threshold mechanoreceptors (A-β fibers) (65,74). Also, more intense prick-induced itch sensations in the surroundings, "hyperknesis," have been reported following histamine iontophoresis in healthy volunteers (62).

The existence of central sensitization for itch can greatly improve our understanding of clinical itch. Under the conditions of central sensitization leading to punctuate hyperknesis, normally painful stimuli are perceived as itching. This phenomenon has already been described in patients suffering from atopic dermatitis, who perceive normally painful electrical stimuli as itching when applied inside their lesional skin (75). Furthermore, acetylcholine provokes itch instead of pain in patients with atopic dermatitis (76,77), indicating that pain-induced inhibition of itch might be compromised in these patients.

Recently, it has been reported that normally painful electrical, chemical, mechanical, and thermal stimuli are perceived as itching when applied in or close to lesional skin of atopic dermatitis patients (78). Another example of sensitization to itch is shown in Figure 3. Histamine prick tests in non-lesional skin

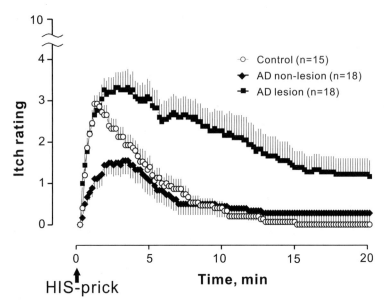

Figure 3 Intensity of itch ratings, following a histamine prick test in forearm skin of healthy volunteers (control), in visually healthy skin of patients with atopic dermatitis (AD non-lesion) and in lesional skin of patients with atopic dermatitis (AD lesion). *Abbreviation*: AD, Alzheimer's disease. *Source*: From Ref. 78.

of atopic dermatitis patients provoked less intense itching as compared with healthy controls. However, when applied inside their lesions, itch ratings were enhanced and lasted very long.

In contrast, the axon reflex erythema still was smaller as compared to the controls, suggesting reduced activation of peripheral pruriceptors (65,79). A reduced central "itch perception threshold" could be assumed in these patients, which might be induced by ongoing activity of peripheral pruriceptors (Fig. 4).

Ongoing activity of pruriceptors has already been confirmed microneurographically in a patient with chronic pruritus (80). In addition, lasting activation of pruriceptors by histamine has been shown to experimentally induce central sensitization for itch in healthy volunteers (78). Thus, there is emerging evidence for a role of central sensitization for itch in chronic pruritus. As there are many mediators and mechanisms which are potentially algogenic in inflamed skin (81), many of them could provoke itch in a sensitized patient. Thus, a therapeutic approach that targets only a single pruritic mediator does not appear to be promising for patients with chronic itching diseases, for example, atopic dermatitis. In contrast, the main therapeutic implication of this phenomenon is that a combination of centrally acting drugs counteracting the sensitization and topically acting drugs counteracting the inflammation should be more promising in ameliorating pruritus (Fig. 5).

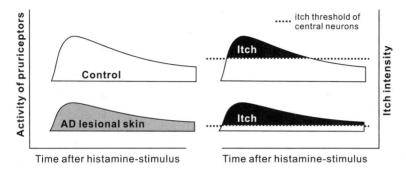

Figure 4 Schematic view of the activity of peripheral pruriceptors (*left panel*) and perceived itch intensity (black area, *right panel*). Even under the condition of reduced activation of peripheral pruriceptors, a more intense itch sensation can be generated, if the central itch threshold is lowered. *Source*: From Ref. 78.

EXPERIMENTAL MODELS FOR ITCH

Traditionally, acute applications of pruritugens such as histamine, serotonin, or mast-cell-degranulating substances have been used as human itch models (82–84). In rodents, histamine is generally less effective (85,86) and causes scratch responses only in selected mouse strains (87). Intradermal injection of SP is one of the most commonly used models in rodents (88,89). In rodents, cutaneous application of serotonin is a well-established itch model, which has been used for both electrophysiology and behavioral studies (90–93).

Subacute Models for Itch

Instead of focusing on a single mediator, recent approaches try to mimic pathophysiology of pruritic diseases more directly. It is well known that dry skin is a

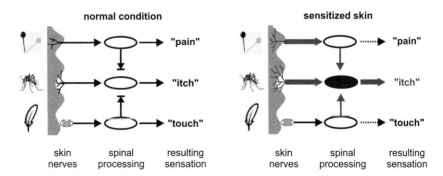

Figure 5 Schematic view of the peripheral and central sensitization processes, which lead to increased itch sensation. Under normal conditions, painful stimuli and touch can suppress itch by a spinal interaction (*left panel*). In the sensitized state, normally painful stimuli can induce the sensation of itch and also touch can provoke itch (*right panel*).

major cause of itch in humans In a mouse model of itch, dry skin was induced by cutaneous treatment with the irritant sodium lauryl sulfate (SLS). The resulting increase of scratch behavior could be reduced by naloxone treatment (94), suggesting that this new approach might correlate to clinical itch conditions. Similarly, an allergic model of itch has been developed in the rat (95) and the induced scratching was not mediated by serotonin. Another example of more clinically relevant animal models of itch are IL-4 overexpressing mice (96) which resemble aspects of atopic dermatitis.

Also in humans, there are some attempts to combine inflammation and itch models. Application of pruritics in inflamed skin (SLS irritation) has recently been studied (84,97). Moreover, lesional skin of atopic dermatitis patients has been investigated with classical psychophysical methods (78,98). Thus, the experimental models to clarify the pathophysiology of itch are being further developed and are beginning to fill the gap between acute animal models and clinical itch conditions.

REFERENCES

1. Schmelz M, Schmidt R, Bickel A, Handwerker HO, Torebjörk HE. Specific C-receptors for itch in human skin. J Neurosci 1997; 17:8003–8008.
2. Andrew D, Schmelz M, Ballantyne JC. Itch-mechanisms and mediators. In: Dostrovsky JO, Carr DB, Koltzenburg M, eds. Progress in Pain Research and Management. Seattle: IASP Press, 2003:213–226.
3. Schmelz M, Schmidt R, Weidner C, Hilliges M, Torebjork HE, Handwerker HO. Chemical response pattern of different classes of C-nociceptors to pruritogens and algogens. J Neurophysiol 2003; 89:2441–2448.
4. Weidner C, Schmelz M, Schmidt R, Hansson B, Handwerker HO, Torebjörk HE. Functional attributes discriminating mechano-insensitive and mechano-responsive C nociceptors in human skin. J Neurosci 1999; 19:10184–10190.
5. Schmidt R, Schmelz M, Weidner C, Handwerker HO, Torebjork HE. Innervation territories of mechano-insensitive C nociceptors in human skin. J Neurophysiol 2002; 88:1859–1866.
6. Andrew D, Craig AD. Spinothalamic lamina 1 neurons selectively sensitive to histamine: a central neural pathway for itch. Nat Neurosci 2001; 4:72–77.
7. Giannetti A, Girolomoni G. Skin reactivity to neuropeptides in atopic dermatitis. Br J Dermatol 1989; 121:681–688.
8. Petersen LJ, Winge K, Brodin E, Skov PS. No release of histamine and substance P in capsaicin-induced neurogenic inflammation in intact human skin in vivo: a microdialysis study. Clin Exp Allergy 1997; 27:957–965.
9. Sauerstein K, Klede M, Hilliges M, Schmelz M. Electrically evoked neuropeptide release and neurogenic inflammation differ between rat and human skin. J Physiol 2000; 529:803–810.
10. Andoh T, Nagasawa T, Satoh M, Kuraishi Y. Substance P induction of itch-associated response mediated by cutaneous NK1 tachykinin receptors in mice. J Pharmacol Exp Ther 1998; 286:1140–1145.

11. Heyer G, Hornstein OP, Handwerker HO. Reactions to intradermally injected substance P and topically applied mustard oil in atopic dermatitis patients. Acta Derm Venereol 1991; 71:291–295.
12. Greaves MW, Wall PD. Pathophysiology of itching. Lancet 1996; 348:938–940.
13. Wallengren J, Hakanson R. Effects of substance P, neurokinin A and calcitonin gene-related peptide in human skin and their involvement in sensory nerve-mediated responses. Eur J Pharmacol 1987; 143:267–273.
14. Cappugi P, Tsampau D, Lotti T. Substance P provokes cutaneous erythema and edema through a histamine-independent pathway. Int J Dermatol 1992; 31:206–209.
15. Hägermark O, Hokfelt T, Pernow B. Flare and itch induced by substance P in human skin. J Invest Dermatol 1978; 71:233–235.
16. Weidner C, Klede M, Rukwied R, et al. Acute effects of substance P and calcitonin gene-related peptide in human skin—a microdialysis study. J Invest Dermatol 2000; 115:1015–1020.
17. Schmelz M, Petersen LJ. Neurogenic inflammation in human and rodent skin. News Physiol Sci 2001; 16:33–37.
18. Fjellner B, Hägermark O. Studies on pruritogenic and histamine-releasing effects of some putative peptide neurotransmitters. Acta Derm Venereol 1981; 61:245–250.
19. Foreman JC, Jordan CC, Oehme P, Renner H. Structure–activity relationships for some substance P-related peptides that cause wheal and flare reactions in human skin. J Physiol (Lond) 1983; 335:449–465.
20. Barnes PJ, Brown MJ, Dollery CT, Fuller RW, Heavey DJ, Ind PW. Histamine is released from skin by substance P but does not act as the final vasodilator in the axon reflex. Br J Pharmacol 1986; 88:741–745.
21. Kessler W, Kirchhoff C, Reeh PW, Handwerker HO. Excitation of cutaneous afferent nerve endings in vitro by a combination of inflammatory mediators and conditioning effect of substance P. Exp Brain Res 1992; 91:467–476.
22. Lorenz D, Wiesner B, Zipper J, et al. Mechanism of peptide-induced mast cell degranulation: translocation and patch-clamp studies. J Gen Physiol 1998; 112:577–591.
23. Ferry X, Brehin S, Kamel R, Landry Y. G-protein-dependent activation of mast cell by peptides and basic secretagogues. Peptides 2002; 23:1507–1515.
24. Noveral JP, Grunstein MM. Tachykinin regulation of airway smooth muscle cell proliferation. Am J Physiol 1995; 269:L339–L343.
25. Lambert RW, Granstein RD. Neuropeptides and Langerhans cells. Exp Dermatol 1998; 7:73–80.
26. Parenti A, Amerini S, Ledda F, Maggi CA, Ziche M. The tachykinin NK1 receptor mediates the migration-promoting effect of substance P on human skin fibroblasts in culture. Naunyn Schmiedebergs Arch Pharmacol 1996; 353:475–481.
27. Weber M, Birklein F, Neundorfer B, Schmelz M. Facilitated neurogenic inflammation in complex regional pain syndrome. Pain 2001; 91:251 257.
28. Church MK, Clough GF. Human skin mast cells: in vitro and in vivo studies. Ann Allergy Asthma Immunol 1999; 83:471–475.
29. Blunk JA, Schmelz M, Zeck S, Skov P, Likar R, Koppert W. Opioid-induced mast cell activation and vascular responses is not mediated by micro-opioid receptors: an in vivo microdialysis study in human skin. Anesth Analg 2004; 98:364–370.
30. Rukwied R, Lischetzki G, McGlone F, Heyer G, Schmelz M. Mast cell mediators other than histamine induce pruritus in atopic dermatitis patients: a dermal microdialysis study. Br J Dermatol 2000; 142:1114–1120.

31. Rajka G. Latency and duration of pruritus elicited by trypsin in aged patients with itching eczema and psoriasis. Acta Derm Venereol 1969; 49:401–403.
32. Hägermark O. Influence of antihistamines, sedatives, and aspirin on experimental itch. Acta Derm Venereol 1973; 53:363–368.
33. Steinhoff M, Vergnolle N, Young SH, et al. Agonists of proteinase-activated receptor 2 induce inflammation by a neurogenic mechanism. Nat Med 2000; 6:151–158.
34. Vergnolle N, Bunnett NW, Sharkey KA, et al. Proteinase-activated receptor-2 and hyperalgesia: a novel pain pathway. Nat Med 2001; 7:821–826.
35. Vergnolle N, Wallace JL, Bunnett NW, Hollenberg MD. Protease-activated receptors in inflammation, neuronal signaling and pain. Trends Pharmacol Sci 2001; 22:146–152.
36. Kawabata A, Kawao N, Kuroda R, Tanaka A, Itoh H, Nishikawa H. Peripheral PAR-2 triggers thermal hyperalgesia and nociceptive responses in rats. Neuroreport 2001; 12:715–719.
37. Corvera CU, Dery O, McConalogue K, et al. Thrombin and mast cell tryptase regulate guinea-pig myenteric neurons through proteinase-activated receptors-1 and -2. J Physiol (Lond) 1999; 517:741–756.
38. Hoogerwerf WA, Zou L, Shenoy M, et al. The proteinase-activated receptor 2 is involved in nociception. J Neurosci 2001; 21:9036–9042.
39. Coelho AM, Vergnolle N, Guiard B, Fioramonti J, Bueno L. Proteinases and proteinase-activated receptor 2: a possible role to promote visceral hyperalgesia in rats. Gastroenterology 2002; 122:1035–1047.
40. Kawagoe J, Takizawa T, Matsumoto J, et al. Effect of protease-activated receptor-2 deficiency on allergic dermatitis in the mouse ear. Jpn J Pharmacol 2002; 88:77–84.
41. Jarvikallio A, Naukkarinen A, Harvima IT, Aalto ML, Horsmanheimo M. Quantitative analysis of tryptase- and chymase-containing mast cells in atopic dermatitis and nummular eczema. Br J Dermatol 1997; 136:871–877.
42. Steinhoff M, Neisius U, Ikoma A, et al. Proteinase-activated receptor-2 mediates itch: a novel pathway for pruritus in human skin. J Neurosci 2003; 23:6176–6180.
43. Gough L, Schulz O, Sewell HF, Shakib F. The cysteine protease activity of the major dust mite allergen Der p 1 selectively enhances the immunoglobulin E antibody response. J Exp Med 1999; 190:1897–1902.
44. Wakita H, Furukawa F, Takigawa M. Thrombin and trypsin induce granulocyte-macrophage colony-stimulating factor and interleukin-6 gene expression in cultured normal human keratinocytes. Proc Assoc Am Physicians 1997; 109:190–207.
45. Pastore S, Giustizieri ML, Mascia F, Giannetti A, Kaushansky K, Girolomoni G. Dysregulated activation of activator protein 1 in keratinocytes of atopic dermatitis patients with enhanced expression of granulocyte/macrophage-colony stimulating factor. J Invest Dermatol 2000; 115:1134–1143.
46. D'Andrea MR, Rogahn CJ, Andrade-Gordon P. Localization of protease-activated receptors-1 and -2 in human mast cells: indications for an amplified mast cell degranulation cascade. Biotech Histochem 2000; 75:85–90.
47. Bar-Shavit R, Maoz M, Yongjun Y, Groysman M, Dekel I, Katzav S. Signalling pathways induced by protease-activated receptors and integrins in T cells. Immunology 2002; 105:35–46.
48. Cremer B, Heimann A, Dippel E, Czarnetzki BM. Pruritogenic effects of mitogen stimulated peripheral blood mononuclear cells in atopic eczema. Acta Derm Venereol (Stockh) 1995; 75:426–428.

49. Lippert U, Hoer A, Moller A, Ramboer I, Cremer B, Henz BM. Role of antigen-induced cytokine release in atopic pruritus. Int Arch Allergy Immunol 1998; 116:36–39.
50. Grothe C, Heese K, Meisinger C, et al. Expression of interleukin-6 and its receptor in the sciatic nerve and cultured Schwann cells: relation to 18-kD fibroblast growth factor-2. Brain Res 2000; 885:172–181.
51. Nordlind K, Chin LB, Ahmed AA, Brakenhoff J, Theodorsson E, Liden S. Immuno-histochemical localization of interleukin-6-like immunoreactivity to peripheral nerve-like structures in normal and inflamed human skin. Arch Dermatol Res 1996; 288:431–435.
52. Wahlgren CF, Tengvall Linder M, Hägermark O, Scheynius A. Itch and inflammation induced by intradermally injected interleukin-2 in atopic dermatitis patients and healthy subjects. Arch Dermatol Res 1995; 287:572–580.
53. Darsow U, Scharein E, Bromm B, Ring J. Skin testing of the pruritogenic activity of histamine and cytokines (interleukin-2 and tumour necrosis factor-alpha) at the dermal–epidermal junction. Br J Dermatol 1997; 137:415–417.
54. Chi KH, Myers JN, Chow KC, et al. Phase II trial of systemic recombinant inter-leukin-2 in the treatment of refractory nasopharyngeal carcinoma. Oncology 2001; 60:110–115.
55. Hägermark O, Strandberg K, Hamberg M. Potentiation of itch and flare responses in human skin by prostaglandins E2 and H2 and a prostaglandin endoperoxide analog. J Invest Dermatol 1977; 69:527–530.
56. Woodward DF, Nieves AL, Hawley SB, Joseph R, Merlino GF, Spada CS. The prur-itogenic and inflammatory effects of prostanoids in the conjunctiva. J Ocul Pharmacol Ther 1995; 11:339–347.
57. Neisius U, Olsson R, Rukwied R, Lischetzki G, Schmelz M. Prostaglandin E2 induces vasodilation and pruritus, but no protein extravasation in atopic dermatitis and con-trols. J Am Acad Dermatol 2002; 47:28–32.
58. Nilsson HJ, Levinsson A, Schouenborg J. Cutaneous field stimulation (CFS): a new powerful method to combat itch. Pain 1997; 71:49–55.
59. Brull SJ, Atanassoff PG, Silverman DG, Zhang J, LaMotte RH. Attenuation of exper-imental pruritus and mechanically evoked dysesthesiae in an area of cutaneous allo-dynia. Somatosens Mot Res 1999; 16:299–303.
60. Simone DA, Nolano M, Johnson T, Wendelschafer-Crabb G, Kennedy WR. Intrader-mal injection of capsaicin in humans produces degeneration and subsequent reinner-vation of epidermal nerve fibers: correlation with sensory function. J Neurosci 1998; 18:8947–8954.
61. Nolano M, Simone DA, Wendelschafer-Crabb G, Johnson T, Hazen E, Kennedy WR. Topical capsaicin in humans: parallel loss of epidermal nerve fibers and pain sen-sation. Pain 1999; 81:135–145.
62. Atanassoff PG, Brull SJ, Zhang J, Greenquist K, Silverman DG, LaMotte RH. Enhancement of experimental pruritus and mechanically evoked dysesthesiae with local anesthesia. Somatosens Mot Res 1999; 16:291–298.
63. Bromm B, Scharein E, Darsow U, Ring J. Effects of menthol and cold on histamine-induced itch and skin reactions in man. Neurosci Lett 1995; 187:157–160.
64. Mizumura K, Koda H. Potentiation and suppression of the histamine response by raising and lowering the temperature in canine visceral polymodal receptors in vitro. Neurosci Lett 1999; 266:9–12.

65. Heyer G, Ulmer FJ, Schmitz J, Handwerker HO. Histamine-induced itch and alloknesis (itchy skin) in atopic eczema patients and controls. Acta Derm Venereol (Stockh) 1995; 75:348–352.
66. Sugiura H, Omoto M, Hirota Y, Danno K, Uehara M. Density and fine structure of peripheral nerves in various skin lesions of atopic dermatitis. Arch Dermatol Res 1997; 289:125–131.
67. Urashima R, Mihara M. Cutaneous nerves in atopic dermatitis—a histological, immunohistochemical and electron microscopic study. Virch Arch Int J Pathol 1998; 432:363–370.
68. Grewe M, Vogelsang K, Ruzicka T, Stege H, Krutmann J. Neurotrophin-4 production by human epidermal keratinocytes: increased expression in atopic dermatitis. J Invest Dermatol 2000; 114:1108–1112.
69. Toyoda M, Nakamura M, Makino T, Hino T, Kagoura M, Morohashi M. Nerve growth factor and substance P are useful plasma markers of disease activity in atopic dermatitis. Br J Dermatol 2002; 147:71–79.
70. Kinkelin I, Motzing S, Koltenzenburg M, Brocker EB. Increase in NGF content and nerve fiber sprouting in human allergic contact eczema. Cell Tissue Res 2000; 302:31–37.
71. Romero MI, Rangappa N, Li L, Lightfoot E, Garry MG, Smith GM. Extensive sprouting of sensory afferents and hyperalgesia induced by conditional expression of nerve growth factor in the adult spinal cord. J Neurosci 2000; 20:4435–4445.
72. Shu XQ, Mendell LM. Neurotrophins and hyperalgesia. Proc Natl Acad Sci USA 1999; 96:7693–7696.
73. Bickford RGL. Experiments relating to itch sensation, its peripheral mechanism and central pathways. Clin Sci 1938; 3:377–386.
74. Simone DA, Alreja M, LaMotte RH. Psychophysical studies of the itch sensation and itchy skin ("alloknesis") produced by intracutaneous injection of histamine. Somatosens Mot Res 1991; 8:271–279.
75. Nilsson HJ, Schouenborg J. Differential inhibitory effect on human nociceptive skin senses induced by local stimulation of thin cutaneous fibers. Pain 1999; 80:103–112.
76. Vogelsang M, Heyer G, Hornstein OP. Acetylcholine induces different cutaneous sensations in atopic and non-atopic subjects. Acta Derm Venereol 1995; 75:434–436.
77. Groene D, Martus P, Heyer G. Doxepin affects acetylcholine induced cutaneous reactions in atopic eczema. Exp Dermatol 2001; 10:110–117.
78. Ikoma A, Rukwied R, Stander S, Steinhoff M, Miyachi Y, Schmelz M. Neuronal sensitization for histamine-induced itch in lesional skin of patients with atopic dermatitis. Arch Dermatol 2003; 139:1455–1458.
79. Heyer G, Hornstein OP, Handwerker HO. Skin reactions and itch sensation induced by epicutaneous histamine application in atopic dermatitis and controls. J Invest Dermatol 1989; 93:492–496.
80. Schmelz M, Hilliges M, Schmidt R, et al. Active "itch fibers" in chronic pruritus. Neurology 2003; 61:564–566.
81. Reeh PW, Kress M. Effects of classical algogens. Semin Neurosci 1995; 7:221–226.
82. Fjellner B, Hägermark O. Experimental pruritus evoked by platelet activating factor (PAF-acether) in human skin. Acta Derm Venereol 1985; 65:409–412.

83. Woodward DF, Nieves AL, Spada CS, Williams LS, Tuckett RP. Characterization of a behavioral model for peripherally evoked itch suggests platelet-activating factor as a potent pruritogen. J Pharmacol Exp Ther 1995; 272:758–765.

84. Thomsen JS, Sonne M, Benfeldt E, Jensen SB, Serup J, Menne T. Experimental itch in sodium lauryl sulphate-inflamed and normal skin in humans: a randomized, double-blind, placebo-controlled study of histamine and other inducers of itch. Br J Dermatol 2002; 146:792–800.

85. Thomsen JS, Petersen MB, Benfeldt E, Jensen SB, Serup J. Scratch induction in the rat by intradermal serotonin: a model for pruritus. Acta Derm Venereol 2001; 81:250–254.

86. Jinks SL, Carstens E. Responses of superficial dorsal horn neurons to intradermal serotonin and other irritants: comparison with scratching behavior. J Neurophysiol 2002; 87:1280–1289.

87. Inagaki N, Nagao M, Igeta K, Kawasaki H, Kim JF, Nagai H. Scratching behavior in various strains of mice. Skin Pharmacol Appl Skin Physiol 2001; 14:87–96.

88. Andoh T, Kuraishi Y. Nitric oxide enhances substance P-induced itch-associated responses in mice. Br J Pharmacol 2003; 138:202–208.

89. Andoh T, Honma Y, Kawaharada S, Al Akeel A, Nojima H, Kuraishi Y. Inhibitory effect of the repeated treatment with Unsei-in on substance P-induced itch-associated responses through the downregulation of the expression of NK (1) tachykinin receptor in mice. Biol Pharm Bull 2003; 26:896–898.

90. Carstens E. Responses of rat spinal dorsal horn neurons to intracutaneous microinjection of histamine, capsaicin, and other irritants. J Neurophysiol 1997; 77:2499–2514.

91. Yamaguchi T, Nagasawa T, Satoh M, Kuraishi Y. Itch-associated response induced by intradermal serotonin through 5-HT2 receptors in mice. Neurosci Res 1999; 35:77–83.

92. Thomsen JS, Simonsen L, Benfeldt E, Jensen SB, Serup J. The effect of topically applied salicylic compounds on serotonin-induced scratching behaviour in hairless rats. Exp Dermatol 2002; 11:370–375.

93. Nojima H, Carstens E. Quantitative assessment of directed hind limb scratching behavior as a rodent itch model. J Neurosci Meth 2003; 126:137–143.

94. Miyamoto T, Nojima H, Shinkado T, Nakahashi T, Kuraishi Y. Itch-associated response induced by experimental dry skin in mice. Jpn J Pharmacol 2002; 88: 285–292.

95. Nojima H, Carstens E. 5-Hydroxytryptamine (5-HT)2 receptor involvement in acute 5-HT-evoked scratching but not in allergic pruritus induced by dinitrofluorobenzene in rats. J Pharmacol Exp Ther 2003; 306:245–252.

96. Chan LS, Robinson N, Xu L. Expression of interleukin-4 in the epidermis of transgenic mice results in a pruritic inflammatory skin disease: an experimental animal model to study atopic dermatitis. J Invest Dermatol 2001; 117:977–983.

97. Thomsen JS, Benfeldt E, Jensen SB, Serup J, Menne T. Topically applied aspirin decreases histamine-induced wheal and flare reactions in normal and SLS-inflamed skin, but does not decrease itch. A randomized, double-blind and placebo-controlled human study. Acta Derm Venereol 2002; 82:30–35.

98. Kobayashi H, Kikuchi K, Tsubono Y, Tagami H. Measurement of electrical current perception threshold of sensory nerves for pruritus in atopic dermatitis patients and normal individuals with various degrees of mild damage to the stratum corneum. Dermatology 2003; 206:204–211.

4

Ethnic Sensitive Skin

Manisha J. Patel

Department of Dermatology, Wake Forest University Health Sciences Center, Winston-Salem, North Carolina, U.S.A.

Gil Yosipovitch

Department of Dermatology, Neurobiology, and Anatomy, Wake Forest University Health Sciences Center, Winston-Salem, North Carolina, U.S.A.

The diversification of the world's population and global marketing raises the importance of understanding issues of ethnic sensitive skin and also begs the elucidation of the role of ethnic variation. Variations in skin properties inherent to specific races may explain the disparities seen in dermatologic diseases between different ethnic groups.

Despite the exponential growth of medical research and information, very little data have been published on the biology of ethnic skin. Racial differences in skin have been minimally investigated by objective measures and, historically, these investigations have primarily focused on the differences between black and white skin (1,2). More recently, a heightened sensitivity among Asian populations versus Caucasians has been suggested, though not substantiated by reliable evidence. Foy et al. investigated two matched panels of Caucasian and Japanese women volunteers to determine their topical irritant reaction, both acute and cumulative, to a range of materials. Although the acute irritant response to stronger irritants tended to be greater in the Japanese panel, reaching statistical significance, cumulative irritation, albeit to weaker irritants, rarely reached significance between the two cohorts (3).

Jourdain et al. conducted an epidemiological survey to examine the possible ethnic variations in perception of sensitive skin with four different ethnic groups (Afro-Americans, Asians, Euro-Americans, and Hispanics). Although no statistical difference between the ethnic groups in terms of sensitive skin prevalence was noted, this limited study revealed some general trends that may be quite relevant at the population level (4). This lack of concurrent studies makes racial differences in skin sensitivity one of the more confounding issues in dermatology.

Recent consumer marketing surveys have shown that the number of female consumers assessed as having sensitive skin has been rising, thus highlighting the need to formulate a clear definition, identify reliable and valid objective measures, and further clarify racial variations to best tailor individual care (5). The introduction of new products and ingredients into the marketplace requires skin-safety testing. A risk-assessment process is required to insure skin compatibility under a variety of potential exposure conditions. In an age of global market economies, dermatologists and industry are charged with elucidating whether diverse human populations differ with respect to their susceptibility to adverse skin reactions when exposed to identical chemical and physical insults. This chapter reviews the data to date on racial variations in skin sensitivity.

Conflicting data have been published on the inherent differences in skin surface properties among various ethnic groups, though there is a widespread perception that differences exist (6). Armed with tools to assess variation, one must seek to explain the etiology for ethnic variation in skin sensitivity. Studies examining skin properties have sought to explain the similarities and differences seen between various racial groups. Objective methods studied have included numerous measures including transepidermal water loss (TEWL), blood-vessel reactivity, and epidermal pH. Other physiologic measurements evaluated are listed in Table 1. Berardesca and Maibach (7) highlight that the interpretation of pathophysiologic phenomena should consider not only anatomic and functional characteristics of ethnic groups but also socioeconomic, hygienic, and nutritional differences. Hygienic and cosmetic practices are often delineated by one's cultural environment and, thereby, add a variable into the equation that is difficult to assess as a potential cause of racial variation in skin sensitivity.

BIOPHYSICAL PARAMETERS

The presumption that there are physiological differences between the races and these presumed differences account for variations in perceived skin sensitivity have led to several studies comparing properties used to assess barrier function. Initial studies dating back to the early 1900s used erythema as the endpoint to quantify irritation. Four studies between 1919 and 1982 concluded that using erythema as a measure of irritation showed that blacks are less reactive than Caucasians to irritants (1,8–10). If, however, the stratum corneum was removed, black and Caucasian subjects had no significant difference in irritation

Table 1   Main Structural and Functional Properties Used to Study Barrier Function[a]

TEWL
Blood vessel reactivity/laser Doppler velocimetry
Stratum corneum thickness
Number of cell layers and resistance to stripping (22)[a]
Lipid content (23)[a]
Water content measured by skin capacitance, conductance, impedance, and resistance
Electrical resistance (24)[a]
Desquamation (25)[a]
Corneocyte size
Amount of ceramides (26)[a]
Recovery after stripping
Sebum production
Epidermal pH

[a]Differences shown between black and Caucasian skin.
Abbreviation: TEWL, transepidermal water loss.
Source: From Ref. 7.

as measured by erythema (11). This led many researchers to evaluate anatomical and physiological differences of the stratum corneum. Table 2 highlights anatomical differences discovered between black and Caucasian skin. However, inherent problems exist with these conclusions. Visual scoring of erythema is quite subjective and notoriously difficult to measure in darker skin (2). This limitation led researchers to then look for structural differences in the stratum corneum that would account for differences in irritation responses in blacks and Caucasians.

TEWL reflects the integrity of the barrier function of the stratum corneum. TEWL has been measured under basal conditions in whites, Hispanics, and blacks to assess whether melanin content could induce changes in skin biophysical properties. Berardesca et al. (12) found that no racial differences in TEWL exists either on the volar or dorsal forearms. Several smaller scale studies comparing TEWL between Asians and Caucasians, in addition to the different Asian subgroups—Chinese, Malays, and Indians—did not demonstrate any significant differences (13,14). However, the correlation of this information to variations in skin sensitivity is difficult given that most researchers agree that basal measurements of TEWL do not correlate with the ability of the stratum corneum to function under conditions of skin irritation and adverse occupational environments (15).

SKIN IRRITATION

Studies conducted by Robinson assessing racial differences in acute and cumulative skin irritation caused by occluded patch test exposure between Caucasians and Asian populations (Chinese and Japanese) underscored that although it

Table 2   Structural Differences Between Black and White Skin

Structure	Black skin	White skin
Epidermal melanosome	Large, membrane-bound, and distributed primarily singly inside keratinocytes; numerous even in stratum corneum	Small and distributed primarily in aggregates
Hair follicle melanosomes	In outer root sheath and in bulb of vellus hairs	Neither in outer root sheath nor in bulb of vellus hair follicles
Fibroblasts	Numerous and large; many binucleated and multinucleated ones	Variable numbers; some binucleated and multinucleated ones
Blood vessels (superficial)	Numerous, mostly dilated	Sparse to moderate numbers
Lymphatic vessels	Numerous	Moderated numbers
Mixed eccrine, apocine glands	Many	Variable
Stratum corneum thickness	Same	Same

Source: From Ref. 27.

may be possible to detect differences in individual studies, repeat testing often fails to confirm a consistent trend (16,17). After sodium lauryl sulphate testing between Japanese and German women, Aramaki et al. (13) found no significant differences in the barrier function in the stratum corneum; they, however, noted significant subjective sensory differences. Their group concluded that perhaps Japanese women complain about stronger sensations, reflecting a different cultural behavior rather than measurable differences in skin physiology.

NERVE FIBER

Researchers have sought to elucidate if variations in perception of skin irritation can be accounted for by differences in nerve fiber networks. As a first line of defense, the skin is equipped with a complex and interactive nerve fiber system to detect irritants and maintain homeostasis. In a study conducted by Reilly et al. (18), no apparent difference in innervation was observed between European Caucasian and Japanese/Chinese skin at the architectural or biochemical level (18). The presence, properties, and biochemical content of fibers between various ethnic skin types was similar in all cases tested.

   Variations in ethnic skin have also been explored by studying the perception of pain, and one could extrapolate sensitivity in dermatologic patients using a psychophysical, computerized, quantitative, thermal, sensory-testing device.

The study included a total of 20 Chinese, 14 Malay, and 15 Indian subjects. Using the method of limits, experimental pain perception threshold was measured on the forehead and volar aspect of the forearm. The measurements were repeated after skin-barrier perturbation with adhesive tape stripping of the stratum corneum. Thermal pain thresholds were similar in all three ethnic groups before and after tape stripping (19).

Many researchers and policy makers argue against the use of racial categories in medicine, saying that classifying people according to race reinforces existing social divisions in society or leads to discriminatory practices (20). Modern concepts of race and ethnicity have been cast as largely social constructions (21). However, advances in genetics and developments in pharmacogenetics have renewed the historical emphasis on biology in concepts of race and ethnicity. As the pendulum swings again to emphasize biological differences between races, we cannot ignore modern conceptions of race that emphasize social and political heritage. By focusing on biological factors as the explanation for differences in skin sensitivity between ethnic groups, researchers risk ignoring possible environmental, psychosocial, and economic factors that are important in producing sensitive skin.

REFERENCES

1. Anderson KE, Maibach HI. Black and white human skin differences. J Am Acad Dermatol 1976; 276–282.
2. Modjtahedi SP, Maibach HI. Ethnicity as a possible endogenous factor in irritant contact dermatitis: comparing the irritant response among Caucasians, Blacks, and Asians. Contact Dermatitis 2002; 47(5):272–278.
3. Foy V, Weinkauf R, Whittle E, Basketter DA. Ethnic variation in the skin irritation response. Contact Dermatitis, 2001; 45(6):346–349.
4. Jourdain R, Lacharriere O, Bastien P, Maibach HI. Ethnic variations in self-perceived sensitive skin: epidemiological survey. Contact Dermatitis 46(3):162–169.
5. Willis CM, Shaw S, De Lacharriere O, Baverel M, Reiche L, Jourdain R, et al. Sensitive skin: an epidemiological study. Br J Dermatol 2001; 145(2):258–263.
6. Grimes P, Edison BL, Green BA, Wildnauer RH. Evaluation of inherent differences between African, American and white skin surface properties using subjective and objective measures. Cutis 2004; 73(6):392–396.
7. Berardesca E, Maibach H. Ethnic skin: overview of structure and function. J Am Acad Dermatol 2003; 48(suppl 6):S139–S142.
8. Buckley CE III, Lee KL, Burdick DS. Methacholine-induced cutaneous flare response: bivariate analysis of responsiveness and sensitivity. J Allergy Clin Immunol 1982; 69(1 Pt 1):25–34.
9. Marshal EK, Lynch V, Smith HW. On dichlorethylsulphide (mustard gas) II. Variations in susceptibility of the skin to dichlorethylsulphide. J Pharmacol Exp Therapy 1919; 12:291–301.
10. Weigand DA, Mershon MM. The cutaneous irritant reaction to agent O-chlorobenzylidene (CS). Report No. EB-TR-4332, 1970.

11. Weigand DA, Gaylor JR. Irritant reaction in Negro and Caucasian skin. South Med J 1974; 67(5):548–551.
12. Berardesca E, de RJ, Leveque JL, Maibach HI. In vivo biophysical characterization of skin physiological differences in races. Dermatologica 1991; 182(2):89–93.
13. Aramaki J, Kawana S, Effendy I, Happle R, Loffler H. Differences of skin irritation between Japanese and European women. Br J Dermatol 2002; 146(6):1052–1056.
14. Goh CL, Chia SE. Skin irritability to sodium lauryl sulphate—as measured by skin water vapour loss—by sex and race. Clin Exp Dermatol 1988; 13(1):16–19.
15. Yosipovitch G, Theng C. Asian skin: its architecture, function and differences from Caucasian skin. Cosmet Toiletries 2000; 117(9):57–62.
16. Robinson MK. Population differences in acute skin irritation responses: race, sex, age, sensitive skin and repeat subject comparisons. Contact Dermatitis 2002; 46(2):86–93.
17. Robinson MK. Racial differences in acute and cumulative skin irritation responses between Caucasian and Asian populations. Contact Dermatitis 2000; 42(3):134–143.
18. Reilly DM, Ferdinando D, Johnston C, Shaw C, Buchanan KD, Green MR. The epidermal nerve fibre network: characterization of nerve fibres in human skin by confocal microscopy and assessment of racial variations. Br J Dermatol 1997; 137(2):163–170.
19. Yosipovitch G, Meredith G, Chan YH, Goh CL. Do ethnicity and gender have an impact on pain thresholds in minor dermatologic procedures? A study on thermal pain perception thresholds in Asian ethnic groups. Skin Res Technol 2004; 10(1):38–42.
20. Lee SS, Mountain J, Koenig BA. The meanings of "race" in the new genomics: implications for health disparities research. Yale J Health Policy Law Ethics 2001; 1:33–75.
21. Bhopal R. Glossary of terms relating to ethnicity and race: for reflection and debate. J Epidemiol Commun Health 2004; 58(6):441–445.
22. Robinson MK. Population differences in skin structure and physiology and the susceptibility to irritant and allergic contact dermatitis: implications for skin safety testing and risk assessment. Contact Dermatitis 1999; 41(2):65–79.
23. Rienerston RP, Wheatley VR. Studies on the chemical composition of human epidermal lipids. J Invest Dermatol 1959; 32:49–51.
24. Johnson LC, Corah NL. Racial differences in skin resistance. Science 1963; 139:766–769.
25. Corcuff P, Lotte C, Rougier A, Maibach HI. Racial differences in corneocytes: a comparison between black, white and oriental skin. Acta Derm Venereol 1991; 71(2):146–148.
26. Sugino K, Imokawa G, Maibach H. Ethnic difference of stratum corneum lipid in relation to stratum corneum function. J Invest Dermatol 1993; 100:597.
27. Stephens TJ, Oresajo C. Ethnic sensitive skin. Cosmetic and Toiletries 1994; 109(2):75–80.

5

Ethnic Differences in Skin Sensitivity and Responses to Topically Applied Products

Enzo Berardesca

San Gallicano Dermatological Institute, Rome, Italy

Howard I. Maibach

Department of Dermatology, University of California, San Francisco, California, U.S.A.

Racial differences in skin physiology and reaction to environmental stimuli are more and more described (1). Besides changes in biological behavior, many factors such as exposure, hygiene, and socioeconomical levels may play a role. This chapter reviews the more consistent differences reported between racial groups and their implications in determining different responses after use of topical products.

SKIN PERMEABILITY

Stratum corneum is equally thick in black and white skin (2,3). However, Weigand et al. (4) demonstrated that the stratum corneum in blacks contains more cell layers and requires more cellophane tape strips to remove than the stratum corneum of Caucasians. They found great variance in values obtained from black subjects, whereas data from white subjects were more homogeneous. No correlation existed between the degree of pigmentation and the number of cell layers. These data could be explained by greater intercellular cohesion in blacks resulting in an increased number of cell layers and an increased resistance to stripping. This mechanism may involve lipids, because the lipid content of the stratum corneum ranges from 8.5% to 14%, with higher values in blacks (5). This result was confirmed by Weigand et al. (4) who showed that delipidized specimens of stratum corneum were equal in weight in the two races. Johnson and Corah (6) found the mean electrical resistance of adult black skin to be twice that of adult white skin, suggesting an increased cohesion or thickness of the stratum corneum.

Corcuff et al. (7) investigated the corneocyte surface area and spontaneous desquamation and found no evidence of differences among black, white, and Oriental skin. However, an increased desquamation (up to 2.5 times) was found ($P < 0.01$) in blacks. They concluded that the differences may be related to a different composition of the intercellular cement of the stratum corneum. Sugino et al. (8) found significant differences in the amount of ceramides in the stratum corneum, with the lowest levels in blacks followed by Caucasians, Hispanics, and Asians. In this experiment, ceramide levels were inversely correlated with transepidermal water loss (TEWL) and directly correlated with water content. These data may partially explain the controversial findings in the literature on the mechanisms of skin sensitivity.

Kompaore et al. (9) evaluated TEWL and lag time after the application of a vasoactive compound before and after the removal of the stratum corneum. They found a significantly higher TEWL after stripping in blacks and Asians than in whites. In particular, after stripping, Asians showed the highest TEWL and, at the same time, an increased permeability (compared with the other races) obtained immediately after a few strips.

In contrast, Reed et al. (10) found differences in the recovery of the barrier between subjects with skin type II/III compared with skin type IV, but no differences between Caucasians, in general, and Asians. Darker skin recovered faster after barrier damage induced by tape stripping.

BIOPHYSICAL PARAMETERS

TEWL, skin conductance, and skin mechanical properties have been measured under basal conditions in whites, Hispanics, and blacks to assess whether skin color (melanin content) could induce changes in skin biophysical properties (11). Differences appear in skin conductance, but are more marked in biomechanical features such as skin extensibility, skin elastic modulus, and skin recovery. They differ in dorsal and ventral sites according to races and highlight the influence of solar irradiation on skin and the role of melanin in maintaining it unaltered.

No racial differences in TEWL exist either on the volar or the dorsal forearms. However, water content is increased in Hispanics on the volar forearm and decreased in whites (compared only to blacks) on the dorsal forearm. These findings partially confirm previous observations (12,13). Skin lipids may play a role in modulating the relation between stratum corneum water content and TEWL, resulting in higher conductance values in blacks and Hispanics.

Racial differences in skin conductance are difficult to interpret in terms of stratum corneum water content, because other physical factors, such as the skin surface or the presence of hair, can modify the quality of the skin–electrode contact. In all races, significant differences exist between the volar and the dorsal forearms (11). These results are in apparent contrast to the TEWL recordings. Indeed, increased stratum corneum water content correlates with a higher TEWL (14). The data may be explained on the basis of the different intercellular cohesion or lipid composition. A greater cell cohesion with a normal TEWL could result in increased skin water content.

Racial variability should be considered in terms of different skin responses to topical and environmental agents. Race provides a useful tool to investigate and compare the effects of lifetime sun exposure. It is evident that melanin protection decreases sun damage; differences between sun-exposed and sun-protected areas are not detectable in races with dark skin.

However, TEWL studies are characterized by a large inter-individual variability and biased by environmental effects and eccrine sweating. To bypass these influences, an in vitro technique for measuring TEWL was used to compare TEWL in two racial groups (blacks and whites) (15). Black skin had a significantly higher mean TEWL than white skin. In both groups, a significant correlation between skin temperature and increased TEWL was found ($P < 0.01$). The data confirm differences between races found in in vivo studies (12,13).

SKIN DISEASE AND COSMETIC PROBLEMS

Irritant and Allergic Contact Dermatitis

In 1919, Marshall et al. (16) investigated cutaneous reactions to 1% dichloroethylsulfide in whites and blacks. A drop on the forearm elicited erythema in 58% of whites but only 15% of black subjects, suggesting a decreased susceptibility to cutaneous irritants in blacks. Weigand and Mershon (17) studied patch test reactions to *ortho*-chlorobenzylidene malononitrile. The results indicated that blacks were more resistant and required a significantly longer exposure to develop an irritant reaction. Subsequently, Weigand and Gaylor (18) measured minimal perceptible erythema in blacks and whites after applying dinitrochlorobenzene to intact skin and to skin after the stratum corneum was largely removed by tape stripping. The results confirmed that blacks were generally less susceptible to cutaneous irritants. However, this difference was not detectable when the stratum corneum was removed. They also observed that the range of reactions in normal skin in both races was wider than in stripped skin, suggesting that the stratum corneum may modulate the different racial responses to skin irritants.

Irritation, as measured by TEWL (12,13) revealed a different pattern of reaction in whites after chemical exposure to sodium lauryl sulfate. Blacks and Hispanics developed stronger irritant reactions after exposure.

Stinging may occur in the nasolabial folds and on cheeks after an irritant is applied. Frosch and Kligman (19) reported that most "stingers" were light-complexioned persons of Celtic ancestry who sunburned easily and tanned poorly. Later, however, Grove et al. (20) found no skin-type propensity to sting-ing; they applied 10% lactic acid to the nasolabial folds and cheeks of volunteers and noted that increased stinging was related mainly to the person's history of sensitivity to soaps, cosmetics, and drugs.

Conflicting findings have been reported on the incidence of allergic contact dermatitis in blacks. Kenney (21) reported a decreased rate (5% in black patients). Marshall and Heyl (22) reported that the incidence of industrial contact dermatitis in South Africa is less in darkly pigmented blacks. Bantus showed a 7.4% prevalence (23). Scott (24) noted that contact dermatitis was less frequent in Bantus handling detergents, waxes, and fuels. Despite a previous report describing an increased sensitization rate in whites, Kligman and Epstein (25) found no significant difference in the two races after testing many topical materials. Fisher (26) reported an approximately equal incidence of contact der-matitis in blacks and whites. Paraphenylenediamine, nickel, and potassium bichromate appeared to be the most common allergens.

In Nigeria, nickel was the most frequent sensitizer, with an incidence of 12.3% (27) compared with 11% in North America. In Lagos, the female:male ratio is 1:1, whereas Fregert et al. (28) recorded a ratio of 6:1. In North America, the ratio is 3:1 and in Stockholm, it is 7:3.

Clinically, acute contact dermatitis with exudation, vesiculation, or bullae is more common in whites, whereas blacks more commonly develop disorders of pigmentation and lichenification. Hypopigmentation has been described from contact with phenolic detergents (29), alkylphenols, and monobenzylether of hydroquinone (30).

Acne is believed to be the commonest dermatologic disease in black patients. The most dramatic difference between black and white skin is the inflammatory reaction resulting in postinflammatory hyperpigmentation which is more pronounced in black skin. This condition occurs as darkly pigmented spots or macules, which may persist for months or years after the resolution of acne lesions (31).

EFFECTS OF TOPICALLY APPLIED PRODUCTS

A proneness of blacks to "pomade acne" has been demonstrated. This eruption, consisting mainly of comedones on the forehead and temporal area, seems to be a peculiar response of black skin to topical agents because this reaction can be detected in black children from one to 12 years of age (32). Plewig et al. (33) examined 735 blacks and found that 70% of long-term users of pomades had a form of acne. The more elaborate formulations induced pomade acne more fre-quently and more intensively than simpler preparations such as mineral oil and petroleum jelly. The distribution of the lesions corresponded to the area of contact. Comparable data for whites are lacking. Keratolytics and other chemicals used in acne therapy often cause hyperpigmentation in blacks.

Kaidbey and Kligman (34) studied race-dependent cutaneous reactivity to topical coal. There was a strikingly different response in the two groups: in whites, the response was primarily inflammatory, with development of papules and papulopustules in about two or three weeks, whereas in blacks the inflammatory response was largely absent and, after about 14 days, an eruption of small open comedones appeared. The follicles of white subjects responded early, with rupture of the wall and outpouring of follicular contents in the dermis, whereas in blacks, the first response was proliferative with production and retention of horny cells. That is, in blacks, the skin reacts to a comedogenic compound with hyperkeratoses rather than with the disintegration of follicles, suggesting a greater resistance to irritants.

EFFECTS OF BLEACHING AGENTS AND EXOGENOUS OCHRONOSIS

Ochronosis is a gray discoloration of connective tissue and can be induced by the accumulation of homogentisic acid (HGA) into the skin. In particular, HGA binds to fibrillar collagen, resulting in such discoloration. Besides the endogenous form resulting from the absence of the enzyme HGA oxidase, exogenous ochronosis can be induced in pigmented skin as a consequence of the use of some topical compounds such as pycric acid, phenol, resorcinol, and hydroquinone. Usually, when induced by hydroquinone (which is a phenolic compound similar to HGA), the discoloration appears within few months of application (35). In the U.S. population, the condition has been described to appear in pigmented skin (blacks and Hispanics) after the use of topical hydroquinone at concentrations of 2% or higher for months or years. In these subjects, hydroquinone was applied continuously as a bleaching agent, in order to treat dark pigmentation or dark skin discoloration such as melasma or postinflammatory pigmentation (36). Nevertheless, exogenous ochronosis is not as frequent in the U.S. as in some African populations and countries. This appears to be due to the high concentrations of hydroquinone available in skin-lightening products prior to 1984 in South Africa (average 6–8%) (37). Other compounds capable of inducing irreversible depigmentation, such as *t*-butyl alcohol and mercury, were included in skin-care products in South Africa until 1986. Resorcinol, used in some African countries in cosmetic products for acne, has also been related to the onset of exogenous ochronosis. Hydroquinone and resorcinol are also used simultaneously to achieve a faster depigmentation (37). Furthermore, alcoholic lotions and vehicles used in lightening and acne products can increase the percutaneous absorption of hydroquinone (38).

From a clinical point of view, exogenous ochronosis can be classified into three stages (39):

- Stage I involves erythema and mild pigmentation of the face and the neck.
- Stage II is characterized by the appearance of papules and mottled pigmentation.
- Stage III includes papulonodules and inflammation.

The etiology of hydroquinone and other bleaching agent–induced ochronosis is still uncertain. Although low concentrations of hydroquinone inhibit tyrosinase, higher ones can increase melanin synthesis apparently as a consequence of tyrosinase stimulation (40). Melanocytes can be involved in the process of ochronosis, as it does not appear in the areas affected by vitiligo. The role of sun exposure is still debated, as well (41). Indeed, the condition is often limited to sun-exposed areas.

The treatment of exogenous ochronosis is difficult. Avoidance of exposure to the causative agent may slowly improve the condition. Chemical peels, cryotherapy, and retinoic acid have been used with poor results.

REFERENCES

1. Berardesca E, Maibach H. Racial differences in skin pathophysiology. J Am Acad Dermatol 1996; 34:667–672.
2. Freeman RG, Cockerell EG, Armstrong J, et al. Sunlight as a factor influencing the thickness of epidermis. J Invest Dermatol 1962; 39:295–297.
3. Thomson ML. Relative efficiency of pigment and horny layer thickness in protecting the skin of European and Africans against solar ultraviolet radiation. J Physiol (Lond) 1955; 127:236.
4. Weigand DA, Haygood C, Gaylor JR. Cell layers and density of Negro and Caucasians stratum corneum. J Invest Dermatol 1974; 62:563–565.
5. Rienertson RP, Wheatley VR. Studies on the chemical composition of human epidermal lipids. J Invest Dermatol 1959; 32:49–51.
6. Johnson LC, Corah NL. Racial differences in skin resistance. Science 1963; 139: 766–769.
7. Corcuff P, Lotte C, Rougier A, Maibach H. Racial differences in corneocytes. Acta Derm Venereol (Stockh) 1991; 71:146–148.
8. Sugino K, Imokawa G, Maibach H. Ethnic difference of stratum corneum lipid in relation to stratum corneum function. J Invest Dermatol 1993; 100:597.
9. Kompaore F, Marty JP, Dupont CH. In vivo evaluation of the stratum corneum barrier function in Blacks, Caucasians and Asians with two noninvasive methods. Skin Pharmacol 1993; 6:200–207.
10. Reed JT, Ghadially R, Elias PM. Effect of race, gender and skin type on epidermal permeability barrier function. J Invest Dermatol 1994; 102:537.
11. Berardesca E, de Rigal J, Leveque JL, Maibach HI. In vivo biophysical characterization of skin physiological differences in races. Dermatologica 1991; 182:89–93.
12. Berardesca E, Maibach HI. Racial differences in sodium lauryl sulphate induced cutaneous irritation: black and white. Contact Dermatitis 1988; 18:65–70.

13. Berardesca E, Maibach HI. Sodium lauryl sulphate induced cutaneous irritation: comparison of white and Hispanic subjects. Contact Dermatitis 1988; 19:136–140.
14. Rietschel RL. A method to evaluate skin moisturizers in vivo. J Invest Dermatol 1978; 70:152–155.
15. Wilson D, Berardesca E, Maibach HI. In vitro transepidermal water loss: differences between black-and-white human skin. Br J Dermatol 1988; 119:647–652.
16. Marshall EK, Lynch V, Smith HV. Variation in susceptibility of the skin to dichloroethylsulfide. J Pharmacol Exp Ther 1919; 12:291–301.
17. Weigand DA, Mershon GE. The cutaneous irritant reaction to agent O-chlorobenzylidene malonitrile (CS): quantitation and racial influence in human subjects. Edgewood Arsenal Technical Report 4332, February 1970.
18. Weigand DA, Gaylor JR. Irritant reaction in Negro and Caucasian skin. South Med J 1974; 67:548–551.
19. Frosh P, Kligman AM. A method for appraising the stinging capacity of topically applied substances. J Soc Cosmetic Chem 1981; 28:197.
20. Grove GL, Soschin DM, Kligman AM. Adverse subjective reactions to topical agents. In: Drill VA, Lazar P, eds. Cutaneous Toxicology. New York: Raven Press, 1984.
21. Kenney J. Dermatoses seen in American Negroes. Int J Dermatol 1970; 9:110–113.
22. Marshall J, Heyl T. Skin diseases in the Western Cape Province. S Afr Med J 1963; 37:1308.
23. Dogliotti M. Skin disorders in the Bantu: a survey of 2000 cases from Baragwanath Hospital. S Afr Med J 1970; 44:670.
24. Scott F. Skin diseases in the South African Bantu. In: Marshall J, ed. Essays on Tropical Dermatology. Amsterdam: Excerpta Medica, 1972.
25. Kligman AM, Epstein W. Updating the maximization test for identifying contact allergens. Contact Dermatitis 1975; 1:231.
26. Fisher AA. Contact dermatitis in black patients. Cutis 1977; 20:303–320.
27. Olumide YM. Contact dermatitis in Nigeria. Contact Dermatitis 1985; 12:241–246.
28. Fregert S, Hjorth N, Magnusson B, et al. Epidemiology of contact dermatitis. Trans St John's Hosp Dermatol Soc 1969; 55:17.
29. Fisher AA. Vitiligo due to contactants. Cutis 1976; 17:431–437.
30. Kahn G. Depigmentation caused by phenolic detergent germicides. Arch Dermatol 1970; 102:177–187.
31. Taylor S. Cosmetic problems in skin of color. Skin Pharmacol Appl Skin Physiol 1999; 12:139–143.
32. Verhagen AR. Pomade acne in black patients. Arch Dermatol 1974; 110:465.
33. Plewig G, Fulton JE, Kligman AM. Pomade acne. Arch Dermatol 1970; 101:580.
34. Kaidbey KH, Kligman AM. A human model for coal tar acne. Arch Dermatol 1974; 109:212–215.
35. Levin CY, Maibach H. Exogenous ochronosis: an update on clinical features, causative agents and treatment options. Am J Clin Dermatol 2001; 2:213–217.
36. Touart D, Sau P. Cutaneous deposition diseases, Part II. J Am Acad Dermatol 1998; 39:527–544.
37. Burke P, Maibach H. Exogenous ochronosis: an overview. J Dermatol Treatment 1997; 8:21–26.
38. Bucks D, McMaster J, Guy R, et al. Percutaneous absorption of hydroquinone in humans: effect of 1-dodecylazacycloheptan-2-one (azone) and the 2-ethylhexylester

of 4-(dimethylamino)benzoic acid (Escalol 507). J Toxicol Environ Health 1988; 24:279–289.

39. Dogliotti M, Leibowitz M. Granulomatous ochronosis: a cosmetic-induced skin disorder in blacks. S Afr Med J 1979; 56:757–760.

40. Chen Y, Chavin W. Hydroquinone activation and inhibition of skin tyrosinase. In: Riley V, ed. Proceedings of the 9th International Pigment Cell Conference, New York: Karger, 1976:105–112.

41. O'Donoghue M, Lynfield Y, Derbes V. Ochronosis due to hydroquinone. J Am Acad Dermatol 1983; 8:123–125.

6

The Complex Problems of Sensitive Skin

Marie C. Marriott, David A. Basketter, and Karen J. Cooper

*Safety and Environmental Assurance Centre,
Unilever Colworth, Bedford, U.K.*

INTRODUCTION

It is widely reported that there is a substantial proportion of the population who have, or believe themselves to have, "sensitive skin." Willis et al. (1) reported that approximately 50% of women and 40% of men surveyed regarded themselves as having sensitive skin. Loffler et al. (2) suggest that the perception of sensitive skin is possibly influenced by the media, as published data suggest no correlation between objective skin findings and complaints about sensitive skin, yet there are findings to suggest that sensitive skin is a real issue (3). However, the concept of sensitive skin remains an elusive, complex issue for dermatologists and industry alike, which makes it difficult to investigate.

Sensitive skin is generally defined as a reduced tolerance to frequent or prolonged use of cosmetics and toiletries (4). This intolerance can manifest itself with a variety of symptoms that range from objective signs of irritation such as erythema, dryness, and scaling, to subjective effects such as itching, stinging, and burning. These effects may be a result of allergic or irritant contact dermatitis, urticaria, eczema, psoriasis, etc. This wide variability in symptoms and reactivity presents difficulties when attempting to investigate the phenomenon of sensitive skin or when formulating personal-care products for people with sensitive skin. There exists a range of test protocols which are employed in an attempt to investigate sensitive skin patients and to assess the irritancy of products (5–8), many of which in reality investigate different skin endpoints. However, it is currently unclear whether an individual having a low threshold to one irritant

61

stimulus is also susceptible to all other types of irritant stimuli. To address this question, it is first important to investigate the relationships between the different irritant stimuli. There has been limited work to investigate the relationship between non-immunologic skin reactions, such as stinging, urticaria, and contact dermatitis from surfactants, which has reported conflicting results, suggesting that any correlation between reactivities to these types of irritant endpoints is at best weak (3,6,8–14).

REACTIVITY TO DIFFERENT SENSORY IRRITANTS

Subjective (sensory) irritation following application of a cosmetic is a common complaint from people who consider themselves to have sensitive skin (1). There is evidence to suggest that people with self-perceived sensitive skin are more likely to respond to the effects of lactic acid in a sting test, and this test is often suggested as a good screening method to identify people with sensitive skin (5,7). However, there is evidence to suggest that sensitivity to lactic acid is not necessarily predictive of sensitivity to other irritants (11,12), nor those which cause other sensory responses or visible irritation. In a recent study (13), four chemicals reported to induce different sensory effects (lactic acid, stinging; capsaicin, burning; menthol, cooling; ethanol, a mixture of burning and stinging) were used to investigate various aspects of sensitivity to sensory irritation. A sensory perception test was conducted at defined intervals, whereby the materials were applied to the nasolabial fold for eight minutes, during which volunteers were asked to describe any sensory irritation they may have experienced. The data showed that there was a great deal of variation in the reactivity to the four materials and, generally, heightened reactivity to one material was not predictive of an elevated level of response to another. From a panel of 58 volunteers, four recorded a significant sensory response to all four chemicals; thus it would appear that a small number of individuals were broadly sensitive. Yet, it was not possible to predict who these individuals were from their responses to just one of those irritants, as they were not necessarily the strongest responders to each of the four chemicals. Those findings concurred with previous work conducted by Green and Shaffer (15) who found that individuals differed greatly in their response to just two chemicals and endorse the view (10) that a selection of chemicals should be used to gauge sensitivity rather than one chemical alone.

It has been demonstrated that the chemosensory irritation produced by the sensory irritants mentioned above is not unidimensional (10,13). In a recent study (13), the four aforementioned chemicals were chosen for use in the sensory perception test, as they are reported to induce specific sensations when applied to the skin. Panelists reported a variety of sensory responses and on the basis of the response to the specific sensations alone, fewer panelists would have been classified as sensitive to the chemical than if all sensory reactions to each material were taken into account. It is suggested by Loffler et al. (2) that individuals with sensitive skin are those who have an increase in unpleasant skin sensations rather than true irritation as measured by objective methods. It is reasonable to assume that people who experience a slight-to-moderate itching sensation find that chemicals cause an unpleasant effect when in contact with the skin, but those experiencing a stronger sensation, such as moderate-to-severe burning, are more likely to be "sensitive" to that chemical and skin contact with that chemical is intolerable to those people.

OBJECTIVE IRRITATION

People with sensitive skin may present with heightened objective irritation, such as erythema, to an irritant, along with subjective effects. It would be reasonable to assume that an individual with sensitive skin will have heightened reactivity to any irritant applied to the skin, particularly those from the same class of chemicals that are thought to act via similar mechanisms, for example, different surfactants. Reactivity to sodium dodecyl sulfate (SDS) is often used when investigating the phenomenon of sensitive skin (11–15), and dermatitis to surfactants is widely reported. In a recent study (13), a panel was exposed to three different surfactants, an anionic surfactant SDS, an amphoteric surfactant, cocamidopropyl betaine (CAPB), and a cationic surfactant, benzalkonium chloride (BKC). Anionic surfactants can be potent skin irritants, some cationics are at least equally irritating, whereas amphoterics are reputed to be relatively non-irritating to the skin (16). As would be expected from this evidence, CAPB elicited a lower number of strong irritant responses than either BKC or SDS. Thus, it could be argued that the individuals who developed an irritant response to CAPB were more sensitive than those who did not. However, some of the individuals who developed a strong response to CAPB did not also develop a similarly strong response to the other two surfactants tested. Thus, even when testing chemicals which elicit irritation via a similar mechanism, an irritation response to one chemical is not necessarily indicative of a response to another chemical, even one which has a similar mode of action. This is further supported by the evidence that strong reactivity to one non-immunologic urticant is not necessarily predictive of the degree of response to other such urticants (12,13,16).

RELATIONSHIP BETWEEN SENSORY AND OBJECTIVE IRRITATION

It has been suggested by some that there may be a relationship between sensitivity to sensory irritants and physical irritants. However, others have reported minimal correlation between objective skin findings and subjective effects (2). The relationship between reactivity in the sting test and the irritant response elicited by SDS has been investigated previously. Lammintausta et al. (11) reported an increase in laser Doppler blood flow velocity values elicited by sodium lauryl sulfate (24-hour patch application) in stingers compared with non-stingers, however, when they provoked open, cumulative irritation to SDS, they found no differences between the stingers and non-stingers as measured by transepidermal water loss. The relationship between stinging potential and skin irritation elicited by SDS has been disputed by others; Basketter and Griffiths (14) found no correlation between the two, and in a recent study conducted by Marriott et al. (13), there was little correlation between the level of response to 10% lactic acid and three different surfactants (including SDS) in a 2 × 23 hour covered patch test.

Some have suggested that urticants produce a greater urticarial response in stingers. Lammintausta et al. (11) demonstrated an increased reactivity to sorbic acid and benzoic acid in "stingers" compared with "non-stingers." However, in a study conducted by Coverly et al. (12) and a recent study conducted by Marriott et al. (13), heightened reactivity to urticants was not recorded in stingers compared with non-stingers, supporting the view that stinging and urticaria are not closely related.

From the evidence presented, it is quite clear that, overall, sensitivity to one stimulus is not necessarily predictive of susceptibility to another. Marriott et al. (13) reported a weak relationship between sensory irritation, urticaria, and contact dermatitis to surfactants, with both binomial probability and Chi-squared tests, suggesting that there was some evidence that the different tests conducted were not independent of each other. Others have also demonstrated some evidence for a weak relationship between the different endpoints, although some of the data are conflicting, but the evidence presented would indicate that there is a very small subset of individuals who will react to any stimulus applied under any test conditions. Whether these individuals are those more likely to react to personal-care products in a normal use scenario remains to be shown.

REFERENCES

1. Willis CM, Shaw S, Lacharriere ODE, Baveral M, Reiche L, Jourdain R, Bastein P, Wilkinson J. Sensitive skin: an epidemiological study. Br J Dermatol 2001; 145:258–263.
2. Loffler H, Aramaki J, Effendy I, Maibach H. Sensitive skin. In: Zhai H, Maibach H, eds. Dermatotoxicology. New York: CRC Press, 2004:123–135.
3. Draelos Z. Sensitive skin: perception, evaluation and treatment. Am J Contact Dermatitis 1997; 8:67–78.
4. Chew A, Maibach HI. Sensitive skin. In: Loden M, Maibach HI, eds. Dry Skin and Moisturizers—Chemistry and Function. New York: CRC Press, 2000:429–440.
5. Simion FA, Rau AH. Sensitive skin: what it is and how to formulate for it. Cosmet Toilet 1994; 109:43–49.
6. Frosch P, Kligman AM. Method for appraising the sting capacity of topically applied substances. J Soc Cosmet Chem 1977; 28:197–209.
7. Soschin D, Kligman AM. Adverse subjective responses. In: Kligman AM, Leyden JJ, eds. Safety and Efficacy of Topical Drugs and Cosmetics. New York: Grune & Stratton, 1982:377–388.

8. Agner T, Serup J. Quantification of the DSMO-response: a test for the assessment of sensitive skin. Clin Exp Dermatol 1989; 14:214–217.

9. Beradesca E, Fideli D, Gabba P, Cespa M, Rabbiosi G, Maibach H. Ranking of surfactant skin irritancy in vivo in man using the plastic occlusion stress test (POST). Contact Dermatitis 1990; 23:1–5.

10. Green BG, Bluth J. Measuring the chemosensory irritability of human skin. J Toxicol Cutan Ocul Toxicol 1995; 14:23–48.

11. Lammintausta K, Maibach HI, Wilson D. Mechanisms of subjective (sensory) irritation: propensity to non-immunologic contact urticaria and objective irritation in stingers. Dermatosen in Beruf und Umwelt 1988; 36:45–49.

12. Coverly J, Peters L, Whittle E, Basketer DA. Susceptibility to skin stinging, non-immunologic contact urticaria and skin irritation—is there a relationship? Contact Dermatitis 1997; 38:90–95.

13. Marriott M, Holmes J, Peters L, Cooper K, Rowson M, Basketter DA. The complex problem of sensitive skin. Contact Dermatitis 2005; 53:93–99.

14. Basketter DA, Griffiths HA. A study of the relationship between susceptibility to skin stinging and skin irritation. Contact Dermatitia 1993; 29:185–188.

15. Green BG, Shaffer GS. Psychological assessment of the chemical irritability of human skin. J Soc Cosmetic Chem 1992; 43:131–147.

16. Effendy I, Maibach HI. Surfactants and experimental irritant contact dermatitis. Contact Dermatitis 1995; 33:217–225.

7

Surface Stripping Techniques and Sensitive Skin

Marc Paye

Colgate-Palmolive R&D, Milmort, Belgium

Gérald E. Piérard

Department of Dermatopathology, University Hospital Sart Tilman, Liège, Belgium

INTRODUCTION

Sensitive skin (SSK) is a multifactorial condition characterized by hyperreactivity to irritant stimuli, which may be expressed as objective and/or subjective reactions (1,2). Objective reactions may be visible (e.g., erythema and xerosis) or measurable (e.g., changes in the barrier permeability of the skin or in its water-holding capacity). Subjective reactions are usually tightness, itching, stinging, burning of the skin, or pain, and may or may not be accompanied by clinically observable reactions.

Because of this complexity, the mechanism underlying SSK is not well understood. In many cases, an alteration of the skin-barrier function is suspected (2,3), which allows irritants to penetrate more easily into the skin and cause quicker and more intense reaction than in the "normal" population. Differences in the neuronal influx transmission or in the cytokine cascade have also been advanced to explain, respectively, increased sensitivity in subjective signs and increased reactivity by clinical signs (4).

The causes for skin sensitivity are also multiple and have been tentatively grouped into four subcategories (5): contact, environmental, lifestyle, and menstrual cycle–related SSK. Finally, regional differences in skin have also been reported (6) as a very influential factor in defining and characterizing SSK, and talking about sensitive hands is often totally different than talking about facial SSK (7).

Integrating all these variables (type of response × underlying mechanism × cause × skin area) may easily explain why so many diagnostic procedures for SSK have been described in the literature (8) and mainly why some of them have been so controversial.

Most of the screening techniques have been explained in other chapters of this book. This chapter essentially focuses on skin surface stripping (SSS) methods which have recently been introduced in the investigation of SSK. The SSS methods entail the collection of superficial corneocytes to analyze their organization, structure, or responsiveness to external stimuli. It is thus obvious that they will not detect changes in neuronal influx propagation, in cytokine receptor densities on keratinocytes or endothelial cells, or deep phenomena involved in the syndrome of SSK. SSS techniques are thus used for detecting SSK related to superficial stratum corneum (SC) changes and/or due to alteration of the barrier function.

SKIN SURFACE STRIPPING TECHNIQUES

Tape Stripping

Tape stripping is a harvesting method for the most superficial desquamating layer of the SC (9). The adhesive discs (e.g., D-SQUAME® discs, CuDerm, TX, U.S.A.) are applied onto the skin under controlled pressure. A short application time (15 seconds) enables the harvesting of the superficial corneocytes and a long application time (one hour) enables the collection of a thicker layer of corneocytes (10). Guidelines for tape-stripping analysis have been published by the European Group for the Efficacy Measurement of Cosmetics and Other Topical Products (EEMCO) (11). SC tape strippings may be rated by visual examination after placing the sample on a black surface, by weighing, by optical measurement with or without specific staining, by image analysis, and by morphometry. Other procedures involve the biochemical analysis of enzymes (e.g., catalase and proteases) collected with the corneocytes (12).

A specific assessment method for tape stripping has been defined as squamometry (SQM) (9). SQM is a non-invasive, protein-dependent, colorimetric evaluation of the level of alteration in the desquamating corneocyte layer able to detect fine xerotic and irritant changes in the SC. After stripping, the discs are stained for 30 seconds with a solution of toluidine blue and basic fuschin [polychrome multiple stain (PMS); Delasco, IA, U.S.A.]. Tape strippings are placed on a transparent microscope slide which itself is placed on the calibration white plate of a Chromameter® (Chromameter, Minolta, Japan). Measurement of the color of the stripping is made in the $L^*a^*b^*$ mode and the Chroma C^* value is calculated after $(a^{*2} + b^{*2})^{1/2}$. This parameter combines the values of the red and blue chromacities, predominant colors of the PMS. The Chroma C^* value has been shown to be related to the amount of SC harvested in a xerotic situation. SC tape stripping may also be examined under a microscope and scored for morphological or cohesiveness changes (13).

Cyanoacrylate Skin Surface Stripping

A sheet of SC (usually three to five corneocytes layers) is collected from the volar forearms of human volunteers by placing a drop of cyanoacrylate adhesive on a terephthalate polymer sheet, pressing it on the skin of the donor, and removing it after a brief contact (30 seconds to one minute) (14). The harvested SC is usually homogenous and may be used to investigate the interaction of consumer products with their first target on skin.

A specific application of cyanoacrylate SSS is called corneosurfametry (CSM) and allows investigation of the interaction of surfactants with the SC (15,16). Briefly, diluted test products are sprayed onto the skin surface samples or, as a variant, the skin samples are incubated into a solution of the products. After a contact of two hours, residues of surfactants are rinsed off under running tap water and skin samples are allowed to dry. Damages caused to the SC by the products are determined by staining the SC for three minutes with PMS, followed by extensive rinsing under running tap water. Irritated SC fixes more dye than non-irritated SC. Staining is quantified by means of the Chromameter as for SQM. Results are expressed by the Chroma C^* value or by a colorimetric index of mildness (CIM $= L^* - C^*$). The higher the CIM, the milder the product.

SKIN BARRIER FUNCTION, SENSITIVITY, AND SQUAMOMETRY

SQM measures the alterations of corneocytes after application of surfactants. The more altered the corneocytes, the more the staining of the harvested SC. The method is extremely sensitive and is able to detect effects on the SC even after very short and non-occlusive contact times (16,17). Collecting successive tape stripping, under controlled pressure and conditions, on the same site allows determining how deeply the surfactant has penetrated into the SC and has damaged the corneocytes (18,19). The deeper the SC strippings that are stained, the less effective is the protective skin barrier. The method is thus able to detect SSK that is due to poorly effective barrier function and for which the permeation of chemicals and irritants through the horny layer is accelerated. This is, for instance, often the case for subjects with sensitive hands due to occupational insults.

Another case where tape stripping was found useful in detecting SSK is shown by a survey on "sensitive hands" (20). A survey on 150 healthy Caucasian women, 20 to 55 years old, showed that those self-perceiving their hands as being sensitive had corneocytes showing much less intercellular cohesion on the tapes than subjects self-perceiving their hands as being non-sensitive.

SKIN BARRIER FUNCTION, SENSITIVITY, AND CORNEOCYTE SIZE

Corneocyte size is believed to reflect the SC turnover (21) and was suggested to be related to self-perceived facial SSK, probably through an effect on skin barrier function (22). In their investigations, the authors selected three groups of subjects perceiving themselves as non-sensitive, often sensitive, or always sensitive. After tape stripping of all subjects, the harvested corneocytes were transferred to a glass slide, the adhesive removed, and the cells stained with a solution of gentian violet and brilliant green. Thirty cells were randomly selected per sample and their size determined by image analysis. The average projected area of corneocytes (APAc) was measured, which reflected the level of skin sensitivity. A correction factor was furthermore introduced in the APAc value for function of the age of the subject and of the season, factors known to influence skin sensitivity. The "corrected APAc" decreased with increasing sensitivity of the cheek skin, reflecting a decrease in corneocyte size with increasing skin sensitivity. By this method, the authors were able to detect 80% of the self-perceived SSK subjects from their population, whereas other screening methods did not reach such a level (e.g., 50% of the self-perceived SSK subjects detected with the stinging test).

ATOPIC DERMATITIS AND CORNEOSURFAMETRY

Patients with atopic dermatitis are among the individuals with high SSK that are more readily reacting to chemical and physical insults, due to defective barrier function (3).

CSM performed with a reference surfactant (1% sodium lauryl sulfate) on SC sheets collected from atopic patients showed a more intense staining than on SC sheets collected from normal non-sensitive individuals (10,23). The CSM was significantly lower in atopic persons, indicating a higher susceptibility to irritation induced by surfactants or other products.

CORNEOSURFAMETRY TO DIFFERENTIATE BETWEEN DIFFERENT TYPES OF SENSITIVE SKIN

As explained in "Introduction," SSK may be subdivided into different categories, depending on the cause of symptoms. In a prospective study, Goffin et al. (24) selected three groups of 15 subjects displaying differences in skin sensitivity. The first group was self-perceived as non-sensitive, the second as sensitive to environmental factors or to fabrics, and the third to detergent-based products. Each subject served as a donor of cyanoacrylate SSS. The SSSs were used for a CSM study where four dishwashing liquids and four household products were tested. It was clear from this study that the overall responsiveness of the SC to the products was higher in the detergent-SSK group than in the other two groups. This observation was explained by the fact that detergent-SSK subjects could have a weakened resistance of their SC to surfactants or detergent-based products. This study suggests that the biochemical basis of the skin sensitivity would be different in function, depending on the specific intolerance to external threats of the subjects. Furthermore, CSM could be used as a useful diagnosing tool to select specific panels of surfactant-SSK volunteers for clinical testing programs of hygiene or cleaning products intended for such a population.

Another advantage of CSM is that for a given population of donors, which may be among detergent-SSK subjects, the alterations induced to the SC may be compared for different products and the most appropriate products for their skin condition can thus be selected and proposed.

USE OF SQUAMOMETRY TO SELECT SURFACTANT-BASED PRODUCTS FOR SENSITIVE SKIN SUBJECTS

Many body cleansers and hand-dish products are targeted to consumers complaining of SSK. Such products must be very mild for the skin and, even in very exaggerated experimental application conditions, induce minimal irritation of the skin. Methods used to compare the mildness to skin of those SSK-designed products must then be able to detect faint changes of the skin surface, which are even not always visible by the naked eye. This is one of the numerous advantages of the bioengineering methods developed to measure skin surface, such as evaporimetry (25), skin surface electrical properties measurements (26), laser Doppler velocimetry (27), and others. SQM has also been described as a method able to detect subclinical alterations of the SC due to surfactant-based products (17–19,28) that are not visible and even, in certain cases, not detected by the earlier methods. This allows SQM to be a method of choice to compare the interaction with skin of either regular products that are applied to skin for a short period of time or of extremely mild products designed for SSK.

USE OF SKIN SURFACE STRIPPING METHODS FOR TESTING BARRIER PROTECTANTS FOR SENSITIVE SKIN SUBJECTS

Barrier creams or barrier protectants are often recommended to subjects with SSK due to impaired skin barrier. SQM has been successfully used to demonstrate the beneficial effect of a skin-barrier protectant against irritation due to SLS (29). Forearms of the volunteers were pretreated or not with tannic acid (skin protectant). SLS was applied (10 μL) at different doses and 30 minutes later, the sites were covered for 24 hours with cotton and paper tape. Thirty minutes after tape removal and site rinsing and drying, tape strippings were collected and processed for SQM analysis. Measured staining of the discs (Chroma C^*) clearly demonstrated a reduction in skin surface damages where the forearms had been pretreated with the barrier protectant.

Similarly, CSM is a well-suited in vitro procedure to evaluate the efficacy of skin-barrier creams (10,30). For that purpose, a controlled amount of the barrier cream is applied onto a cyanoacrylate SSS before applying a reference surfactant such as SLS. The more efficacious the barrier cream, the less the staining of the SC sheet.

CONCLUSION

This chapter has reviewed two SSS methods, SQM and CSM, and has explained how useful they are in the diagnosis of SSK and in the selection of very mild products especially appropriate for such a population target. However, it remains that SSSs are investigating skin changes or phenomena happening at the level of the superficial SC. SSK is very complex and involves all layers of the skin, not only SC. From the different underlying mechanisms of SSK, it appears that an impairment of the skin-barrier function seems to be best detected by SSS. From the various types of SSK, SSS seems to identify best those subjects who are sensitive to surfactant-based products.

In conclusion, SSS methods appear to be excellent complementary techniques for screening SSK persons but often have to be used in conjunction with other methods.

REFERENCES

1. Simion AF, Rau AH. Sensitive skin: what it is and how to formulate for it. Cosmet Toiletries 1994; 109:43–50.
2. Frosch P, Kligman AM. A method for appraising the stinging capacity of topically applied substances. J Soc Cosmet Chem 1977; 28:197–209.
3. Tupker RA, Pinnagoda J, Coenraads PJ, Nater JP. Susceptibility to irritants: role of barrier function, skin dryness and history of atopic dermatitis. Br J Dermatol 1990; 123:199–203.
4. Misery L. La neuro-cosmétique. Proceedings XX Journées Eur Dermocosmetol, Lyon, 16–17 November 2000, 16–23.
5. Morizot F, Guinot C, Lopez S, Le Fur I, Tschachler E. Sensitive skin: analysis of symptoms, perceived causes and possible mechanisms. All Cosm Toiletries 2000; 115(11):83–89.
6. Henry F, Goffin V, Maibach HI, Piérard GE. Regional differences in stratum corneum reactivity to surfactants. Contact Dermat 1997; 37:271–275.
7. Morrison BM Jr, Paye M. A characterization of sensitive skin. Am Acad Dermatol Meeting, New Orleans, 4–9 February 1995.
8. Primavera B, Carrera M, Berardesca E, Tests for sensitive skin. In: Paye M, Barel AO, Maibach HI, eds. Handbook of Cosmetic Science and Technology, 2nd ed. Boca Raton: CRC Press, Taylor and Francis group, 2006:733–743.
9. Piérard GE, Piérard-Franchimont C, Saint-Léger S, Kligman AM. Squamometry: the assessment of xerosis by colorimetry of D-Squame adhesive discs. J Soc Cosmet Chem 1992; 47:297–305.

10. Piérard GE, Piérard-Franchimont C. Drug and cosmetic evaluations with skin strippings. In: Maibach HI, ed. Dermatologic Research Techniques. Boca Raton, FL: CRC Press, 1996:133–149.
11. Piérard GE. EEMCO guidance for the assessment of dry skin (xerosis) and icthyosis: evaluation by stratum corneum strippings. Skin Res Technol 1996; 2:3–11.
12. Redoules D, Tarroux R, Assalit MF, Perié JJ. Characterization and assay of five enzymatic activities in the stratum corneum using tape stripping. Skin Pharmacol Appl Skin Physiol 1999; 12:182–192.
13. Paye M, Goffin V, Cartiaux Y, Morrison BM Jr, Piérard GE. D-Squame strippings in the assessment of intercorneocyte cohesion. Allergologie 1995; 18:S462–S463.
14. Marks R, Dawber RPR. Skin surface biopsy: an improved technique for the examination of the horny layer. Br J Dermatol 1971; 84:117–122.
15. Piérard GE, Goffin V, Piérard-Franchimont C. Corneosurfametry: a predictive assessment of the interaction of personal care cleansing products with human stratum corneum. Dermatology 1994; 189:152–156.
16. Piérard GE, Goffin V, Piérard-Franchimont C. Squamometry and corneosurfametry in rating interactions of cleansing products with stratum corneum. J Soc Cosmet Chem 1994; 45:269–277.
17. Paye M, Cartiaux Y. Squamometry: a tool to move from exaggerated to more and more realistic application conditions for comparing the skin compatibility of surfactant-based products. Int J Cosmet Sci 1999; 21:59–68.
18. Charbonnier V, Morrison BM, Paye M, Maibach HI. Open application assay in investigation of sub-clinical irritant dermatitis induced by SLS in man: advantage of squamometry. Skin Res Technol 1998; 4:244–250.
19. Charbonnier V, Paye M, Maibach HI. Determination of subclinical changes of barrier function. In: Zhai H, Maibach HI, eds. Dermatotoxicology. 6th ed. Boca Raton, FL: CRC Press, 2004:937–955.
20. Paye M, Dalimier Ch, Cartiaux Y, Chabassol C. Consumer perceived sensitive hands: what is behind? Skin Res Technol 1999; 5:28–32.
21. Lévêque JL, Porte G, de Rigal J, Corcuff P, François AM, Saint-Léger D. Influence of chronic sun exposure on some biophysical parameters of the human skin: an in vivo study. J Cut Ag Cosmet Dermatol 1988; 1:123.
22. Ota N, Horiguchi T, Fujiwara N, Kashibuchi N, Hirai Y, Mori F. Identification of skin sensitivity through corneocytes measurements. IFSCC Mag 2001; 4(1):9–14.
23. Goffin V, Piérard GE. Corneosurfametry and the compromised atopic stratum corneum. Arch Dermatol Res 1996; 288:489–491.
24. Goffin V, Piérard-Franchimont C, Piérard GE. Sensitive skin and stratum corneum reactivity to household cleaning products. Contact Dermat 1996; 34:81–85.
25. Rogiers V, The EEMCO Group. EEMCO guidance for the assessment of transepidermal water loss in cosmetic sciences. Skin Pharmacol Appl Skin Physiol 2001; 14: 117–128.
26. Berardesca E, The EEMCO Group. EEMCO guidance for the assessment of stratum corneum hydration: electrical methods. Skin Res Technol 1997; 3:126–132.
27. Pierard GE. EEMCO guidance for the assessment of skin colour. J Eur Acad Dermatol Venereol 1998; 10:1–11.

28. Charbonnier V, Maibach HI, Morrison BM Jr, Paye M. Quantification of non-erythematous irritant dermatitis. In: Maibach HI, ed. Toxicology of Skin. Philadelphia, PA: Taylor & Francis, 2001:31–37.
29. Shimizu T, Maibach HI. Squamometry: an evaluation method for a barrier protectant (tannic acid). Contact Dermat 1999; 40:189–191.
30. Goffin V, Piérard-Franchimont C, Piérard GE. Shielded corneosurfametry and corneo-xenometry: novel bioassays for the assessment of skin barrier products. Dermatology 1998; 196:434–437.

8

Technical Bases of Biophysical Instruments Used in Sensitive Skin Testing

Maria Breternitz and Joachim W. Fluhr

Department of Dermatology and Allergology, Friedrich-Schiller University,
Jena, Germany

Enzo Berardesca

San Gallicano Dermatological Institute, Rome, Italy

INTRODUCTION: WHAT IS SENSITIVE SKIN?

The definition of sensitive skin is still evolving (1). In recent years, the term "sensitive skin" has been used with greater frequency, owing to a large proportion of the population complaining of a peculiar susceptibility, for example, when applying commonly used skin-care products. Their complaints do not fall under the classical definitions of irritation, allergic contact dermatitis, or photobiological phenomena (phototoxicity or photoallergy). These patients report subjective complaints such as burning, stinging, itching, and a tight feeling, following various environmental stimuli, such as climate, skin-care products, detergents, and sunscreen application (2). These symptoms can be noticed immediately following product applications or delayed by minutes, hours, or days. Symptoms may only result following cumulative product applications or in combination with concomitant products (3).

Owing to the lack of objective signs, the phenomenon of sensitive skin is difficult to assess (4). There is a growing awareness that some individuals exhibit skin sensitivity and have a high incidence of adverse reactions to cosmetics and toiletries. Dermatologists are increasingly recognizing the concept of "sensitive skin." On the basis of the current understanding, sensitive skin can be defined as a reduced tolerance to frequent or prolonged use of cosmetics and toiletries, with symptoms ranging from visible signs of irritation (e.g., erythema and scaling) to more subjective neurosensory forms of discomfort (e.g., stinging, burning, itching, and tightness) (5). Many people experience high facial reactivity when exposed to external factors. Approximately 40% of the population claims to suffer from this condition. Models to define this condition are not standardized and its boundaries are neither well defined nor extensively investigated. Nevertheless, the stinging response after local application of lactic acid in the so-called stinging test is widely used as a marker of skin sensitivity (6). The reason why some patients react with skin symptoms without having any visible skin signs is still under discussion (7). No consensus about definition and recognition of the biological basis of sensitive skin has been achieved (8). Mills and Berger (1) suggest that the term "sensitive skin" applies to the following four categories: (*i*) those individuals with obvious skin disease, (*ii*) those individuals with subclinical (mild) or atypical clinical signs of disease, (*iii*) those individuals with past insults to the skin, and (*iv*) those individuals who do not fit into one of these three categories and appear to be "normal." To define sensitive skin in a broad sense, one may need to perform skin profiles regarding biophysical, non-invasive parameters of these patients. In this chapter, we would like to give an overview of the non-invasive biophysical measurements and their technical bases used in the assessment of sensitive skin.

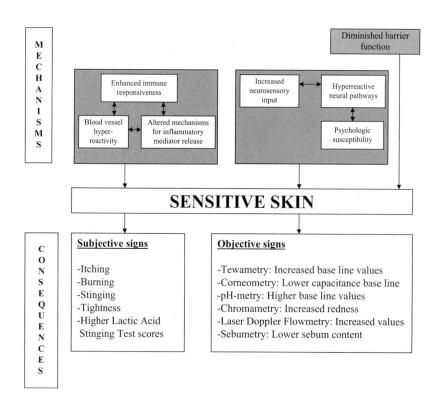

Epidemiology

Despite the significance of sensitive skin, only little epidemiological evidence exists with respect to its prevalence (5). In 2001, Willis et al. (5) published an epidemiological study in the U.K. to assess the prevalence of sensitive skin in the population and to examine possible factors that may be associated with sensitive skin. They found that sensitive skin is a common phenomenon in the U.K., with about 50% of women and 40% of men regarding themselves as having sensitive skin. Ten percent of women and 5.8% of men described themselves as having very sensitive skin. Jourdain et al. (9) reported that 52% of women between 18 and 45 years of age agreed with the statement: "I have sensitive facial skin." Approximately 30% of the total population strongly agreed with this statement. The incidence of about 50% self-assessed sensitive skin mirrors the prevalence in findings obtained in the previous epidemiological study of Willis et al. and in the investigations of Johnson and Paige (10). Draelos (3) reported that approximately 40% of the population considers themselves to possess the characteristics of sensitive skin, creating a sizable market for products designed to minimize skin sensitivity. Consumer studies in all races identify a complex entity containing one-quarter to one-half of the adult population. Therefore, the sensitive skin problem is far from being a rarity (11). However, these studies are still unable to answer the question of whether sensitive skin has increased over the past decades or the socio-cultural background has changed. Such a change would reflect the influence of mass media (e.g., through advertising of the cosmetic industry) and/or an increased self-body perception. Additionally, social and environmental factors such as education and pollution might influence the self-perceived sensitive skin.

Pathomechanism

The physiology of facial skin hyperirritability is not completely defined (12), and although the pathomechanism still remains unclear, several factors are believed to influence sensory irritation. The quality and concentration of the exposing agent and regional variations in reactivity, as well as microanatomical differences such as density of hair follicles and sweat glands, elaborate network of nerves, skin sebum content, and density of blood vessels appear to be contributory. Physiological differences such as hyperreactive neural pathways, blood vessel hyperreactivity, and altered mechanisms for inflammatory mediator release have been implicated. Some sensory irritation is believed to be a form of subclinical contact urticaria (12–17).

Willis et al. (5) compared women with sensitive skin with women with non-sensitive skin and showed a statistically overrepresentation of certain features and characteristics in the former group. Burning, itching, and stinging occurred more commonly in sensitive skin, confirming the link between increased neurosensory discomfort and the self-perception of sensitive skin. Why, in physiological terms, some individuals have a greater predilection for this type of response is not fully understood. The results from Willis et al. (5) are consistent with the data of provocation studies showing self-perceived sensitive skin is significantly more susceptible to the neurogenic effects of chemical irritants such as lactic acid (4,18).

Draelos (19) reported that physiologically, sensitive skin possesses one or more of the following anatomic cutaneous characteristics: heightened neurosensory input, enhanced immune responsiveness, and/or diminished barrier function. Substances that are tolerated by most people, such as lactic acid, cause extreme stinging in people showing an increased neurosensory response. In addition, persons with sensitive skin might suffer from multiple allergies to food, inhaled agents, and topical allergens reflecting an enhanced immune responsiveness. Substances that have a negative impact on barrier function, whether endogenous or exogenous, increase both irritant and allergic contact dermatitis (20). Thus, sensitive skin is thought to be due to a thin and defective stratum corneum barrier or a direct neuronal influence (1,4,14).

Lammintausta and Maibach (21) showed an increased frequency of stingers in the following groups: infants, women, elderly, persons with skin type I, patients with history of atopic dermatitis and dry skin. These stingers are thought to have a defective stratum corneum barrier and a lower skin pH than control persons after topical application of lactic acid (4). Seidenari et al. (12) described the skin of sensitive subjects as less supple, less hydrated and more erythematous and telangiectatic when compared with the skin of normal subjects. A trend towards an increase in transepidermal water loss (TEWL), pH, and colorimetric a^* values (redness) and a decrease in capacitance (stratum corneum hydration), sebum, and colorimetric L^* values on the face of subjects with sensitive skin was described. Muizzuddin et al. (18) reported that skin sensitivity is due to a combination of a disrupted barrier and a tendency to hyperreact to topical agents. Distante et al. (6) revealed that sensitive skin showed higher TEWL values, higher values in laser Doppler flowmetry (LDF), and lower stratum corneum hydration values in different facial sites when compared with a group with non-sensitive skin. These findings support the hypothesis that defects in barrier function, stratum corneum structure, and vascular dynamics may induce a higher transcutaneous penetration in subjects with sensitive skin, leading to increased skin hyperreactivity. Altered permeability barrier functions and vessel dynamics may contribute to the susceptibility of sensitive skin to various stimuli. Patients with sensitive skin are unusually susceptible to the induction of inflammatory and/or neurosensory symptoms by various exogenous triggers, for example, natural and synthetically derived chemical irritants, contact allergens, ingested foods, climatic conditions, sun exposure, and incorrect skin care (22).

Alterations of baseline biophysical parameters, representing a trend towards barrier impairment, support the hypothesis that skin hyperreactivity to water-soluble irritants in panelists with subjective irritation is induced by increased transcutaneous penetration of water-soluble chemicals and a greater amount of absorbed irritants (15). Finally, cutaneous vascular hyperreactivity has been demonstrated by an increased blood flow assessed by LDF after the application of irritant substances to the skin of sensitive subjects (14), and corresponds to variations in baseline colorimetric measurements (12).

Association with Diseases and Other Skin Disorders

The investigations of Willis et al. (5) showed that atopic diathesis was more prevalent among women who regarded themselves as suffering from sensitive skin. About 50% reported a personal history of atopic eczema and/or asthma/ hay fever, compared with 27% in the non-sensitive group. Although the association between atopy and skin susceptibility to irritation is established, a predictive link between atopic diathesis and sensitive skin is not evident. The presence of atopy does not lead, in all cases, to sensitive skin. Half of the sensitive skin group had no history of atopy and one-third of atopic women regarded themselves as having non-sensitive skin.

Other skin disorders, such as rosacea and acne, have been linked to increased skin reactivity (1). Willis et al. (5) described that over one-third of the total sample population reported skin problems other than those covered in their questionnaire. Their study also confirmed the association between sensitive skin and both dry skin and the propensity for blushing/flushing. These characteristics, respectively, indicate a tendency to barrier impairment and heightened vascular reactivity (12,19). Dry skin was more prevalent in those who perceived themselves as having sensitive skin, as was the tendency to blush or flush readily (5). Inherent structural features of the epidermis and stratum corneum may influence susceptibility of the skin to irritation from exogenous chemicals (23). Hyperreactors may have a thinner stratum corneum with a reduced corneocyte area (23), causing a higher transcutaneous penetration of water-soluble chemicals, which makes them more susceptible to exogenous factors (15). Neural pathways and blood vessel hyperresponsivity may be contributory (14).

Draelos (20) gave an overview of diseases that predispose to sensitive skin:

- Allergic contact dermatitis
- Atopic dermatitis
- Comedogenic acne
- Contact urticaria (immunologic and non-immunologic)
- Eczematous dermatitis
- Irritant contact dermatitis
- Papular or pustular acne
- Perioral dermatitis
- Psoriasis
- Rosacea
- Seborrheic dermatitis

Draelos stated that many patients with sensitive skin have underlying dermatological conditions that play a role in the development of allergic reactions.

These skin conditions should be treated before any further evaluation of sensitive skin is undertaken (20).

Furthermore, in certain cases, it is important that dermatologists recognize a common group of patients with dermatological non-disease. These patients have significant symptomatology, but no objective evidence of disease. Cotterill (24) investigated a group of patients presenting dermatological complaints in the face, but no significant objective dermatological pathology (11). Their complaints were burning, intense itching, and hirsute. Among these patients, disturbed body image (dysmorphophobia) and depression were common. Those patients who are anxiously preoccupied with their skin may be managed by psychotherapy and/or antidepressants (11,24).

ASSESSMENT WITH NON-INVASIVE BIOPHYSICAL INSTRUMENTS

Self-assessment is not always an accurate parameter for categorizing skin as sensitive or non-sensitive, although it can be valuable. Thus, it might be important to assess sensitive skin by more objective parameters (18). There are various established methods for investigating skin irritation, for example, conventional patch tests, exaggerated use tests, and repeated open application tests (ROAT) (25–27). In contrast, methods for most other types of skin reactions, including urticaria, burning, itching, and stinging, are less established (28).

Lactic Acid Stinging Test

A lot of people complain about symptoms such as burning, stinging, itching, and a tight feeling when applying commonly used skin-care products. Furthermore, they report these sensations following various environmental stimuli, such as climate, detergents, and sunscreen application (2). Frosch and Kligman (13) investigated skin responses to different irritants and observed a 14% incidence of sensitive skin in a normal population.

The lactic acid stinging test (LAST) is used to diagnose the sensory irritation component of the sensitive skin syndrome. The stinging test is accepted as a marker of sensitivity and employed for the selection of subjects experiencing subclinical cutaneous irritation. However, this test is based on self-perceived assessment. Although difficult to quantify, the stinging test is employed for the identification of sensitive subjects (12). In practice, only the stinging test first described by Frosch and Kligman (13) has gained widespread use in the identification of products with a potential to elicit sensory responses. This assay has been investigated in some detail and has undergone several modifications over the years (14,29). However, the sting test neither provides a surrogate for a wider range of sensory effects nor is it useful as a general indicator of sensitivity or sensitive skin (30,31).

LAST provides practicing dermatologists with the most widely accepted clinical method for testing susceptibility to chemically induced neurosensory skin irritation. In the hands of clinical investigators, LAST provided a useful experimental strategy for research on the pathophysiology of the sensitive skin syndrome. Details of the test methodology vary considerably. Sensitivity is increased and specificity is lost as the concentration of lactic acid (ranging from 3% to 30%) is raised (22). A typical published LAST protocol follows (14,32,33).

After cleaning the area below the eyes with soap and water, facial sweating is induced by exposure to a commercial facial sauna (e.g., Silhouet-Tone 50126, Canada) for 15 minutes. A solution of 5% lactic acid in water is then applied with a swab in a gentle rotating motion to one side of the cheek from the side of the upper lip upwards across the cheek. Water is applied as a placebo control in the same manner to the contralateral side. After two, four, and five minutes, the panelists are requested to describe the presence and intensity of skin sensation in the test areas. The following ordinal four-point scale is used: 0 = no stinging, 1 = slight, 2 = moderate, 3 = severe. If the cumulative score at two, four, and five minutes of skin sensations is 3 or more, the subject is considered to be a "stinger" (7). Ten percent of the general population are stingers after application of 5% or 10% lactic acid on facial skin (34).

The facial LAST is the most popular test to investigate the subclinical aspects of sensitive skin. We recommend the following two methods to perform the test:

1. Application of a 10% aqueous solution of lactic acid at room temperature to the nasolabial fold (the test is usually carried out on the nasolabial fold, a site richly innervated with sensory fibers) and cheek, using brisk rubbing strokes of a cotton tipped applicator dipped in the lactic acid solution.
2. Conditioning the patient to a state of profuse sweating by exposure to a facial sauna for a period of 15 minutes followed by a brisk application of 5% aqueous lactic acid to the nasolabial fold and cheek (once).

Unfortunately, reproducibility of data from one testing population at given time points remains critical. Christensen and Kligman (29) have proposed dividing stingers into mild, moderate, and severe on the basis of application of 10% racemic DL lactic acid in a 1.7 cm Hilltop chamber to the malar bone for 10 minutes. The time to initial stinging is noted along with the peak stinging intensity. This test revision might improve reproducibility owing to its utilization of more sensitive facial skin with a larger area of lactic acid application.

The feeling of stinging is induced at the nasolabial folds. The extreme sensitivity of this region is a reflection of its microanatomy, including high density of hair follicles, sweat glands, elaborate network of the nerves, and permeable stratum corneum. Therefore, the disintegrated barrier function of stratum corneum will increase the quantity of lactic acid permeating through the skin and thus increasing the degree of stinging. Wu et al. (35) investigated the correlation between stinging, TEWL, and stratum corneum hydration (capacitance). They found tendencies of decrease in baseline capacitance and increase in baseline TEWL, which are in accordance with increased clinical scores at five minutes. Moreover, they found that the subjects with lower capacitance and higher TEWL have a shorter onset time of stinging, with a negative correlation between the baseline of capacitance and clinical score at five minutes in a 3% lactic acid test. This demonstrates the relationship between the degree of stinging and epidermal permeability barrier function. Wu et al. (35) concluded that Tewameter® and Corneometer® could be used as objective methods for evaluating the susceptibility of skin.

Marriott et al. (28) found a slight trend for females to be more sensitive to the application of lactic acid when compared with males, statistically significant at five minutes. It has been suggested that women are generally more sensitive and therefore more likely to develop stinging responses than men, although this difference has not been conclusively demonstrated (29).

The stinging test is widely used in various modified forms, and many different factors have been identified as potentially influencing the sensitivity of this test, including the anatomical region to which the test material is applied (28). Stinging has been shown as a predominantly facial phenomenon (13,30). Marriott et al. (28) detected that the nasolabial fold and forehead gave higher levels of stinging responses than the chin and malar bone.

Sinaiko and Maibach (22) reported that the characteristics of facial skin, especially of the nasolabial fold, give rise to the stinging response to chemicals such as lactic acid, which include presumed thin stratum corneum, an elaborate network of sensory nerves, high density of skin appendages, and high epidermal permeability (36). Additional factors that may favor the likelihood of a positive LAST include time of the year (increased stinging is reported in winter months) (37), physical trauma to stratum corneum, such as scratching or stripping with cellophane tape (38), chemical delipidization of stratum corneum, for example, with acetone (38), co-existing skin disease, such as rosacea (7), and co-existence of certain other pain syndromes, notably, facial symptoms related to computer display use (33) and possibly, interstitial cystitis (39).

TEWL Measurement

TEWL is one of the most important parameters to evaluate the epidermal permeability barrier function of the skin. A low TEWL, therefore, is a characteristic feature of a healthy skin.

TEWL measurement, also called evaporimetry when performed with an open-loop system, can be used to assess barrier, indirectly predicting the influence of topically applied substances at the skin surface.

Measurement of TEWL is used for the characterization of the permeability barrier function in clinical contact dermatitis as well as in irritant and allergic patch test reaction (40). It is typically used to assess barrier function objectively

(40,41). There are different methods for TEWL measurement: the unventilated chamber (closed) method, the ventilated chamber method, and the method using an open chamber (42). The unventilated chamber methods are incapable of continuous measurement and might potentially occlude the skin. Ventilated chambers, using dry or moistened carrier gas, are capable of continuous TEWL measurements. Both methods interfere with the microclimate near the skin surface, influencing the water loss to varying extents. Thus, these methods have certain inherent drawbacks. The open chamber, water vapor evaporation, gradient estimation method provides continuous measurement in ambient air, with little alteration of the water vapor boundary layer overlying the skin (43). As a consequence of these different measuring principles, results obtained with different methods cannot be directly compared yet (40). Recent research shows the importance of adequate calibration systems (42) that are introduced for two of the commercially available devices, namely the Tewameter 300® and the Aquaflux® (Fig. 1A–C). In this chapter, we focus on open chamber system because all publications on sensitive skin are performed with these devices.

To perform accurate and reliable measurements, several factors and sources of variation need to be known and taken into account. Variations are mainly related to (*i*) the panelists, (*ii*) the environment, and (*iii*) the instrument.

1. Individual-related variables that may influence TEWL measurement are age, anatomical sites, the intra- and inter-individual variation, physical, thermal, or emotional sweating, and skin surface temperature (40,41).

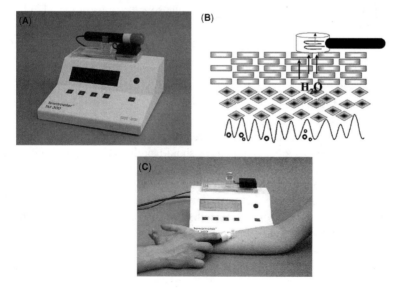

Figure 1 (**A**) Tewameter 300®. (**B**) Measuring principle of the Tewameter. (**C**) Measurement with a Tewameter.

2. Environment-related variables that may have an influence on TEWL measurement are air convection, ambient air temperature and humidity, direct light, diurnal variation, seasonal variation, and geographical variation (40,41). Sweating and skin surface temperature may also influence the TEWL values. Thus, a pre-measurement acclimatization of 15 to 30 minutes in the measurement room with an ambient air temperature regulated to about $20°C$ $(20-22°C)$ is recommended (40,41,44). During summer, subjects may even have to acclimatize for a longer period in order to avoid the influence of sweating. The ambient air humidity and air temperature are complex and important variables in TEWL measurements and may influence the measurements. Climatized facilities should be available and the relative humidity regulated to about 40%. Recently, technical advances have been made with preheated measurement sessions in order to minimize or possibly avoid the influence of climatic variations (45). Direct light has a possible influence on TEWL measurement; thus, measurements under direct light sources or close to windows with direct sunlight should be avoided (40).
3. The instrument-related variables with possible influence on TEWL measurement are zero drift (especially in older devices), the surface plane, contact pressure, the use of the probe protection covers, intra- and inter-instrumental variability, and inaccuracy. The control of these variables is essential for accurate, reliable, and reproducible measurements. Variations in the contact pressure between the probe head and the surface of the skin may cause alterations in the TEWL. Thus, a constant light pressure of the probe against the skin should be maintained (40,41).

The practical guidelines are summarized as follows (40,41):

-   During long-term experiments, medical treatment, cosmetics, and products that could disturb TEWL measurements should be avoided.
-   TEWL measurements of a single experiment should, whenever possible, be completed within one season. Measurements during hot summer and freezing winter days should preferentially be avoided, with the exception, of course, when the aim of the study asks for this kind of environmental conditions.
-   Individuals should acclimatize for 15 to 30 minutes before TEWL measurements, with the skin at the measuring site left uncovered. The test person should not eat or consume caffeine-containing drinks just before and during the measurements.
-   Measurement of skin temperature of the test person on the test site is recommended.
-   Only TEWL values from the same (or close-by) anatomical area are expected to be comparable.

- Relative humidity and temperature of the measuring room should be recorded during TEWL measurements and stated in the report.
- If a climate room facility is available, the ambient room temperature should be regulated to 20 to 22°C, and the relative humidity lower than 60%.
- TEWL should not be measured under direct light sources.
- The measuring surface should be placed horizontally and the probe applied parallel to this surface.
- The contact pressure of the probe on the skin should be kept low and constant.
- The measuring probe itself should not be touched before and during measurements and can be handled with the electrical wire or a coating or by wearing gloves.
- TEWL values should be registered 30 to 45 seconds after application of the probe to the skin, preferably using a computer. With newer models, the time to reach a steady state is considerably shorter.
- TEWL measurements should be as short as possible in order to avoid occlusion. Before each measurement, the zero value should be displaced.
- The use of the protection covers should be clearly stated in the protocol and publication (40,41).

TEWL can be considered a parameter indicative of the functional state of the epidermal barrier. One of the characteristics of healthy skin is the proportionality between TEWL and hydration (46). The results of several studies show a relationship between sensory irritation and the skin barrier, as manifested by changes in TEWL (12,34,35). Trends towards higher baseline TEWL values measured on the nasolabial fold and cheek were reported in stingers when compared with non-stingers (12,34,35). These subjects also showed higher LAST scores and an increased TEWL at sites of experimentally induced acute irritant dermatitis (12,34,35).

Wu et al. (35) showed an increase in TEWL in subjects with lower LAST scores than in subjects with higher LAST scores (5% lactic acid). This correlation was statistically significant. They also reported a statistically insignificant trend towards higher baseline TEWL measured at the nasolabial fold in subjects with higher LAST scores. Distante et al. (6) studied the intra- and inter-individual differences in sensitive skin. They included 20 healthy females, 10 of them with sensitive skin. They selected evaluation sites at 10 anatomically defined facial areas and reported that the comparison of TEWL values between a sensitive skin group and a non-sensitive group showed higher mean values for TEWL in all sites in the sensitive skin group. The comparison of all tested facial areas within individuals to investigate intra-individual differences in TEWL showed a similar pattern of distribution in both groups (6).

Measurement of Stratum Corneum Hydration

Water plays an important role in the physical properties of the stratum corneum, and reliable quantification of water in the corneum is essential for understanding skin physiology. Commercially available biophysical methods for assessing skin moisture are based on measuring impedance or its reciprocal, conductance, as a function of one or more different stimulations. In this chapter, we consider the corneometry method for the measurement of hydration of the stratum corneum and the Dermalab based on the same principle. A Corneometer® (Courage & Khazaka, Cologne, Germany; CM 820 and CM 825) is described as being a capacitance-based measuring device operating at low frequency (40–75 Hz), which is sensitive to relative dielectric changes of material placed in contact with the electrode surface. The stratum corneum is a dielectric medium dependent on its water content (Fig. 2A–C). The probe exerts a constant pressure on the skin surface of 3.5 N and covers an area of 49 mm^2. It estimates water content in the epidermis to an approximate depth ranging between 60 and 100 μm (47). The results are strongly influenced by the quality of the skin surface, including surface roughness.

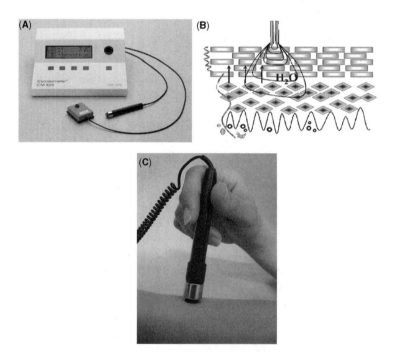

Figure 2 (**A**) Corneometer 825®. (**B**) Measuring principle of the Corneometer. (**C**) Measurement with a Corneometer.

   To perform accurate and reliable measurements, several factors and sources of variation need to be known and taken into account. The probe should be placed perpendicular to the skin surface with slight pressure, just sufficient to start the measurement process. Substances present between the electrodes and the skin, such as hair or remnants of emollients, may affect the results (48). When necessary, shaving or clipping the hairs is recommended before starting the measurement. A different position of the probe can cause unreliable readings. Several measurements of the same site might cause occlusion, which results in an increase in displayed values. Therefore, we recommend to wait for at least five seconds before repeating a measurement at the same site. It is advisable to measure at least three times, once at each of three different but nearby sites. Measuring errors may occur if the skin or probe surface is wet, for instance, by sweating or if the surface is contaminated by dirt particles, oil, grease, or cosmetic products. Cleaning of the probe is recommended between measurements. It is also important to consider environmental influences. Measurements should be performed under appropriate ambient conditions, keeping the temperature low enough to minimize sweat production (20–22°C) and, ideally, relative humidity between 40% and 60% (48). Measurement under direct light sources should be avoided. The volunteers are measured relaxed and acclimatized to the measuring environment for 10 to 20 minutes. The instrument itself should also be acclimatized during the same time. The test site should be exposed to the ambient air for at least 10 minutes prior to the start of measurements.

   There are some variables that have a possible influence on the measurement. Individual-related variables are regional differences in stratum corneum water content, the influence of body hair, and the effect of age (49). There are also some environment-related variables, with a possible influence on measurement. Temperature and relative humidity influence the water content of stratum corneum. Therefore, room humidity should be kept constant (49).

   Seidenari et al. (12) demonstrated lower baseline electrical capacitance of the right cheeks of individuals self-reporting sensitive skin and with a propensity towards higher LAST scores when compared with a self-reported non-sensitive group with lower LAST scores. A correlation between baseline capacitance values and subjective responses after the washing test could be demonstrated. Dehydration might be the basis for subjective sensations after exposure to water and soap (12). Wu et al. (35) stated that LAST score is negatively correlated with baseline capacitance of the nasolabial skin. The latter study also reported that 5% lactic acid application increased local capacitance to a lesser degree in subjects with higher LAST scores than in subjects with lower LAST scores. Distante et al. (6) compared capacitance values between a sensitive group and a non-sensitive group (6). They reported lower capacitance values in all sites in the sensitive group. However, the differences between the two groups were not statistically significant.

   As evidenced by its comparatively reduced electrical capacitance, the skin of stingers is less well hydrated than that of non-stingers (12,35). Considering the hypothesis that stingers have an increased stratum corneum permeability, one might speculate that skin of stingers becomes dehydrated as water migrates more rapidly from the stratum corneum to the surface and evaporates (22).

Skin Surface pH Measurement

The acidity of the skin varies physiologically within a pH range of about 4.3 to 5.5, depending on the skin area and the age of the individual. The acidic pH is attributed to the presence of buffering substances in the skin, which are able to buffer small quantities of acid or alkali applied to the skin and to reduce their irritancy. The acidic pH is necessary to maintain bacteriological, chemical, and mechanical resistances of the skin. A mixture of buffering substances controls cutaneous acidic pH, in order that small amounts of alkalinic or acidic compounds can be applied without modifying it. The larger the buffering capacity, the smaller the cutaneous pH changes (4). The buffering capacity is due to several systems: (*i*) lactic acid/lactate system provided by sweat glands, (*ii*) free amino acids of the stratum corneum, (*iii*) proteins of the stratum corneum, and (*iv*) carbon dioxide/bicarbonate system (from plasma) (50). In general terms, the pH value at the surface of the skin is the product of water-soluble substances in the stratum corneum, of secreted and processed sweat and lipids, and of carbon dioxide diffusion (48).

Fluhr and Elias (51) proposed a classification for factors that influence skin surface pH:

1. endogenous factors, unrelated to pathological features (e.g., developmental changes in pH),
2. endogenous factors, related to clinical pathological situations (e.g., increased pH in atopic dermatitis),
3. exogenous factors (e.g., influence of detergents on pH).

Endogenous or physiological factors, unrelated to pathological features and influencing skin pH are race, anatomical site, gender, age, and circadian rhythm (51). Other features with a possible influence are sweating, skin temperature, and sebum on the skin. It is usually admitted that skin surface pH is relatively similar in different body sites except in areas with higher moisture, such as the intertriginous areas, which have a slightly higher pH (neutral to alkaline) than other body areas (51,52). Similarly, gender is considered to have no significant effect (except perhaps due to different cosmetic habits) (52,53). It is important to control precisely the time of investigation and the site of measurement and to equilibrate subjects in a climatized room before determining the pH in order to minimize the effect of eccrine sweating. Age-related pH changes can be divided into:

1. newborn period with the formation of an acid mantle within the first weeks after birth,
2. childhood period with elevated stratum corneum (SC) pH values,

3. adult period with lowest SC pH values over lifetime, and
4. aging period with an increase in SC pH values (51).

Skin pH has been reported to vary with race and genetic background. Black people have a lower skin surface pH than Caucasians (54). It seems that the differences in skin pH between different races are primarily related to pigmentation (51). The influence of circadian rhythms is relatively moderate (48).

Exogenous factors significantly affect the measured skin surface pH. Washing procedures have an alkalizing effect on the skin surface pH, independent of the pH of the washing solution. Skin washing with detergents and cleansing products can have a temporary effect. The use of alkaline soap increases skin surface pH. Depending on the product, topical application of cosmetic products is able to influence moderately the stratum corneum pH. Thus, the use of a neutral or acidic cleanser is less harmful to the surface pH than alkaline soap (55). Many parameters involved with seasonal changes may affect the skin surface pH (48,51).

For the specific requirements of skin pH measurements, a planar electrode was developed with a single unit containing active and reference electrodes. The contact site between the electrode and the skin covers an area of approximately 10 mm in diameter, and its use is non-invasive. Any commercialized pH meter devices fitted with a planar electrode can be used for the measurement of skin surface pH (56).

For a correct measurement of skin surface pH, it is recommended to follow all practical operating conditions. Care must be taken in identifying the skin site, the time of day of the measurement, and the environmental conditions. Subjects should receive precise instructions before the test, mainly in terms of hygiene procedure or the use of topical products (4).

Some practical or experimental considerations should be taken into account (Fig. 3A,B):

- The electrolyte liquid (3 mol/L solution of potassium chloride) level in the external electrode sheath (reference electrode) should be higher than the level in the measuring internal electrode.
- The electrode face (membrane) should not be brought into contact with hard objects. During short intervals between measurements, the electrode (or rather the electrode face) is best immersed in a KCl solution or in distilled water.
- The elastic electrode covering should be filled constantly with a KCl solution.
- Any kind of contamination of the electrode (e.g., by fats or proteins) should be monitored and eliminated.
- The pH meter must be calibrated prior to measurements, using standard buffer solutions with known and stable pH values (e.g., pH 4.0 and pH 7.0). Before application to the skin, the electrode must be dipped into distilled water to moisten the surface. Then, the flat electrode top is placed on the skin with slight pressure during the measurement.

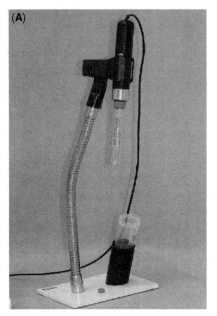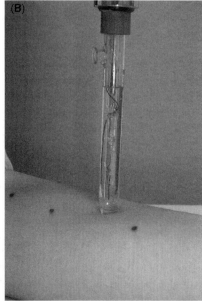

Figure 3   (**A**) pHmeter 900®. (**B**) Measurement with a pH meter®.

- A regular calibration of the electrode is required, not only for each new electrode, but also every 5 to 15 days, depending on the use and the state of the electrodes.
- The volume of applied water may affect the concentration of extracted material at the measurement site. Hence, we recommend to standardize the volume of applied water (e.g., 20 μL).
- The pressure exerted on the probe does not influence the values if the pressure is slight to moderate. Excessive pressure should be avoided.
- Ambient temperature and sweating may affect the pH measurements. It is desirable to perform measurements under controlled conditions, keeping the ambient temperature low enough to minimize sweat production (e.g., 20–22°C) and the relative humidity between 40% and 60%. Volunteers should be relaxed and acclimatized to the measuring environment for at least 15 to 20 minutes. The pH meter itself should also be equilibrated for at least the same time.
- Care should be taken that no cosmetic residue or excessive sebum is left on the surface of the skin. In both cases, gentle dry wiping is advised for the removal. Cleaning must be avoided as it will greatly affect pH measurements (even pure water).
- A minimum period of three to six hours should be awaited between the personal hygiene procedures of the subject and the measurements. This

is the reason why conditions of washing and personal hygiene should be specified in the study protocol.

- In order to minimize the effect of cosmetic products and/or dirt, we suggest the removal of the uppermost stratum corneum layer with a single application of adhesive tapes (e.g., D-Squames®, Scotch tape®, Tesafilm®) and a gentle removal.

Issachar et al. (4) investigated whether there is an objective sign of cutaneous sensitivity by measuring the decrease and recovery of skin pH after a single application of lactic acid. Lactic acid was rubbed on the nasolabial folds and on the ventral forearm of a preselected population versus a control population. The participants were classified as sensitive or non-sensitive by a single application on the nasolabial fold of 0.05 mL of a 10% lactic acid solution. The physiological cutaneous pH values measured on the ventral forearm and on the nasolabial fold were 5.5 for both sensitive skin and normal skin without any significant difference. After the application of 10% solution of lactic acid, the skin surface pH decreased dramatically on both sites. There was no significant difference between forearm and nasolabial fold immediately after the application, but the decrease was longer on the forearm (pH remained at low values for seven hours), whereas on the nasolabial fold, skin pH increased quickly. The large number of eccrine sweat glands on the face ($350 \pm 50/cm^2$, but only $225 \pm 25/cm^2$ on the forearm) could be responsible for this shift (4). In their study, when lactic acid was applied to sensitive skin, it penetrated quickly, thus stimulating the sensory nerve network triggering stinging (4), whereas it remained on the surface of normal skin. The skin surface pH remained lower and no stinging occurred. The investigators made the conclusion that sensitive skin represents an easily and rapidly identifiable subpopulation with a more general tendency to have skin reactions. Study of the cutaneous pH after lactic acid stimulation could be an objective test to predict cosmetic-related cases of adverse reactions (4). A trend towards higher baseline skin surface pH values was noted in subjects with self-reported sensitive skin and higher LAST scores, compared with a non-sensitive group with lower LAST scores (12).

Skin Color Assessed by Chromametry

Chromametry is used to assess color changes in the skin. Our perception of skin color and redness due to inflammation is highly subjective and may be influenced by a number of variables, including pigmentation and desquamation (57).

Measurement of skin color can be made by using two different principles: (i) Spectrophotometric, using either broadband or selected wavelengths in the visible range with the measurement of adsorbance and reflectance, gives detailed information about physical skin color properties, but scanners are cumbersome to use routinely, (ii) Tristimulus (blue, red, green) analysis of light reflected from skin structures.

Two types of convenient instruments, a narrowband spectrophotometer (DermaSpectrometer®, Cortex Technology, Hadsund, Denmark) and a tristimulus colorimeter (Minolta Chroma Meter®, Osaka, Japan), are used commonly today for quantification of skin color and erythema. Both instruments are portable and easy to handle.

To describe color, the CIE-color space is widely accepted. The color is expressed in a 3-dimensional space. The L^* value (luminance) gives the relative brightness, ranging from total black ($L^* = 0$) to total white ($L^* = 100$). The a^* value represents the color range from red (positive values) to green (negative values), whereas the b^* value ranges from yellow to blue. One unit in this space represents a difference, which the human eye can separate.

Hemoglobin and melanin are the two dominant chromophores of the skin. Hemoglobin shows specific and high absorption of light in the green spectral range and minimal absorption in the red range. Melanin absorbs without peaks over the whole visual spectrum, increasingly with shorter wavelengths. With increase in erythema, a greater amount of green light is absorbed with less reflections. Skin optics do not simply depend on the content of chromophores located either as melanin in the basal epidermis or as hemoglobin more deeply in the dermis. Light reflection from the skin depends on scattering of the air/stratum corneum interface and backscattering from deep structures, particularly the dermis. Longer wavelengths (red) penetrate skin more deeply and undergo proportionally greater absorption in the tissue. Thus, deeper structures, such as arteries and veins, may be dominated by the contrast color and their blue aspect (57).

To perform accurate measurements, several factors and sources of variation must be known. There are different individual-related variables that may influence the measurement. Fullerton and Serup (58,59) described differences for basal a^* and b^* levels between males and females in different age groups. They concluded that aged skin may be less colored. They also found male skin redder than female skin. Differences in pigmentation among races, for example, blacks and Caucasians, is a major color variable. Visual estimation of erythema in pigmented skin may be misleading, because redness is influenced by the red component of the brown color. Thus, measurement of color and erythema is difficult in races with more pigmented skin. Regional variation of skin color at different anatomical sites is considerable and needs to be taken into account. When measuring hairy test sites, such as the scalp and beard region, interference may occur. Minor growth of hair will not influence measurements. Changes in skin surface properties, such as white scales or larger flakes, may cover underlying redness and influence measurements (60). Furthermore, treatment of skin surface with drugs or cosmetics may influence measurements (57). Intra-individual reproducibility of repeated measurements on untreated and treated skin has shown only small variations (57). Greater variability has been found when comparing day-to-day variation of untreated skin (61,62). Owing to diurnal variation, repeated measurements should be performed at the same time of the day (63). Physical and mental activities have an influence on skin color. Exercise, for example, strongly influences cutaneous blood flow (CBF) and color. Mental stress and adrenergic system activation are associated with vasoconstriction, pale skin, and sweating. Influence on blood flow and color may be excessive (57). Smoking and caffeine intake >500 mg per day (approximately five cups of coffee) may influence skin color in the corticosteroid vasoconstriction test and are recommended to be avoided in the Food and Drug Administration guideline on the blanding test (64). Furthermore, the use of vasoactive medications that could modulate blood flow may also influence the skin color and these panelists should be excluded. Alcohol is known as a cutaneous vasodilatator (65). Owing to the influence of the orthostatic position on skin color, it is recommended that subjects take up a standardized position during color measurement, fixed relative to the heart level (57).

Skin color measurement may also be influenced by environment-related variables. Temperature changes induce blood vessel dilatation or constriction, thus influencing skin color. The normal skin surface temperature is about 30 to 32°C. Local heating results in vasodilatation and redness, which is maximal at about 40°C where the perfusion is of arterial character. Both local skin temperature and core temperature are variables of major importance in skin color (66). Ambient light was found not to influence chromameter measurements (62). However, direct sunlight should be avoided when measuring with this instrument, as excessive changes in measurement conditions and false light coming into the sensor system may cause an error message on the display. Tan in the summer and xerosis in the winter may influence skin color measurements, depending on degree and severity (57).

Instrument-related variables may have an influence on the measurement of skin color. The contact pressure between chromameter probe and skin may influence measurements. Thus, the instrument should be placed gently onto the skin, strictly avoiding excess pressure, and measurements should be performed swiftly (57). Intra- and inter-instrument variabilities may also have an influence on the measurement of skin color (Fig. 4A,B).

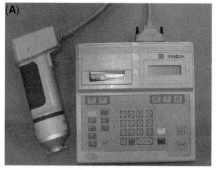 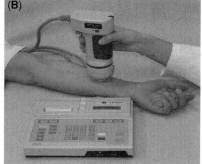

Figure 4   (**A**) Chromameter 300®. (**B**) Measurement with the Chromameter 300.

Some practical considerations should be taken into account (57):

- Before starting measurements, test sites are left uncovered and motion-less for at least five minutes.
- Measurements should be performed within reasonable temperature ranges in the laboratory, preferably 19 to 23°C, avoiding measurements in direct sunlight.
- Before starting each measuring series, the chromameter should be reca-librated. Calibration and measurements should always be performed under the same conditions.
- The position of the test subject should be standardized during the study (especially if it is performed on the extremities) to eliminate orthostatic variation.
- Skin color varies spontaneously during the day and repeated measure-ments should, therefore, be done at the same time of the day.
- Always a representative untreated reference skin site or a placebo for-mulation reference site adjacent to the test sites should be measured.
- The instrument should be gently placed vertically on the skin, avoiding excess pressure. Measurements should be performed rapidly.
- Three measurements within each test site should be taken and the mean value should be used as the result.
- After measurement of a subject, the measuring head should be cleaned.

In the clinical evaluation published by Seidenari et al. (12), the skin of sen-sitive subjects was described as more erythematous and teleangiectatic. Signifi-cant differences were present for erythema at all three assessed skin areas. In the investigation of baseline biophysical parameters, they observed an increase in colorimetric a^* values (evidencing a stronger red component) and a decrease in colorimetric L^* values on the face of subjects self-reporting sensitive skin with higher LAST scores when compared with subjects with non-sensitive skin with lower LAST scores. The clinical evaluation of erythema corresponded to an increase in a^* values (12).

Laser Doppler Flowmetry

The assessment of skin microcirculation is of great interest in dermatology and cosmetology in the quantification of skin irritation, sun protecting factor, and the efficacy of anti-redness treatments (67). Several techniques such as laser Doppler velocimetry, laser Doppler imaging, photoplethysmography, thermal conductance, thermography, and xenon washout techniques can be used to inves-tigate the flow in cutaneous microcirculation. Laser Doppler velocimetry and laser Doppler imaging are the most widely used techniques for the assessment of microcirculation (Fig. 5A–C) (67). Studies have shown that skin blood flow, objectively assessed by laser Doppler velocimetry, may have to be raised three to four times before the naked eye can detect changes (68).

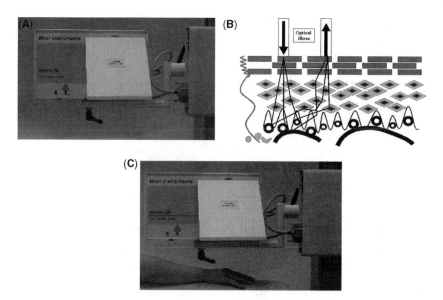

Figure 5 (**A**) Laser Doppler Imager®. (**B**) Measuring principle of LDF. (**C**) Measurement with LDF. *Abbreviation*: LDF, laser Doppler flowmetry.

LDF has been used for studying the microcirculation in many tissues, including skin. It is a continuous and non-invasive recording of microvascular tissue perfusion (2). Many different LDF instruments are commercially available, for example, Moor LDI. LDF is an optical technique for the estimation of microcirculation, based on the Doppler principle. When the laser beam is directed towards the tissue, reflection, transmission, absorption, and scattering occur. Laser light backscattered from moving particles, such as erythrocytes, is shifted in frequency according to the Doppler principle, whereas radiation back-scattered from non-moving structures remains at the same frequency. Laser Doppler blood flowmeters are handy and relatively easy to use. However, as for other measuring methods, sources of variation need to be known and taken into consideration. Because the cutaneous microcirculation is a dynamic system with many functions, for example, thermoregulation and metabolism, many environmental and, even more importantly, individual factors influence the CBF (69).

There are some individual-related variables that must be taken into account, such as age range, excluding the neonatal period (CBF decreases in the first weeks after birth) where CBF as measured by LDF is not age dependent (70,71). Huether and Jacobs (72) could not find significant sex-related differences in CBF at any of the test sites (72). Agner (73) reported no sex-related difference in the basal CBF. However, in an experiment of CBF on the forearms, significantly higher values were measured in males (74). Thus, at present, the findings regarding sex and CBF are contradictory (69), but no major differences in CBF between both sexes have been reported. No significant differences in the basal CBF between racial groups should be expected (69). The regional variation of CBF is considerable and needs to be taken into account (69).

CBF itself is a physiological parameter subject to regulation and rapid variations. In the basal state, the vessels are in a relative contracted position, with a limited potential for contraction but a wide potential for dilatation and increase of flow. One reason for the conflicting results may be the small size of the measuring area and the problem of exact repositioning of the probe. It is important to examine individuals in the same position, as CBF is dependent on position. Long-term studies should be performed with repetitive measurements at the same time of the day because of circadian and ultradian rhythmicity for basal CBF (75). Physical and mental activities may have an influence on CBF. Hence, performing measurements in a quiet environment with a minimum of audiovisual and other mental stimuli is recommended (69). The intake of all potentially vasoactive agents, such as vasodilatating and anti-inflammatory drugs, the consumption of nicotine, caffeine, and alcohol should be avoided (69). Smoking has been demonstrated to reduce forearm CBF and alcoholic ingestion to increase CBF (76,77).

Environment-related variables that influence the measurement of blood flow are air convection, humidity, as well as ambient and local temperatures. Therefore, it is advisable to measure CBF at constant environmental conditions and to protect the panelists against air draughts, for example, from air conditioning. In order to prevent undesired effects of ambient or local temperature changes on CBF, adaptation of 20 to 30 minutes of the subject to the room conditions is recommended. This includes the removal of heavy clothing to circumvent later adaptive vasoconstriction in response to lower ambient temperature. At the usual ambient temperatures of 20 to 25°C in a draught-free environment, CBF is relatively stable (69).

Technique-related variables might influence the measurement of blood flow. The range of flowmetry instruments and the range of applications and modifications, together with the popularity of the method, make it impossible to develop a universal standard. Guidelines for good laboratory practice and for good clinical practice have been published by the EC and the FDA, in order to improve the level of documentation (78,79). Each researcher or laboratory needs to establish their own standard operating procedure, including validation under their specific practical conditions (69).

For measurement of CBF, using LDF, some practical or experimental considerations must be taken into account (69):

- Allow the flowmeter to warm up for at least 15 minutes. Apply the probe to the measuring site with no special pressure. It has been shown that skin blood flow is reduced dramatically by slight (<15 mmHg) pressure of the probe to the skin (80).

- The test subject should not take any food or drugs, which might influence CBF. Avoid any topical treatment of the test site prior to study unless it is part of the experiment.
- The test subject should not deliberately exercise, be exposed to unusual temperatures, or be under mental stress immediately before CBF measurements.
- Allow the test subject to rest for 15 minutes or more under quiet conditions, preferably in the laboratory room in the position in which recordings are going to be obtained, that is, sitting, and with the test site uncovered for at least 30 minutes (67).
- Take 1 to 2 recordings and average them if the flowmeter operates within a small measuring field, that is, 1 to 3 mm^2. Avoid movement of the optical cable (69).
- Control the laboratory room and the measuring conditions, particularly with respect to temperature and convection of air and noise. Avoid measurements under direct light, including sunshine, which might influence skin temperature. Perform measurements with the site studied at a standardized level relative to the level of the heart (69).
- Little effect on CBF was present at room temperatures from 24 to 30°C, so the measurements should be taken in a room with a temperature in this range.

Issachar et al. (2) in their study investigated the permeability of the vasodilatator methyl nicotinate in a sensitive skin group versus a normal control group. Subjects with sensitive skin showed an increased reaction to methyl nicotinate, assessed with laser Doppler perfusion imaging during the first 30 minutes following application. During the 40 minutes following methyl nicotinate application, sensitive skin blood flow values were higher when compared with the control group. However, they decreased more quickly after reaching the maximum. Sensitive skin blood flow is higher than normal skin blood flow for 35 minutes. According to Frosch and Kligman (13), who first studied the sensitive skin phenomena, sensitive skin may be due to increased penetration of irritants. This conclusion is reached by arguing that stinging can be elicited in anyone by allowing access to the nerve endings (2). Berardesca et al. (15) detected a correlation between sensitive skin and increased vasodilatation induced by methyl nicotinate. Similarly, Issachar et al. (2) reported that the maximum response in sensitive skin is higher than in the normal skin. However, Issachar et al. (2) observed that returning to baseline required less time in sensitive skin. They hypothesized that stratum corneum barrier function may play an important role in determining skin hyperreactivity. Increased penetration of methyl nicotinate may trigger increased erythema in the sensitive skin group when compared with that of non-reactors. Distante et al. (6) compared the skin flux values of LDF between a sensitive group and a non-sensitive group and showed higher values in all sites in the sensitive skin group, except for one site on the forehead. However, the differences were not statistically significant.

LDF reveals an exaggerated local vasodilatory response in stingers, associated with both non-immunologic contact urticaria induced and acute irritant dermatitis (14). Non-immunologic contact urticaria induced by benzoic acid 1% and sorbic acid 0.5% or 1% appears to produce a more pronounced local increase in skin blood flow velocity in stingers (14). In stingers, the topical application of methyl nicotinate induces a more prominent local vasodilatory effect measured by LDF when compared with that of non-stingers (2).

Assessment of Surface Lipid Content by Semiqualitative Sebumetry

The face is exposed to most of the environmental factors; therefore, it is covered by a lipid film. Sebum is the major component of the lipid film on the forehead. Sebum secretion is a regulated process and it is dependent on the inherited traits of each individual but varies according to age, sex, and topographic body location (81). There are big differences in facial skin types in terms of the amount of secreted sebum. In general, skin can be classified into three types according to each individual's subjective assessment regarding sebum secretion: oily, normal, and dry. However, individual assessments based on subjective criteria tend to be inconsistent. In order to classify the skin type objectively, several methods have been developed to measure sebum secretion (82). The sebum amount present at the skin surface can be assessed non-invasively using one of the several methods on the basis of solvent extraction, cigarette paper pads, photometric assessment, bentonite clay, and lipid-sensitive tapes. Quantitative parameters include sebum casual level, sebum excretion rate, sebum replacement time, instant sebum delivery, follicular excretion rate, density in sebum-enriched reservoirs, and sustainable rate of sebum excretion (83).

The basic principle of the photometric technique relies on the fact that opalescent glass or a sapphire plate of a given opacity to light becomes translucent when its surface is covered with lipids. The photometric procedure is time-saving and highly reproducible (83). The sebum extraction from skin measured by a photometric procedure is called sebumetry. The measuring instrument generally used is called Sebumeter® (Courage & Khazaka). The Sebumeter has gained popularity and is commonly used in dermatology practices and cosmetic companies (84,85) (Fig. 6A–C). Sebum is collected on a piece of opaque plastic strip instead of a sapphire plate. The measuring probe consists of a 0.1 mm thick, matted plastic strip on a roller, which is manually advanced for each measurement. The probe with the plastic foil (standard load and standard area) is pressed against the skin surface with a built-in spring delivering 10 N guaranteeing constant pressure for each measurement. After the probe has been in contact with the skin surface for 30 seconds, measured by an internal timer, it is placed back into the main unit of the Sebumeter. Transparency of the plastic film is measured by a photocell after emitted light passes twice through the strip. The increase in transmission correlates to lipid adherence. The result is evaluated by a microprocessor, using an internal standard (Sebumeter determines sebum

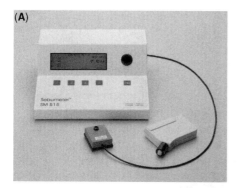
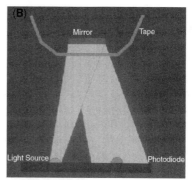
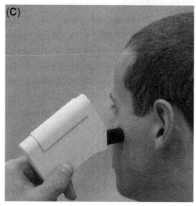

Figure 6 (**A**) Sebumeter 815®. (**B**) Measuring principle of the Sebumeter. (**C**) Measurement with a Sebumeter.

output in μg/cm²). The interpretation of the result divides the different skin types into dry, normal, and oily (86).

It is known that the measurements reflect the actual amount of lipids present on the strip. In fact, it is estimated that an average of about 40% of the total skin surface lipids is absorbed with one sampling. The digital read-out displayed as micrograms per square centimeter gives the estimated total amount of lipids on the skin. However, this extrapolation may be inaccurate when seborrhea is intense due to a saturation effect on the plastic strip. One shortcoming of the Sebumeter is its extrapolated photometric calculating method (83). In spite of this limitation, the recommendations proposed by the manufacturer are commonly used in the classification of skin types (81). Another pitfall is represented by the skin microrelief and roughness, which impairs the close contact between the probe and the entire stratum corneum (83,86).

There are some factors that affect sebum excretion, such as ethnicity, age range, gender, adequate skin profile, and anatomical test area. They must be defined and appropriate for the purpose of the study. The environmental conditions including seasons, relative humidity, and temperature should be controlled. Care should be taken to avoid any chronobiological effect (83).

Another method for measuring sebum excretion is a qualitative method using the microporous, hydrophobic Sebutape®. Sebutape shows the quantity of sebum excreted on the tape after applying on the face for more than an hour (87). Sebutape is simple to use, but the quantification of sebum secretion is difficult (88). These adhesive patches detect sebum (oil) production without the use of any solvents, powders, or chemicals. The method of the adhesive patch is simple: it is a result of the unique combination of an adhesive and microporous film. The film acts as a passive collector of sebum. The gradual displacement of air in the pores of the microporous film changes its appearance. Pores that are filled with sebum are no longer capable of scattering light, so they appear transparent. The lateral spread of sebum in the film is minimized due to the design of the pores. This results in sharp boundaries indicating the location of the active oil glands. The size of the transparent area is a measure of the amount of sebum collected. Patches are placed on a dark background storage card for evaluation by eye or computer image technologies.

Only few data are available on sebum content and sensitive skin. Seidenari et al. (12) described that skin sebum content measured as transparency of an opaque band is lower in stingers than in non-stingers.

Quantitation of Cutaneous Thermal Sensation

Three types of fibers are responsible for thermal sensation. A-beta fibers are myelinated and mediate the touch—vibration and pressure with a conduction velocity of 2 to 30 m/sec. A-delta fibers are smaller and myelinated. They have a conduction velocity of >30 m/sec and mediate cold and pain sensation. C-fibers are small and non-myelinated and mediate warm and itching sensations (89).

Quantitative sensory testing methods have been utilized mainly to study the impairment of somatosensory function in neurological diseases. Particularly in dermatology, thermal sensation testing analysis becomes a more and more utilized quantitative sensory testing method. The threshold of warm and cold sensation as well as hot and cold pain can be measured using this method. The quantitative somatosensory thermotest assesses the function of afferent channels concerned with sensory submodalities served by small caliber fibers (in free nerve endings and in their associated small myelinated and non-myelinated fibers). Measured ramps of ascending or descending temperature are applied to the skin through a Peltier contact thermode, and detection thresholds are recorded as the subject signals the onset of a particular sensation (90).

SUMMARY

Various studies that have employed bioengineering methods have noted important differences in the skin of stingers when compared with that of non-stingers: a relationship between sensory irritation and the epidermal barrier function, manifested by changes in TEWL. Higher baseline TEWL values were reported in stingers when compared with non-stingers. These subjects also showed higher LAST scores and a more exaggerated increase in TEWL at sites of experimentally induced acute irritant dermatitis. The stratum corneum of stingers seems to be less hydrated, as evidenced by lower electrical capacitance values. They may have higher baseline pH values and a lower sebum content. Higher chromometric a^* values likewise indicate hypersensitive vascular responses in stingers. Stingers also appear to have a more reactive cutaneous vasculature. In this chapter, we have summarized the current knowledge of biophysical assessment in identifying and characterizing sensitive skin.

NAMES AND ADDRESSES OF MENTIONED PRODUCTS

Courage & Khazaka electronic GmbH
  Mathias-Brüggen-Straße 91
  D-50829 Köln, Germany
  Phone: +49 221 9564990
  Fax: +49 221 9564991
  Email: info@courage-khazaka.de
  Website: www.courage-khazaka.de

Minolta
  3-91 Daisennishimacki, Sakai
  Osaka 590-8551
  Japan
  Website: www.konicaminolta.com/worldwide/japan/se/

Moor Instruments Ltd.
  Millwey, Axminster,
  Devon, EX 13 5 HU, U.K.
  Phone: +44 (0) 1297 35715
  Fax: +44 (0) 1293 35716
  Email: moorldi@moor.co.uk

Cuderm Corporation
  P.O. Box 797686
  Dallas, Texas 75379-7686, U.S.A.
  Phone: +1 972 248-8095
  Fax: +1927 248-1094
  Website: www.cuderm.com

Cortex Technology ApS
  Smedevaenget 10
  DK-9560 Hadsund, Denmark
  Phone: +45 9857 4100
  Fax: ++45 9857 2223
  Website: www.cortex.dk
  Email: cortex@cortex.dk

REFERENCES

1. Mills OH Jr and Berger RS. Defining the susceptibility of acne-prone and sensitive skin populations to extrinsic factors. Dermatol Clin 1991; 9(1):93–98.
2. Issachar N et al. Correlation between percutaneous penetration of methyl nicotinate and sensitive skin, using laser Doppler imaging. Contact Dermatitis 1998; 39(4):182–186.
3. Draelos ZD. Is this product designed for sensitive skin? Cosmet Dermatol 2002; 15(8):71–78.
4. Issachar N et al. pH measurements during lactic acid stinging test in normal and sensitive skin. Contact Dermatitis 1997; 36(3):152–155.
5. Willis CM et al. Sensitive skin: an epidemiological study. Br J Dermatol 2001; 145(2):258–263.
6. Distante F et al. Intra- and inter-individual differences in sensitive skin. Cosmet Toiletries 2002; 117(7):39–46.
7. Lonne-Rahm SB, Fischer T, Berg M. Stinging and rosacea. Acta Derm Venereol 1999; 79(6):460–461.
8. Goffin V, Pierard-Franchimont C, Pierard GE. Sensitive skin and stratum corneum reactivity to household cleaning products. Contact Dermatitis 1996; 34(2):81–85.
9. Jourdain R et al. Ethnic variations in self-perceived sensitive skin: epidemiological survey. Contact Dermatitis 2002; 46(3):162–169.
10. Johnson AW, Paige DW. Making sense of sensitive skin. Proceedings of the 18th Annual IFSCC Congress, Yokohama; Poster. 1995.
11. Amin S, Engasse P, Maibach HI. Sensitive skin: what is it? 343–349.
12. Seidenari S, Francomano M, Mantovani L. Baseline biophysical parameters in subjects with sensitive skin. Contact Dermatitis 1998; 38(6):311–315.
13. Frosch PJ, Kligman AM. A method for appraising the stinging capacity of topically applied substances. J Cosmetic Chem 1977; 28:197–209.
14. Lammintausta K, Maibach HI, Wilson D. Mechanisms of subjective (sensory) irritation. Propensity to non-immunologic contact urticaria and objective irritation in stingers. Derm Beruf Umwelt 1988; 36(2):45–49.
15. Berardesca E et al. In vivo transcutaneous penetration of nicotinates and sensitive skin. Contact Dermatitis 1991; 25(1):35–38.
16. Rougier A et al. Regional variation in percutaneous absorption in man: measurement by stripping method. Arch Derm Res 1986; 278:465.
17. Amin S, Lathi A, Maibach H. Contact urticaria and the contact urticaria syndrome. In: Marzulli F, Maibach H, eds. Dermatotoxicology. 5th ed. Washington, DC: Taylor and Francis, 1995:485–503.
18. Muizzuddin N, Marenus KD, Maes DH. Factors defining sensitive skin and its treatment. Am J Contact Dermat 1998; 9(3):170–175.
19. Draelos ZD. Sensitive skin: perceptions, evaluation, and treatment. Am J Contact Dermat 1997; 8(2):67–78.
20. Draelos ZD. Treating the patient with multiple cosmetic product allergies. A problem-oriented approach to sensitive skin. Postgrad Med 2000; 107(7):70–72, 75–77.
21. Lammintausta K, Maibach HI. Exogenous and endogenous factors in skin irritation. Int J Dermatol 1988; 27(4):213–222.
22. Sinaiko R, Maibach HI. Bioengineering Correlates of the Sensitive Skin Syndrome. The Sensory Irritation Component.

23. Hamami I, Marks R. Structural determinants of the response of the skin to chemical irritants. Contact Dermatitis 1988; 18(2):71–75.
24. Cotterill JA. Dermatological non-disease: a common and potentially fatal disturbance of cutaneous body image. Br J Dermatol 1981; 104(6):611–619.
25. Jenkins HL, Adams MG. Progressive evaluation of skin irritancy of cosmetics using human volunteers. Int J Cosmetic Sci 1989; 11:141–149.
26. Walker AP et al. Test guidelines for the assessment of skin tolerance of potentially irritant cosmetic ingredients in man. European Cosmetic, Toiletry and Perfumery Association. Food Chem Toxicol 1997; 35(10/11):1099–1106.
27. Nakada T, Hostynek JJ, Maibach HI. Use tests: ROAT (repeated open application test)/PUT (provocative use test): an overview. Contact Dermatitis 2000; 43(1):1–3.
28. Marriott M, Whittle E, Basketter DA. Facial variations in sensory responses. Contact Dermatitis 2003; 49(5):227–231.
29. Christensen M, Kligman AM. An improved procedure for conducting lactic acid stinging tests on facial skin. Journal Soc Cosmet Chem 1996; 47:1–11.
30. Basketter DA, Griffiths HA. A study of the relationship between susceptibility to skin stinging and skin irritation. Contact Dermatitis 1993; 29(4):185–188.
31. Coverly J et al. Susceptibility to skin stinging, non-immunologic contact urticaria and acute skin irritation; is there a relationship? Contact Dermatitis 1998; 38(2):90–95.
32. Hawkins SS et al. Cleansing, moisturizing, and sun-protection regimens for normal skin, self-perceived sensitive skin, and dermatologist-assessed sensitive skin. Dermatol Ther 2004; 17(suppl 1):63–68.
33. Berg M, Lonne-Rahm SB, Fischer T. Patients with visual display unit-related facial symptoms are stingers. Acta Derm Venereol 1998; 78(1):44–45.
34. Lammintausta K, Maibach HI, Wilson D. Susceptibility to cumulative and acute irritant dermatitis. An experimental approach in human volunteers. Contact Dermatitis 1988; 19(2):84–90.
35. Wu Y et al. Correlation between stinging, TEWL and capacitance. Skin Res Technol 2003; 9(2):90–93.
36. Rougier A, Lotte C, Maibach HI. In vivo percutaneous penetration of some organic compounds related to anatomic site in humans: predictive assessment by the stripping method. J Pharm Sci 1987; 76(6):451–454.
37. Soschin D, Kligman AM. Adverse subjective responses. In: Kligman AM, Leyden JJ, eds. Safety and Efficacy of Topical Drugs and Cosmetics. New York: Grune & Stratton, 1982:381.
38. Kobayashi H et al. Measurement of electrical current perception threshold of sensory nerves for pruritus in atopic dermatitis patients and normal individuals with various degrees of mild damage to the stratum corneum. Dermatology 2003; 206(3):204–211.
39. Alagiri M et al. Interstitial cystitis: unexplained associations with other chronic disease and pain syndromes. Urology 1997; 49(5A suppl):52–57.
40. Pinnagoda J et al. Guidelines for transepidermal water loss (TEWL) measurement. A report from the Standardization Group of the European Society of Contact Dermatitis. Contact Dermatitis 1990; 22(3):164–178.
41. Rogiers V. EEMCO guidance for the assessment of transepidermal water loss in cosmetic sciences. Skin Pharmacol Appl Skin Physiol 2001; 14(2):117–128.
42. Fluhr J et al. Assessment of Permeability Barrier Function Measuring Transepidermal Water Loss: Comparing 3 Closed-Loop Systems and 4 Open-Loop Systems In Vivo

and In Vitro Both in Human and Animal Models (Tewameter TM210 and 300, Vap-oMeter, Dermalab, Evaporimeter EP1, HR4300 Evaporimeter and MEECO electro-lytic moisture analyser). (in press).

43. Nilsson GE. Measurement of water exchange through skin. Med Biol Eng Comput 1977; 15(3):209–218.
44. Pinnagoda J et al. Transepidermal water loss with and without sweat gland inacti-vation. Contact Dermatitis 1989; 21(1):16–22.
45. Fluhr J, R S. Calibration standard for open chamber systems. US Symposium of the International Society for Bioengeneering and the skin (ISBS), Orlando, FL, USA. Skin Res Technol 2004; 10(4):1–34.
46. Villarama CD, Maibach H. Sensitive skin and transepidermal water loss. In: Fluhr JW, Elsner P, Berardesca E, Maibach H, eds. Bioengeneering of the Skin: Water and Stratum corneum. 2nd edn. London, New York, Washington, DC: CRC Press, 2004.
47. Barel AO et al. Non-invasive electrical measurements for evaluating the water content of the horny layer: comparison between capacitance and conductance measurements. In: Scott RC et al., ed. Prediction of Pecutaneous Penetration: Methods, Measure-ments, Modelling. London: IBC Technical Services Ltd., 1991:46.
48. Parra JL, Paye M. EEMCO guidance for the in vivo assessment of skin surface pH. Skin Pharmacol Appl Skin Physiol 2003; 16(3):188–202.
49. Berardesca E. EEMCO guidance for the assessment of stratum corneum hydratin: electrical methods. Skin Res Technol 1997; 3:126–132.
50. Robinson S, Robinson AH. Chemical composition of sweat. Physiol Rev 1954; 34(2):202–220.
51. Fluhr JW, Elias PM. Stratum corneum pH: formation and function of the 'acid mantle'. Exogenous Dermatol 2002(1):163–175.
52. Yosipovitch G et al. Skin surface pH in intertriginous areas in NIDDM patients. Poss-ible correlation to candidal intertrigo. Diabetes Care 1993; 16(4):560–563.
53. Wilhelm KP, Cua AB, Maibach HI. Skin aging. Effect on transepidermal water loss, stratum corneum hydration, skin surface pH, and casual sebum content. Arch Derma-tol 1991; 127(12):1806–1809.
54. Berardesca E et al. Differences in stratum corneum pH gradient when comparing white Caucasian and black African-American skin. Br J Dermatol 1998; 139(5):855–857.
55. Bornkessel A et al. Investigation of a washing emulsion for sensitive skin-an appli-cation test. Skin Res Technol 2005; 11.
56. Ehlers C et al. Comparison of two pH meters used for skin surface pH measurement: the pH meter 'pH900' from Courage & Khazaka versus the pH meter '1140' from Mettler Toledo. Skin Res Technol 2001; 7(2):84–89.
57. Fullerton A et al. Guidelines for measurement of skin colour and erythema. A report from the Standardization Group of the European Society of Contact Dermatitis. Contact Dermatitis 1996; 35(1):1–10.
58. Fullerton A, Serup J. Site, gender and age variations in normal skin colour on the back and the forearm. Tristimulus colorimeter (Minolta Chroma Meter CR-200) measure-ments. Skin Res Technol (in press).
59. Fluhr JW, Pfisterer S, Gloor M. Direct comparison of skin physiology in children and adults with bioengineering methods. Pediatr Dermatol 2000; 17(6):436–439.

60. Takiwaki H, Serup J. Measurement of color parameters of psoriatic plaques by narrow-band reflectance spectrophotometry and tristimulus colorimetry. Skin Pharmacol 1994; 7(3):145–150.
61. Wilhelm KP, Maibach HI. Skin color reflectance measurements for objective quantification of erythema in human beings. J Am Acad Dermatol 1989; 21(6):1306–1308.
62. Fullerton A et al. Interlaboratory comparison and validity study of the Minolta Chromameters CR-200 and CR-300. Skin Res Technol 1996.
63. Queille-Roussel C, Poncet M, Schaefer H. Quantification of skin-colour changes induced by topical corticosteroid preparations using the Minolta Chroma Meter. Br J Dermatol 1991; 124(3):264–270.
64. Division of Bioequivalence (F). Guidance: Topical dermatological corticosteroids. In vivo bioequivalence. International Pharmaceutical Regulatory Monitor. Division of Bioequivalence (F), 1995:1–36.
65. Division of Bioequivalence (F). Guidance: Topical dermatological corticosteroids. In vivo bioequivalence. International Pharmaceutical Regulatory Monitor. Appendix B, section B2. 1995:1–36.
66. Ring EFJ. Thermal imaging of skin temperature. Handbook of Non-invasive Methods and the Skin. 1995:457–471.
67. Berardesca E, Leveque JL, Masson P. EEMCO guidance for the measurement of skin microcirculation. Skin Pharmacol Appl Skin Physiol 2002; 15(6):442–456.
68. Wahlberg JE, Nilsson G. Skin irritancy from propylene glycol. Acta Derm Venereol 1984; 64(4):286–290.
69. Bircher A et al. Guidelines for measurement of cutaneous blood flow by laser Doppler flowmetry. A report from the Standardization Group of the European Society of Contact Dermatitis. Contact Dermatitis 1994; 30(2):65–72.
70. Ishihara M et al. Cutaneous blood flow. In: Kligman AM, Takase Y, eds. Tokyo: University of Tokyo Press, 1988:167–181.
71. Bircher A et al. Laser Doppler-measured cutaneous blood flow: effects with age. In: Leveque JL, Agache P, eds. Aging Skin: Properties and Functional Changes. 1993.
72. Huether SE, Jacobs MK. Determination of normal variation in skin blood flow velocity in healthy adults. Nurs Res 1986; 35(3):162–165.
73. Agner T. Basal transepidermal water loss, skin thickness, skin blood flow and skin colour in relation to sodium-lauryl-sulphate-induced irritation in normal skin. Contact Dermatitis 1991; 25(2):108–114.
74. de Boer EM, Bezemer PD, Bruynzeel DP. A standard method for repeated recording of skin blood flow using laser Doppler flowmetry. Derm Beruf Umwelt 1989; 37(2):58–62.
75. Yosipovitch G et al. Circadian and ultradian (12 h) variations of skin blood flow and barrier function in non-irritated and irritated skin-effect of topical corticosteroids. J Invest Dermatol 2004, 122(3).824–829.
76. Waeber B et al. Skin blood flow reduction induced by cigarette smoking: role of vasopressin. Am J Physiol 1984; 247(6 Pt 2):H895-H901.
77. Wilkin JK, Fortner G. Cutaneous vascular sensitivity to lower aliphatic alcohols and aldehydes in Orientals. Alcohol Clin Exp Res 1985; 9(6):522–525.
78. Hirsch AF. Good Laboratory Practice Regulations. 1st edn. 1989.

79. EEC note for guidance: good clinical practice for trials on medicinal products in the European Community. CPMP Working Party on Efficacy of Medicinal Products. Pharmacol Toxicol 1990; 67(4):361–372.
80. Obeid AN et al. A critical review of laser Doppler flowmetry. J Med Eng Technol 1990; 14(5):178–181.
81. Youn SW et al. Evaluation of facial skin type by sebum secretion: discrepancies between subjective descriptions and sebum secretion. Skin Res Technol 2002; 8(3):168–172.
82. Lookingbill DP, Cunliffe WJ. A direct gravimetric technique for measuring sebum excretion rate. Br J Dermatol 1986; 114(1):75–81.
83. Pierard GE et al. EEMCO guidance for the in vivo assessment of skin greasiness. The EEMCO Group. Skin Pharmacol Appl Skin Physiol 2000; 13(6):372–389.
84. Thune P, Gustavsen T. Comparison of two techniques for quantitative measurements of skin surface lipids. Acta Derm Venereol 1984; 134:30.
85. Dikstein S et al. Comparison of the Sebumeter and the Lipometer. Bioeng Skin 1987; 3:197.
86. Rode B, Ivens U, Serup J. Degreasing method for the seborrheic areas with respect to regaining sebum excretion rate to casual level. Skin Res Technol 2000; 6(2):92–97.
87. Serup J. Formation of oiliness and sebum output-comparison of a lipid-absorbant and occlusive-tape method with photometry. Clin Exp Dermatol 1991; 16(4):258–263.
88. Pierard GE, Pierard-Franchimont C, Kligman AM. Kinetics of sebum excretion evaluated by the Sebutape-Chromameter technique. Skin Pharmacol 1993; 6(1):38–44.
89. Archer CB. Functions of the skin. In: Champion RH, Burton JL, Burns DA, Breathnach SM, eds. Textbook of Dermatology, 6th ed. London: Blackwell Science, 1930–1933, 1998.
90. Verdugo R, Ochoa JL. Quantitative somatosensory thermotest. A key method for functional evaluation of small calibre afferent channels. Brain 1992; 115(Pt 3):893–913.

9

Identification of a Sensitive Skin Panel

**Marie C. Marriott, David A. Basketter,
Karen J. Cooper, and Lisa Peters**

*Safety and Environmental Assurance Centre,
Unilever Colworth, Bedford, U.K.*

INTRODUCTION

Epidemiological studies suggest that up to 70% of reported adverse reactions to personal-care products involve irritant rather than allergic reactions (1). The consumers expect personal-care products to be safe, but expectations will be even higher for those products marketed specifically for individuals with sensitive skin. The consumer anticipates that by purchasing items labeled as "hypoallergenic" or "safe for sensitive skin," they are minimizing their risk of experiencing skin irritation to the product, be that an erythematous response or subjective irritation, such as stinging, itching, or burning.

As part of the process to ensure consumer safety, manufacturers of home and personal-care products frequently evaluate topical skin effects in a panel of healthy human volunteers. Specially selected and highly trained sensory panels are widely used to establish a consumer acceptance of a personal-care product in terms of efficacy and its sensory characteristics. It has been suggested that to optimize the safety of personal-care products and to explore margins of safety in terms of skin irritation, identification and use of sensitive skin panels may be an important way forward. The challenge this poses is whether it is possible to select suitable groups of appropriately sensitive individuals.

Research-based publications have suggested that selecting such a sensitive group may not be so easy in practice. How does one define sensitive skin? How can such a group be identified? What type of testing, if any, is most appropriate to distinguish such a group? What mechanism of irritation is most relevant to sensitive skin and what is the best method of measuring such irritation?

This chapter considers why the consumer is drawn to such products and the problems that exist in the definition of sensitive skin. It will also provide a summary of methodologies currently available and a critical evaluation of how/whether a sensitive skin panel can be identified.

DEFINITION OF SENSITIVE SKIN

Many consumers perceive themselves to be "sensitive" to certain types of skin-care products. Questionnaires have been used to gather information on self-perception of sensitive skin and some of which probe for details on the possible psychological aspects that may contribute to the levels of consumer satisfaction perceived (e.g., the role of stress in eczema). For example, Willis et al. (2) surveyed a population of 3800 individuals from Buckinghamshire (3300 women and 500 men), from which 51.4% of women and 38.2% of men considered themselves as having sensitive skin. In fact, 57% of women and 31.4% of men detailed experience of an adverse reaction to a personal-care product. People may also classify themselves as having "sensitive skin" if they consider themselves to be sensitive to common allergens, such as nickel, and to sun exposure or if they currently or have previously experienced a skin disease, such as eczema. Consequently, the meaning of sensitive skin is quite individual for any given consumer and relates to their own experiences and perception of adverse reactions. Certainly, some individuals will perceive themselves to have sensitive skin for reasons quite unrelated to how their skin responds to mechanical and topical irritation as a result of using skin-care products. Hence, it is not surprising that self-assessment of sensitive skin often does not correlate well with objective measures of sensitivity (e.g., skin responses following topical application of certain chemicals) (3–6).

Even when considering those who are sensitive specifically to skin-care products, often individuals tend to be selectively sensitive (e.g., only sensitive to certain product types). From the research into irritant contact dermatitis, many individuals appear to be selectively sensitive and will only react to a small number of stimuli when tested (7).

A common definition of sensitive skin, used by dermatologists and industry alike, is "a reduced tolerance to frequent or prolonged use of cosmetics and toiletries, with symptoms ranging from visible signs of irritation such as erythema and scaling through to more subjective neurosensory forms of discomfort such as stinging, burning, itching, tightness, and smarting" (2). Hence, any skin testing conducted to identify a sensitive skin panel should ideally include both visible and sensory endpoints. Currently, there are several methods to assess these endpoints separately, but there is only very little literature available on a single method that captures both successfully. Indeed, there is some evidence to suggest that visual and sensory irritations do not correlate particularly well (8).

It has been documented that individuals with rosacea and an atopic background appear to be a particularly sensitive population (9,10) and may be a good group from which to recruit a sensitive skin panel. However, in industry, there is a tendency to test skin-care products only on healthy adults, such that the panel mimics the "normal" consumer population. To ensure healthy adults are recruited into studies, individuals are asked pertinent questions regarding their health at the recruitment stage and those with existing skin conditions, such as eczema or psoriasis, would not be recruited onto the study. Indeed, the steroid creams often prescribed for acute skin disease have a tendency to inhibit the immune response and so individuals taking such medication (and indeed, other anti-inflammatory drugs) would not be invited to studies testing such products.

To determine sensitivity of panels of healthy adults, typically, individuals are challenged by topical application of certain chemicals with a known irritation profile. Frequently, positive and negative controls are tested alongside test materials to ensure that the panel is sufficiently sensitive. In a covered patch test, 0.3% sodium lauryl sulfate (SLS) (positive control) and distilled water (negative control) are included (11). In a four-hour patch test, 20% SLS is used to aid classification of chemicals, and numbers of positive reactions are used as a measure to judge whether the panel is sufficiently sensitive to validate the study (12). In the sting test (13), 10% lactic acid has historically been used to determine the sensitivity of volunteers, prior to their testing personal-care products. Indeed, this sting-test method has been used as a means to identify a sensitive skin panel.

Although patch testing and in-use testing are commonly used in industry to assess the acute dermal toxicity of personal-care products following a topical application (using visual assessment and sensory comments as measures of irritation), none of the documented methods for assessing the chemosensory response or topical skin responses (e.g., irritant contact dermatitis and contact urticaria) captures the complexities of sensitive skin. Although research has identified that many unique physiological characteristics exist within individuals with atopic dermatitis, atopic eczema, and atopic rosacea (i.e., clinically defined sensitive subpopulations), such as differing nerve fiber densities (14) and abnormalities in epidermal lipid metabolism of atopics (15), better understanding of how these factors relate to sensitive skin is required. Studies exploring such links may help define sensitive skin more fully at the physiological level and thus aid determination of how best to test for a sensitive skin panel.

TEST METHODS FOR INVESTIGATING SENSITIVE SKIN

Establishing a simple yet robust testing regime to investigate sensitive skin is problematic because of the variability in clinical manifestations and the lack of clarity regarding what constitutes sensitive skin in the first instance. There are a variety of methods that have been developed in an attempt to investigate and identify people with sensitive skin, but no single, widely accepted testing protocol exists at present. Different methods generally investigate one particular endpoint, including sensory responses such as stinging, itching, and burning and objective irritation such as erythema, vasodilation, or a wheal-and-flare response. More recently, bioengineering equipment has been used to determine specific physical parameters such as transepidermal water loss (TEWL) and skin thickness, which may be associated with heightened reactivity (10).

Subjective (Sensory) Irritation

When examining the current literature, the facial lactic acid sting test (13) is generally the method most commonly used to investigate or identify individuals with sensitive skin. It is sometimes reported that this test best correlates with those individuals who demonstrate objective and/or subjective symptoms of sensitive skin (10,13); however, there is some debate about this issue (3,8). The test usually involves the application of 10% lactic acid to the nasolabial fold using a cotton bud to rub the material briskly onto the skin. Stinging is rated by use of a questionnaire prompting the panelists to score the level of stinging they experience at 2.5, 5, and sometimes 8 minutes after application. This is usually done using a four-point scale (0 = none, 1 = slight, 2 = moderate, and 3 = severe). A cumulative stinging score of 3 or more is generally used to classify the individual as a "stinger." In 1977, Frosch and Kligman suggested the nasolabial fold as the region of the face most sensitive to lactic acid; its high sensitivity is related to the high permeability of this region and the high density of hair follicles and sweat glands, which serve as penetration shunts into the dermis, and also to the elaborate sensory nerve network that innervates this area.

   This method has been criticized for having poor reproducibility; it has been investigated in some detail and undergone a certain degree of modification over the years. Different areas of the face have been utilized, including the nasolabial fold, cheek, upper lip, and forehead, with differing sensitivities demonstrated at the different sites (4,16,17). The nasolabial fold and cheek are generally recognized as being the most sensitive to the application of lactic acid; however, wide interindividual differences have been demonstrated (17). It has also been suggested that applying lactic acid under occlusion using a HillTop chamber provides a more reproducible method (12); however, others have found this not to be the case (17).

There are a variety of similar methods that are designed to induce the sensory responses of differing types. The chloroform:methanol (20:80) test is designed to elicit burning, with the mixture applied to the skin, and the time it takes to induce an intense burning response is recorded. Highly sensitive individuals experience burning more rapidly than less sensitive individuals (18). Histamine can be used in a similar way and induces an itching response (19). These tests can be used alongside each other to identify individuals sensitive to itching, stinging, and burning.

More recently, several other chemicals have been investigated and it is suggested that a number of different chemicals that induce different sensory sensations should be used to gauge an individual's sensitivity (20,21); these include capsaicin, menthol, ethanol, and lactic acid. These chemicals are hypothesized to cause sensory irritation via different mechanisms, capsaicin via a specific receptor–ligand interaction, lactic acid via proton-gated channels, and ethanol via a more general membrane-disruption effect (20). The method used is similar to the sting test in that it involves applying the chemicals to the face and asking panelists to identify and rate the intensity of any sensory response they experience. The degree of response and number of chemicals to which individuals respond are analyzed to determine the volunteer's sensitivity (20).

The importance of providing descriptors to panelists to aid them in identifying the particular sensation they experience has been identified. This is also of value in terms of consistency. Some of the more common descriptors previously reported are detailed in Table 1.

There has been some debate on the best way to quantify the intensity of the sensory response experienced. In the original sting-test method developed by Frosch and Kligman (13), a four-point scale was used, which is the most

Table 1   Sensory Descriptors

Sensory response	Definition
Stinging	Sensation that occurs when alcohol is applied to a cut or abrasion
	Sharp sensation similar to those produced by a pinprick or an insect bite (20,21)
Itching	Desire to scratch (20)
Tingle	Lively "pins and needles" sensation (20)
Prickle	Sensation caused by the movement of rough fabrics over the skin (22)
Burning	Painful sensation produced by extreme temperatures or chemical irritants (20)
Numbness	Diffuse sensation produced during the onset or offset of an anesthetic (21)

widely used tool to measure sensory irritation. However, this scale has been criticized for its lack of sensitivity. Recently, the labeled magnitude scale has been used to quantify sensory responses, as it is suggested that this scale provides a much better assessment of the degree of sensory response and the data collected can be more easily analyzed using sensitive parametric statistical tests (23).

Objective Irritation

As well as tests that provoke subjective responses, there are a number of test methods that include objective irritation as the endpoint of concern. The dimethylsulfoxide (DMSO) test produces a whealing response and a strong burning reaction and it measures the diffusional resistance of the horny layer (18). Ninety percent or 100% DMSO is applied to the forearm for five minutes, and the skin response is then graded by a visual assessor (24). Measurements of TEWL, hydration of the superficial epidermis, blood flow, and skin thickness can also be measured and used to determine the degree of response.

The nicotinate test involves the application of methyl nicotinate to the forearm in concentrations between 1.4% and 13.7% for a period of 15 seconds. The vasodilatory effect is assessed by visual observation and laser Doppler flowmetry. This method can also be conducted using SLS (10). SLS attacks the horny layer, making it more permeable to chemicals and also causing inflammation (18). SLS is applied to the surface of the volar forearm in concentrations of 1% and 2.5% (w/v) for 24 hours. The skin is assessed three hours after removal of the SLS solutions and the individuals reacting strongly to the lower concentrations are deemed more sensitive.

The "ammonium hydroxide blistering time" is a test that measures the permeability of the stratum corneum barrier; it works on the rationale that the time taken to raise a blister is a function of the number of cell layers in the horny layer (18). A solution of ammonium hydroxide is placed on the skin inside a plastic well. The skin is carefully observed using a magnifying lens until a tense blister forms in the well. The time taken for the full blister to form is recorded and the individuals with the shorter times are regarded as being more sensitive.

Bioengineering Tools

Bioengineering tools are increasingly used to aid investigation of all aspects of dermatitis, including researching sensitive skin, and tend to be used to add further information regarding physiological changes, which can be detected at very low levels before visible signs of irritation manifest. Techniques that are most often employed include TEWL, skin conductance, skin pH, laser Doppler flowmetry, and chromametry.

Exposure of the skin to chemical irritants can damage the stratum corneum and impair its barrier function, which results in an increase of water loss from the skin, thus TEWL measurements can be used to evaluate the integrity of the stratum corneum. This measurement is often conducted alongside visual assessment when conducting skin irritation studies, as it is capable of measuring damage to the stratum corneum before visual irritation is apparent. There is also some evidence that increased skin sensitivity is related to an increased basal TEWL (18).

Another bioengineering tool that can be used to further evaluate skin irritation reactions include the corneometer, which is used to measure the hydration of the skin. The measurement is based on the difference between the dielectric constant of water (81) and other substances (<7). The measuring capacitor shows changes of capacitance according to skin moisture content. Bioengineering tools can also be used to assess blood-flow alterations using laser Doppler flowmetry, changes in skin color chromametry/colorimetry, and alterations in skin thickness using A-scan ultrasound (18).

Some relationships between different bioengineering parameters and increased skin susceptibility have been suggested. Seidenari et al. (5) showed a significant correlation between colorimetric a^* values and capacitance with increased skin susceptibility. Some studies have shown a relationship between TEWL and sensitive skin (25,26), whereas others have not found such a correlation (27). Thus, more work needs to be done in this area to determine what, if any, parameters are specifically altered in individuals with sensitive skin.

Utilizing Sensitive Skin Populations

All the tests previously discussed may be used in an attempt to identify individuals with sensitive skin, who can then be used to investigate product safety or to further investigate aspects of sensitive skin. The most prevalent methods deployed include patch testing, repeat-insult patch testing, cumulative irritancy testing, modified soap chamber test, and the forearm-controlled application technique (10).

PROBLEMS ASSOCIATED WITH IDENTIFYING A SENSITIVE SKIN PANEL

Variability in the Manifestation of Sensitive Skin

Self-perception of sensitive skin generally does not correlate well with skin sensitivity as measured by skin irritation studies, as discussed earlier, which use topical application of suitable control chemicals to determine the volunteer's level of sensitivity. Hence, questionnaires investigating self-perception of skin sensitivity only have limited value and, where possible, should be supported with suitable controlled testing procedures. Even when this is done, individuals tend to be selectively sensitive and will only react to a small number of stimuli when tested. It has been suggested that atopic individuals are often considered a particularly sensitive group; but again, within this population, there is variability in how the irritation manifests itself (28). Indeed, the varying interpretations of what is meant by the term "atopic" can often complicate matters greatly. Mucosal atopics (i.e., with IgE to common protein allergens) are probably an irrelevant group; skin atopics may be more appropriate, but where there is a likelihood that experimental treatments may precipitate an outbreak of atopic dermatitis, then ethical considerations limit the practical, day-to-day possibilities for testing on such individuals.

As there are a number of different mechanisms for skin irritation, studies monitoring skin sensitivity tend to isolate a single parameter for investigation. As such, there are studies designed to monitor visible irritation (visible signs of contact dermatitis and contact urticaria being the endpoints of concern, such as erythema and dryness), studies that monitor non-visible reactions (such as associated with mild irritation, e.g., subtle changes in skin physiology, and may be measured using bioengineering techniques), and studies that monitor the sensory aspects of irritation specifically. Each parameter has its own complexities and hence the likelihood of designing a study that investigates all parameters is likely to be very elaborate. To address sensitivity of an individual to each of these endpoints, there is a necessity to include several suitable controls into the experiment, and even doing so, large panels would need to be recruited in order to find sufficient individuals that react to a number of different stimuli, at a number of different skin sites (7).

Choice of Chemical Stimuli

For investigation of sensory perception, the sting test with 10% lactic acid has been used historically (13). However, this test looks quite specifically for stinging potential on which to screen a sensitive skin panel. However, for many product types, stinging will not be the predominant sensory comment. Itching is a very common complaint and is thought to result from sensitivity to a specific set of nociceptors (which are thought to be different from those associated with stinging) (20).

Research clearly indicates that sensitivity to lactic acid does not necessarily predict a volunteer's sensitivity to another chemosensory stimulus (7,20). Even a modified method incorporating more than one screening chemical (20) would still only focus on the aspect of sensory irritation. Without including visual assessment to record responses to topically applied materials, even a modified sting test alone may be an inadequate screen for a sensitive skin panel.

SLS is a common surfactant often used as a positive control in patch testing, but, like lactic acid for sensory irritation, use of this chemical alone does not fully address the complexities of irritant contact dermatitis. Data suggest that an individual's reactivity to SLS does not necessarily predict how that individual may react to other irritant chemicals or even to other sur-factants (7,29).

Anatomical Differences in Reactivity

It is frequently noted that visible skin reactivity varies according to the skin site, both in terms of the degree of response (30) and in terms of predicting response (e.g., sensitivity on the forearm is not predictive of sensitivity on the face) (7). This difference is also seen in terms of sensory effects (21,23). The influence of the trigeminal and vagus nerves are noticeable when testing products on the face; the face being far more sensitive in terms of sensory effects than the upper arm or back because of better innervation. Even on the face, certain areas are more receptive than others: the nasolabial fold has been shown to be more sensitive in terms of sensory effects than the chin (13,17). Indeed, the distribution of nociceptors is quite different at different skin sites (23) and this will clearly impact on the numbers of sensory comments recorded.

Other factors related to skin physiology are known to contribute to differences in skin sensitivity. Axillary irritation is a quite unique field of irritation because of the unique nature of the skin physiology of the axilla and the types of glands present (sebaceous, eccrine, apocrine, and apoeccrine glands all exist in this skin site). Consequently, irritation is often expressed by several means (sensory effects, erythema, and dryness effects, even folliculitis may manifest).

Minimizing Individual Differences

Making personal perceptions as standardized as possible is essential when conducting sensory studies. The use of descriptors (Table 1) can aid this, as can testing the individual with specific chemicals known to trigger specific sensory responses (e.g., lactic acid commonly elicits stinging, capsaicin elicits burning, menthol elicits cooling). However, there is always the element of individual differences in perception to contend with. Although primarily associated with stinging, lactic acid is also known to elicit fairly high levels of itching, whereas menthol mainly elicits a cooling sensation, but will also elicit burning in some individuals.

Factors Affecting Reproducibility of Experimental Results

It is well documented that seasonal variation changes skin reactivity. The colder winter months when humidity is lower tend to evoke stronger visible reactions, particularly to products containing surfactants such as shower gels and shampoos, and potentially increasing the number of reactions within a panel quite significantly (31). Stinging response is also known to change in a similar fashion, with more intense responses occurring through the winter months (10). When completing risk assessments of new personal-care products, the effects of seasonal variation on reactivity can be interpreted meaningfully by simply including a positive control such as 0.3% SLS (commonly used in patch testing) to gauge reactivity levels and/or a marketed control product, with a known history in the marketplace, which can be used to benchmark new products.

Age effects are thought to exist, with skin sensitivity becoming somewhat less pronounced from 30 years of age (10). The density of epidermal nerve fibers is also thought to decrease with age (32). Certain skin types are also documented as having increased sensitivity—the pale skin associated with Celtic ancestry is associated with increased stinging sensitivity (10).

There is evidence to suggest that the stage at which a woman is in her menstrual cycle may affect her skin sensitivity. Research, however, has largely been conducted in individuals with atopic dermatitis, and even in this population, information about this topic is limited. Kiriyama et al. (33) observed premenstrual worsening of skin lesions in approximately half of the 286 women interviewed. Again the parameter used for measurement can affect the type of results collected. Harvell et al. (34) also looked for effects of the menstrual cycle, but used TEWL as the primary measurement parameter and found no correlation between maximal progesterone secretion and elevated skin sensitivity.

Chronic stress is known to aggravate the symptoms and increase the skin sensitivity of patients with atopic dermatitis. Lonne-Rahm et al. (14) investigated nerve fiber density in atopics, cortisol levels (as an indicator of stress), and their effect on stinging [using the sting test (13)]. Of the 25 atopics tested (all had histories of stress worsening at the time of testing), 16 (64%) were shown to be stingers compared with only 9 (36%) shown to be "non-stingers." There was a tendency for lower salivary cortisol ratio in the stingers ($P = 0.107$), a low ratio being an indicator of chronic stress. There was also a tendency ($P = 0.066$) for an increase in the numbers of substance P fibers in the papillary dermis of stingers (substance P fibers being linked to the pain response).

Gender Differences

There is the tendency for males to comment much less frequently during clinical testing. When monitoring a three-month hair product use study, females commented on scalp irritation on 343 occasions when compared with only 79 occasions in the same number of male volunteers (35). This may well be due to differing sensory thresholds; the majority of sensory thresholds are thought to be higher in men (36) and the density of epidermal nerve fibers has been recorded as being lower in men when compared with women (32). Obviously, this can have implications when testing to identify a sensitive skin panel and particularly for tests where recording of sensory effects is the prime assessment parameter (e.g., sting test). However, a move to testing for a sensitive skin panel solely in females is generally not recommended, as it excludes a large population of consumers who may well use the personal products in the marketplace (the only time this restriction may be appropriate is when the personal products to be tested in a given sensitive skin panel are designed solely for female use). Also, such gender differences tend not to exist when considering irritant contact dermatitis or contact urticaria (4).

CONCLUSIONS

The evidence presented here demonstrates the difficulties in establishing a testing regime to identify a sensitive skin panel. There are numerous tests used, which investigate both visual and non-visual aspects of skin irritation, but little evidence to suggest a strong relationship between them. One approach to investigate skin sensitivity may be to focus on a single endpoint and to select the test most suitable to identify individuals most sensitive to a particular type of stimulus. Alternatively, multiple screening tests could be conducted on large numbers of individuals to identify a panel with more broadly sensitive skin.

However, even using this approach, it still remains to be shown whether those individuals who are identified as being more sensitive in a skin irritation test have any correlation with people who report an intolerance to normal use of a cosmetic product. In particular, for individuals who are classified as "status cosmeticus," as first defined by Fisher (37), if a sensitive skin panel is identified using any one of the previously mentioned methods, is it likely to be sufficiently representative of this population? The evidence would suggest that these tests are useful, when used appropriately, to identify a representative proportion of the general population who display a heightened irritant response to a chemical irritant(s), rather than specifically for those individuals with dermatological disease, which by its very nature is likely to identify that individual as having sensitive skin.

REFERENCES

1. Simion FA, Allen Rau AH. Sensitive skin: what it is and how to formulate for it. Cosmet Toiletries 1994; 109:43–49.
2. Willis CM, Shaw S, De Lacharriere O, Baverel M, Reiche L, Jourdain R, Bastien P, Wilkinson J. Sensitive skin: an epidemiological study. Br J Dermatol 2001; 145:258–263.
3. Basketter DA, Griffiths HA. A study of the relationship between susceptibility to skin stinging and skin irritation. Contact Dermat 1993; 29:185–188.
4. Lammintausta K, Maibach HI, Wilson D. Mechanisms of subjective (sensory) irritation: propensity to non-immunologic contact urticaria and objective irritation in stingers. Dermatosen in Berut und umwelt 1988; 36:45–49.
5. Seidenari S, Francomano M, Mantovani L. Baseline biophysical parameters in subjects with sensitive skin. Contact Dermat 1998; 38(6):311–315.
6. Loffler H, Dickel H, Kuss O, Diepgen TL, Effendy I. Characteristics of self-estimated enhanced skin susceptibility. Acta Derm Venereol 2001; 81:343–346.
7. Marriott M, Holmes J, Peters L, Cooper K, Rowson M, Basketter DA. The complex problem of sensitive skin. Contact Dermatitis 2005; 53:93–99.
8. Coverly J, Peters L, Whittle E, Basketter DA. Susceptibility to skin stinging, non-immunologic contact urticaria and skin irritation—is there a relationship? Contact Dermat 1998; 38:90–95.

9. Leyden JJ. Biology behind sensitive skin. Skin and Aging 2002; 10:64–66.
10. Draelos ZD. Sensitive skin: perception, evaluation and treatment. Am J Contact Dermat 1997; 8:67–78.
11. Jenkins HL, Adams MG. Progressive evaluation of skin irritancy of cosmetics using human volunteers. Int J Cosmet Sci 1989; 11:141–149.
12. Basketter DA, Whittle E, Griffiths HA, York M. The identification and classification of skin irritation hazard by a human patch test. Food Chem Toxicol 1994; 32(8): 769–775.
13. Frosch P, Kligman AM. Method for appraising the sting capacity of topically applied substances. J Soc Cosmet Chemists 1977; 28:197–209.
14. Lonne-Rahm S, Berg M, Marin P, Nordlind K. Atopic dermatitis, stinging and effects of chronic stress: a pathocausal study. J Am Acad Dermatol 2004; 51(6):899–905.
15. Schafer L, Kragbelle K. Abnormalities in epidermal lipid metabolism in patients with atopic dermatitis. J Invest Dermatol 1991; 96(1):10–15.
16. Christensen M, Kligman AM. An improved procedure for conducting lactic acid stinging tests on facial skin. J Soc Cosmet Chemists 1996; 47:1–11.
17. Marriott M, Whittle E, Basketter DA. Facial variations in sensory responses. Contact Dermat 2003; 49(5):227–231.
18. Chew A, Maibach HI. Sensitive skin. In: Loden M, Maibach HI, eds. Dry Skin and Moisturizers—Chemistry and Function. New York: CRC Press, 2000:429–440.
19. Soschin D, Kligman AM. Adverse subjective responses. In: Kligman AM, Leyden JJ, eds. Safety and Efficacy of Topical Drugs and Cosmetics. New York: Grune and Stratton 1982:377–388.
20. Green BG, Bluth J. Measuring the chemosensory irritability of human skin. J Toxicol Cutans Ocul Toxicol 1995; 14:23–48.
21. Green BG. Regional and individual differences in cutaneous sensitivity to chemical irritants: capsaicin and menthol. J Toxicol Cutan Ocul Toxicol 1996; 15(3):277–295.
22. McMahon SB, Koltzenberg M. Itching for an explanation. Trends Neurosci 1992; 15:497–501.
23. Green BG. Measurement of sensory irritation. Am J Contact Dermat 2000; 11:170–180.
24. Agner T, Serup J. Quantification of the DMSO-response—a test for assessment of sensitive skin. Clin Exp Dermatol 1989; 14:214–217.
25. Muruhata R, Crove D, Roheim J. The use of transepidermal water loss to measure and predict the irritation response to surfactants. Int Cosmet Sci 1986; 8: 225–231.
26. Tupker R, Coenraads P, Pinnagoda J, Nater J. Baseline transepidermal water loss (TEWL) as a prediction of susceptibility to sodium lauryl sulphate. Contact Dermat 1989; 20: 265–269.
27. Paye M, Dalimier Ch, Cartiaux Y, Chabassol C. Consumer perception of sensitive hands: what is behind it? Skin Res Technol 1996; 5:28–32.
28. Basketter DA, Miettinen J, Lahti A. Acute irritant reactivity to sodium lauryl sulphate in atopics and non-atopics. Contact Dermat 1998; 38:253–257.
29. Effendy I, Maibach HI. Surfactants and experimental contact dermatitis. Contact Dermat 1995: 33:217–225.
30. Clarys P, Bareol AO. Comparison of 3 detergents using the patch test and hand/forearm immersion test as measurements of irritancy. J Soc Cosmet Chem 1997; 48:141–149.

31. Basketter D, Griffiths H, Wang X, Wilhelm K-P, McFadden J. Individual ethnic and seasonable variability in irritant susceptibility of skin: the implications for a predictive human patch test. Contact Dermat 1996; 35:208–213.
32. Goransson LG, Mellgren SI, Lindal S, Omdal R. The effect of age and gender on epidermal nerve fiber density. Neurology 2004; 62(5):774.
33. Kiriyama K, Sugiura H, Uehara M. Premenstrual deterioration of skin symptoms in female patients with atopic dermatitis. Dermatology 2003; 206(2):110.
34. Harvell J, Hussonsaeed I, Maibach H. Changes in transepidermal water-loss and cutaneous blood-flow during the menstrual-cycle. Contact Dermat 1992; 27(5):294.
35. Peters L, Whittle E, Rowson M, Marriott M, Basketter D. Scalp dermatitis—what is the background noise? Contact Dermat 2002; 46(suppl 4).
36. Torgen M, Swerup C. Individual factors and physical work load in relation to sensory thresholds in a middle-aged general population sample. Eur J Appl Physiol 2002; 86(5):418.
37. Fisher A. Cosmetic actions and reactions: therapeutic, irritant and allergic. Cutis 1980; 26:22–29.

10

Sensitive Skin Symptoms as Risk Indicators for Hand Eczema

Päivikki Susitaival

*Department of Dermatology, North Karelia Central Hospital,
Joensuu, Finland*

According to epidemiological studies, previous or present widespread atopic dermatitis (AD), previous hand eczema (HE), history of sensitive skin, low-irritant threshold, (history of) metal allergy, history of (job-specific) allergy, and female sex have been connected with increased risk for HE (1–8).

The concept of sensitive skin is complex and by no means clear. In biophysiology, it is considered as a barrier dysfunction causing hyperreactivity to irritants and altered sensory functions. Many more-or-less sophisticated methods exist for the clinical assessment of biophysiological skin parameters such as transepidermal water loss, capacitance, etc. Signs and symptoms of "sensitive skin" include erythema, dryness, flushing, itching, burning, and stinging. Possible host factors in skin irritation include defective barrier function (e.g., atopic skin or subclinical/postdermatitis stage), skin site, sweating, sex, age, race, and menstrual cycle. External factors include manmade chemicals, soaps, cosmetics, dust, earth, friction, plants, foods, water, protective gloves (occlusion), climatic factors (wind, cold, hot, and dry), and fabrics (e.g., wool and acrylics).

Self-assessment of skin sensitivity by reporting signs of sensitive skin is used both in questionnaire studies and in patient interviews. Reporting sensitive skin has had little or no correlation with experimental skin irritation (9,10). Questionnaire results and clinical studies with irritants indicate that skin sensitivity to different stimuli varies greatly between individuals and also within an individual (11,12). Skin stinging and skin irritation do not seem to correlate with each other (13).

Skin sensitivity has mostly been studied from the viewpoint of adverse reactions from cosmetics on facial skin. In a questionnaire survey among 2000 Britons, 51% of women and 38% of men reported a sensitive facial skin (9). Very sensitive skin was reported by considerably less people (10% of women and 6% of men). Atopics constituted only half of those with sensitive skin, and one-third of atopics did not consider their skin sensitive at all (9).

In studies on racial variations of skin sensitivity, the reporting of sensitive skin was similar, but the sensitivity to different irritating stimuli differed by race (10,12). Males were more reactive to irritants in patch tests than females and younger subjects reacted more than older (10).

Nickel allergy or symptoms of metal allergy have been found to associate with HE among women in epidemiological studies, but this association has been diminishing in Denmark where nickel in clothing and jewelry is now controlled (4,7,14,15). In different studies, 30% to 65% of those with symptoms of metal allergy have had a positive patch test to nickel (16,17).

The history of atopic eczema has been shown to at least double the risk of HE in many occupational populations (2,5,6,18). Dry skin type or the so-called atopic skin diathesis has been connected with HE risk in several studies, and it has been estimated that a fifth of occupational HE cases may be ascribed to dry skin diathesis (19–21). Controversial results concerning both these HE risk factors have also been published (20,22).

The criteria for atopic skin diathesis include, among other things, parameters such as intolerance to wool, intolerance to metal, and itch when sweating. Four questions as surrogates for detecting "sensitive skin" have been included in a standard questionnaire used in HE surveys in Finland (23, Tuohilampi questionnaire). The questions are (*i*) Do you suffer from dry skin? (*ii*) Does your skin tend to itch when you sweat? (*iii*) Do you get a rash from jeans buttons, metal fasteners, metal costume jewelry (e.g., earrings), or other metal parts of clothes next to your skin (excluding under the ring)? and (*iv*) Do you feel itchy if you wear wool next to your skin?

Table 1 presents the frequency of positive answers to the earlier questions in four different Finnish working age populations (one female, one mixed, and two male populations). Generally, dry skin was reported by more than half of the women and more than a third of the men. About one-fourth of people reported itching when sweating, which was somewhat more than those reporting the history of AD. Every other person seems to get an itch from wool next to skin. Women have a much higher prevalence of nickel allergy and thus report more "rash from metal."

Figures 1 to 4 present the prevalence of reported HE in the studied populations by atopy (no history of atopy, only respiratory atopy, and skin atopy— "Have you ever had flexural or childhood dermatitis or the so-called AD?")

Table 1 Affirmative Answers to Four Questions for Detecting Sensitive Skin by Dental Nurses (DN, females), Papermill Workers (PW, 70% male), Forest Workers (FW, males), and Metal Workers (MW, males), %

	DN	PW	FW	MW
Dry skin?	64	40	32	41
Itch when sweating?	26	28	21	22
Rash from metal onto skin?	38	17	5	5
Itch from wool onto skin?	48	51	46	na
History of atopic dermatitis[a]?	24	23	20	21

[a]Have you ever had flexural or childhood dermatitis or the so-called atopic dermatitis?
Source: From Refs. 24, 25, 27, 28.

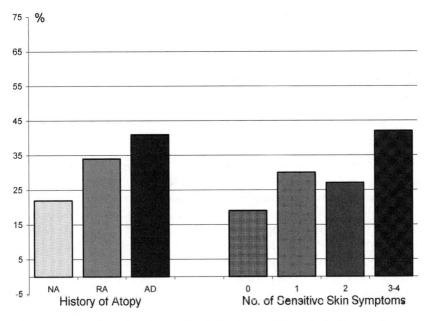

Figure 1 Reporting of hand dermatitis during the past 12 months by history of atopy and the number of reported sensitive skin symptoms (dry skin, itch when sweating, itch from wool next to skin, and symptoms of metal allergy) in 799 dental nurses (all women), %. *Abbreviations*: NA, no history of atopy; RA, only hay fever or asthma; AD, atopic dermatitis—Have you ever had flexural or childhood dermatitis or the so-called AD? *Source*: From Ref. 27.

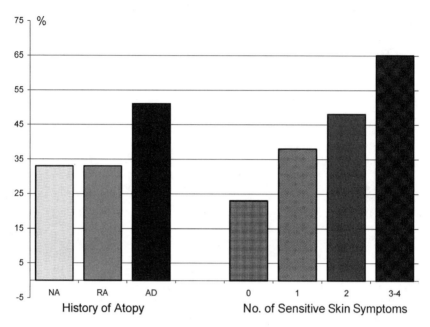

Figure 2 Reporting of hand dermatitis during the past 12 months by history of atopy and the number of reported sensitive skin symptoms (dry skin, itch when sweating, itch from wool next to skin, and symptoms of metal allergy) in 224 papermill workers (70% men), %. *Abbreviations*: NA, no history of atopy; RA, only hay fever or asthma; AD, atopic dermatitis—Have you ever had flexural or childhood dermatitis or the so-called AD? *Source*: From Ref. 25.

and by the number of reported sensitive skin symptoms (from 0 to 3–4). Each sensitive skin symptom seems to increase the HE risk in an additive fashion. The information on sensitive skin symptoms seems to detect more HE risk categories than atopy. Also in logistic modeling, the sensitive skin symptoms have turned out to be a stronger risk for HE than the history of AD (24,25). "Itch when sweating" ($P = 0.001$ to <0.0001) and "rash from metal" ($P = 0.001$–0.0001) correlated best with HE in the studied populations, whereas the weakest correlations were for "itch when wearing wool next to skin."

The correlation of reporting HE to sensitive skin parameters was better among male than among female populations. Women tended to report dry skin more often than men. This can be the result of women being more open to skin-care product marketing. The issue of "dry skin" might also have a cultural component—it is "in" to have sensitive skin. It is possible that men pay less attention to skin dryness and only report it when it is marked.

When looking at how well these questions picked those who also reported the history of AD, the highest sensitivity (0.82–0.44) was for the question on "dry skin" followed by "itch when wearing wool" (0.79–0.32). Highest

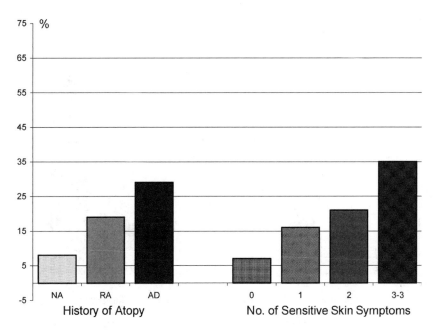

Figure 3 Reporting of hand dermatitis during the past 12 months by history of atopy and the number of reported sensitive skin symptoms (dry skin, itch when sweating, and symptoms of metal allergy) in 646 forest workers (all men), %. *Abbreviations*: NA, no history of atopy; RA, only hay fever or asthma; AD, atopic dermatitis—Have you ever had flexural or childhood dermatitis or the so-called AD? *Source*: From Ref. 24.

specificity, respectively, was for the question on "itch when sweating" (0.78–0.80). In a Japanese study, 84% of atopics have been found to react to their own sweat in the intradermal test, whereas only 11% of the non-atopics reacted (26).

CONCLUSIONS

The four questions on sensitive skin symptoms can be a useful and simple tool in estimating the risk of HE in individuals or groups. History of metal dermatitis (nickel allergy), wool intolerance, itch when sweating, and generally dry skin are markers of sensitive skin and correlate with HE. They are also included in the list of symptoms and signs defining the atopic skin diathesis. It seems that the answers to these questions alone can give a fairly good estimate of the HE risk of the individual. They can be used in epidemiological studies or in practice (e.g., for vocational guidance and job placement) as risk indicators. The combined questions seem to work better as an indicator of HE risk than the history of AD. They deal with present skin symptoms, thus eliminating the memory bias which can affect the information on AD history.

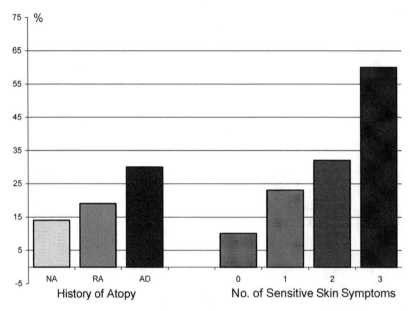

Figure 4 Reporting of hand dermatitis during the past 12 months by history of atopy and the number of reported sensitive skin symptoms (dry skin, itch when sweating, and symptoms of metal allergy) in 810 metal workers (all men), %. *Abbreviations*: NA, no history of atopy; RA, only hay fever or asthma; AD, atopic dermatitis—Have you ever had flexural or childhood dermatitis or the so-called AD? *Source*: From Ref. 28.

REFERENCES

1. Rystedt I. Factors influencing the occurrence of hand eczema in adults with a history of atopic dermatitis in childhood. Contact Dermatitis 1985; 12(4):185–191.
2. Nilsson E, Mikaelsson B, Andersson S. Atopy, occupation and domestic work as risk factors for hand eczema in hospital workers. Contact Dermatitis 1985; 13:216–223.
3. Meding B, Swanbeck G. Epidemiology of different types of hand eczema in an industrial city. Acta Derm Venereol 1989; 69(3):227–233.
4. Nilsson EJ, Knutsson A. Atopic dermatitis, nickel sensitivity and xerosis as risk factors for hand eczema in women. Contact Dermatitis 1995; 33(6):401–406.
5. Susitaival P, Husman L, Horsmanheimo M, Notkola V, Husman K. Prevalence of hand dermatoses among Finnish farmers. Scand J Work Environ Health 1994; 20:206–212.
6. Susitaival P, Kirk J, Schenker MB. Self-reported hand dermatitis in California veterinarians. Am J Contact Dermat 2001; 12:103–108.
7. Meding B, Liden C, Berglind N. Self-diagnosed dermatitis in adults: results from a population survey in Stockholm. Contact Dermatitis 2001; 45(6):341–345.
8. Bryld LE, Hindsberger C, Kyvik KO, Agner T, Menne T. Risk factors influencing the development of hand eczema in a population-based twin sample. Br J Dermatol 2003; 149(6):1214–1220.

9. Willis CM, Shaw S, De Lacharriere O, Baverel M, Reiche L, Jourdain R, Bastien P, Wilkinson JD. Sensitive skin: an epidemiological study. Br J Dermatol 2001; 145(2):258–263.
10. Robinson MK. Population differences in acute skin irritation responses: race, sex, age, sensitive skin and repeat subject comparisons. Contact Dermatitis 2002; 46(2):86–93.
11. Robinson MK. Intra-individual variations in acute and cumulative skin irritation responses. Contact Dermatitis 2001; 45(3):75–83.
12. Jourdain R, Lacharriere O, Bastien P, Maibach HI. Ethnic variations in self-perceived sensitive skin: epidemiological survey. Contact Dermatitis 2002; 46(3):162–169.
13. Basketter DA, Griffiths HA. A study of the relationship between skin stinging and skin irritation. Contact Dermatitis 1993; 29(4):185–188.
14. Mortz CG, Lauritsen JM, Bindslev-Jensen C, Andersen KE. Nickel sensitization in adolescents and association with ear piercing, use of dental braces and hand eczema. The Odense Adolescence Cohort Study on Atopic Diseases and Dermatitis (TOACS). Acta Derm Venereol 2002; 82(5):359–364.
15. Nielsen NH, Linneberg A, Menné T, Madsen F, Frølund L, Dirksen A, Jørgensen T. The association between contact allergy and hand eczema in 2 cross-sectional surveys 8 years apart (the Copenhagen Allergy Study). Contact Dermatitis 2002; 46:71–77.
16. Dotterud LK, Falk ES. Metal allergy in north Norwegian schoolchildren and its relationship with ear piercing and atopy. Contact Dermatitis 1994; 31(5):308–313.
17. Bohm I, Brody M, Bauer R. Comparison of personal history with patch test results in metal allergy. J Dermatol 1997; 24(8):510–513.
18. Coenraads PJ, Diepgen TL. Risk of hand eczema in employees with past or present atopic dermatitis. Int Arch Occup Environ Health 1998; 71(1):7–13.
19. Lammintausta K, Kalimo K. Atopy and hand dermatitis in hospital wet work. Contact Dermatitis 1981; 7(6):301–308.
20. Majoie IM, von Blomberg BM, Bruynzeel DP. Development of hand eczema in junior hairdressers: an 8-year follow-up study. Contact Dermatitis 1996; 34(4):243–247.
21. Dickel H, Briuckner TM, Schmidt A, Diepgen TL. Impact of atopic skin diathesis on occupational skin disease incidence in a working population. J Invest Dermatol 2003; 121(1):37–40.
22. Berndt U, Hinnen U, Iliev D, Elsner P. Role of atopy score and of single atopic features as risk factors for the development of hand eczema in trainee metal workers. Br J Dermatol 1999; 140:922–924.
23. Susitaival P, Kanerva L, Hannuksela M, Jolanki R, Estlander T. Tuohilampi questionnaire for epidemiological studies of contact dermatitis and atopy. People and Work. Research Report 10. Helsinki: Finnish Institute of Occupational Health, 1996.
24. Kallunki H, Kangas J, Laitinen S, Mäkinen M, Ojanen K, Susitaival P. Exposure to and health effects of chemical and biological agents in mechanical wood harvesting (in Finnish). Kuopio: Finnish Institute of Occupational Health, 2002.
25. Susitaival P, Jolanki R, Eskelinen A, Jäppinen P, Estlander T, Talka E, Kanerva L. Skin diseases and allergy risks associated with the production and use of paper, questionnaire study *in Finnish*. Työja Ihminen 2002; 16(4):348–358.
26. Hide M, Tanaka T, Yamamura Y, Koro O, Yamamoto S. IgE-mediated hypersensitivity against human sweat antigen in patients with atopic dermatitis. Acta Derm Venereol 2002; 82:335.

27. Susitaival P, Alanko K, Jolanki R, Kanerva L. Epidemiological study of dermatitis on hands and face in Finnish dental nurses. In: Alanko K, ed. Allergy Risks in Dental Practice (in Finnish). Helsinki: Finnish Institute of Occupational Health, 2000:41–45.
28. Suuronen K, Tuomi T, Alanko K, et al. Unpublished data. Work-related skin and respiratory diseases in metal workers (in Finnish) Report. Finnish Institute of Occupational Health 2005.

11

Objectifying Primary and Acquired Sensitive Skin

Swen Malte John

*Department of Dermatology, Environmental Medicine, Health Theory,
University of Osnabrueck, Osnabrueck, Germany*

PRIMARY AND SECONDARY SENSITIVE SKIN

Skin susceptibility to irritants varies interindividually. It is beyond dispute that individuals with highly sensitive skin do exist (1,2). On the other end of the clinical phenomena, in the spectrum of skin sensitivity, there are individuals with a remarkable cutaneous tolerance to damaging insults (Fig. 1) (1). Using a test battery of various irritants, Frosch (3) identified patterns of individual skin susceptibility; in a group of 44 healthy volunteers, 25% were deemed "hypo-irritable," 61% were "normal," and 14% were "hyperirritable." Tolerance may be pre-existing ("primary"); however, it may also develop—secondarily—in an adaptive response to chronic irritation. Such an adaptive response ("hardening") has been observed in many occupations (4–6). Little is known about this compensatory phenomenon, except that it does not seem to appear in atopics and that it may be irritant specific (2,7).

According to the previously cited experiment of Frosch (3), it is to be assumed that most individuals in a population show a normal skin sensitivity; the extremes occur less likely. However, there seem to be remarkable similarities between hypo-irritability and hyperirritability. Similar to tolerance, hyperirritability may be primary, but it may also develop secondarily in the realm of an acute, ongoing dermatitis (2,7) or even remain after a former dermatitis (8,9). In occupational dermatology, some patients with former, healed dermatitis

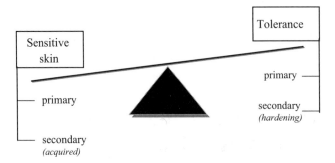

Figure 1 Clinical spectrum of skin sensitivity. It has to be assumed that most individuals in the general population show a normal sensitivity; the extremes occur less likely.

complain of experiencing ongoing increased skin sensitivity. However, in these cases, the clinician cannot detect any skin impairment frequently. This chapter will deal with attempts to assess primary and secondary/acquired sensitive skin and will focus on one particular approach to clinically objectify these phenomena by routine skin irritancy tests, using NaOH, with which we gathered some experience in the recent years. Obviously, these questions are especially salient with regard to work-related dermatoses and it is for these reasons that we have collected data in an occupational setting.

SODIUM HYDROXIDE FOR SKIN SENSITIVITY TESTING

Burckhardt's (10) "alkali resistance test" is the archetype of chemical skin irritation tests. It was introduced in 1947, using 0.5 m sodium hydroxide up to 8×10 minutes under occlusion. The test procedure has been modified in the following years by Burckhardt and co-workers (11–13). They claimed that the test was able to assess the integrity of the epidermal barrier and they recommended it as a screening tool for chemically phenotyping the individual. There were some reports claiming that the technique was useful for pre- or re-employment testing in high-risk professions (14,15). However, the concept was controversial from the start, findings were inconsistent, and the technique fell into oblivion in most countries (2,16–18).

To date, in Germany, in occupational dermatology, alkali resistance tests performed in numerous variations still play an important role for medico-legal evaluations. However, the use of these tests for such purposes in routine diagnostics is controversial (19).

Unlike the popular "model irritant" sodium lauryl sulfate (SLS), for which the standardization process is far advanced (20,21), no such efforts have yet been undertaken concerning NaOH. An interesting aspect, why NaOH may be a candidate for patch testing for skin sensitivity in occupational dermatology, is that the major cause of occupational dermatoses—"wet work"—invariably means to alkalinize the skin. This occupational hazard may be mimicked by the test. The vital importance of a physiological, acidic pH for barrier homeostasis was recently shown (22).

PRIMARY SKIN SENSITIVITY ASSESSED WITH SODIUM HYDROXIDE: SWIFT MODIFIED ALKALI RESISTANCE TEST

Methods

Subjects

A total of 1271 patients from various high-risk professions with a history of previous occupational eczema were seen for medico-legal evaluations in the time period of January 1993 to April 1999 in the Dermatology Department of Osnabrueck University. Of these, 572 patients fulfilled the criteria mentioned subsequently and were accepted for the study (Fig. 2). History-taking and detailed dermatological examination of the complete integument were performed by physicians in specialist's training programs for occupational dermatology or dermatologists. For the most part, there were abundant prior medical records available and assessments from the (former) workplace. Additionally, in most of these patients, epicutaneous patch testing was performed along with prick tests and serologic investigations (e.g., IgE and sIgE) for assessing inhalative atopy.

Irritant Patch Testing

Irritant patch testing was conducted after informed consent was obtained. The study was approved by the Ethical Committee of the University of Osnabrueck.

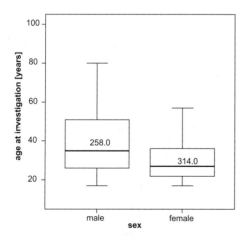

Figure 2 Age and sex distribution of cohort ($n = 572$). Boxplots: bold black lines represent medians and thin squares represent 25% and 75% percentiles.

Measurements were performed only in clinically healthy skin. Skin lesions had to have healed at least three weeks before the investigation. Participants were requested not to use soap or creams/emollients in the areas of investigation 24 hours prior to each examination.

NaOH patch test: Sodium hydroxide (33 μL, 0.5 M) was pipetted to the test site (mid-volar forearm) and covered by a $2.5 \times 3 \times 1.0$ cm^3 glass block, according to Locher (23). The glass block was fixed with non-occlusive tape under slight pressure to assure uniform spreading of the solution. In an adjacent area, 0.9% NaCl (33 μL) served as a control and was covered by a glass block in the same fashion. After 10 minutes, the solution was gently wiped off with a swab. Clinical and biophysical readings were done in the test and control areas, 10 minutes after the end of the provocation phase. Then a second, identical 10-minute provocation phase with consecutive clinical and biophysical assessments after another 10 minutes was conducted. Again, clinical and biophysical readings were done after 24 hours.

Clinical skin changes in the test areas were recorded using a 5-grade ordinal scale: 1, nihil; 2, soap effect; 3, minimal erythema and/or minimal vesiculation and/or maximally one erosion; 4, marked erythema and/or marked edema and/or marked vesiculation and/or two or more erosions; 5, very marked erythema/vesiculation/edema and/or five or more erosions or necrosis.

The test was stopped immediately if after the first provocation phase there were marked clinical skin changes [grade 4 ($n = 51$) or grade 5 ($n = 0$)] or subjective discomfort ($n = 0$).

Skin bioengineering: In a previous pilot study with 92 similar patients, we showed that two 10-minute provocation periods with 0.5 M NaOH provided significant information on individual skin sensitivity (19). Briefly, evaporimetric measurements of skin surface water loss/transepidermal water loss (SSWL/ TEWL) were performed 2 to 10 minutes after the end of NaOH-provocation at two-minute intervals. TEWL allows an estimation of water evaporation through the stratum corneum, providing information on epidermal barrier function (24,25). If evaporimetric measurements are performed immediately after aqueous solutions have been applied to the skin, initially, the SSWL equals excess water loss from skin surface hydration plus TEWL (26). Our experiments revealed that a 10-minute interval, after the end of each of the NaOH-provocation phases, was a suitable time period for clinical and biophysical patch test readings. At this time, excess water loss from skin surface hydration was already minimal so that roughly only TEWL has been estimated.

In the present study, therefore, TEWL as well as relative skin moisture (RSM) was routinely assessed. TEWL was measured using the ServoMed evaporimeter EP1^{TM} (ServoMed, Stockholm, Sweden) in a Perspex incubator, applying the ServoMed gold-plated protection cover (steel grid) and a rubber stopper as an insulating probe holder according to the European Society of Contact Dermatitis guidelines (24). RSM was estimated by capacitance using the corneometer$^®$

C 820 (Courage & Khazaka, Cologne, Germany). Measurements were conducted in triplicate; the median was then taken as the RSM value.

The investigations took place in an air-conditioned laboratory at steady-state conditions (ambient temperature 20–21°C, relative humidity 40–45%). Acclimatization of participants was at least 15 minutes, usually 30 minutes. Measurements were conducted after acclimatization in the prospective test and control areas (ex-ante readings), and then 10 minutes after each provocation phase and finally after another 24 hours.

Relevant Variables

Clinical diagnoses/atopy: Diagnosis of clinical atopy usually had to be made retrospectively, because skin lesions were either healed on investigation or reduced to minor residuals. If florid skin changes were detected on first clinical examination, subjects were asked to return after healing for patch testing. If in the medical records, previous atopic dermatitis ($n = 92$), palmar (plantar) eczema (19) in its various manifestations ($n = 93$), or previous flexural eczema ($n = 208$) were documented, the respective subjects were grouped as "atopic skin disposition" ($n = 248$; note should be made that there were frequent combinations of these skin manifestations). The other main groups of diagnoses were pure "irritant contact dermatitis" (without atopic skin manifestations in the history, $n = 138$) or pure "allergic contact dermatitis" ($n = 130$).

Bioengineering parameters: Δ-TEWL and Δ-RSM, respectively, were calculated in regard to the ex-ante values and the values in the NaCl controls, using the following mathematical term: $\Delta\text{-TEWL}_{\text{NaOH, 10 or 20 min}} = (\text{TEWL}_{\text{NaOH, 10 or 20 min}} - \text{TEWL}_{\text{NaOH, 0 min}}) - |\text{TEWL}_{\text{NaCl, 10 or 20 min}} - \text{TEWL}_{\text{NaCl, 0 min}}|$.

For the second difference ($|\text{TEWL}_{\text{NaCl, 10 or 20 min}} - \text{TEWL}_{\text{NaCl, 0 min}}|$), only the total positive amount was used; this is of relevance, when the second difference is negative. In these $n = 176$ cases ($\text{TEWL}_{\text{NaCl, 10 min}}$) and $n = 102$ cases ($\text{TEWL}_{\text{NaCl, 20 min}}$), respectively, the ex-ante value in the control area was slightly higher than after 10 or 20 minutes of NaCl application. Δ-TEWL and Δ-RSM will be negative, if the difference of values in the NaOH-areas ($\text{TEWL}_{\text{NaOH, 10 min}} - \text{TEWL}_{\text{NaOH, 0 min}}$) is smaller than the respective difference in the control areas. This was only rarely the case in robust skin without skin changes, due to the variance of measurements ($\Delta\text{-TEWL}_{\text{NaOH, 10 min}}$: $n = 37$; $\Delta\text{-TEWL}_{\text{NaOH, 20 min}}$: $n = 46$).

Statistical analyses: Besides descriptive statistical analysis, data evaluation focused on the estimation of a predictive (critical) value of the investigated biophysical parameters; for this purpose, receiver operating characteristic (ROC) curves were developed (27,28). For ROC curves and other investigations, the clinical score (five-point ordinal scale) was dichotomized (clinical grades 1 and 2 vs. grades 3–5). Differences in TEWL and RSM between NaOH and controls were tested using bivariate two-tailed non-parametric tests

(Mann–Whitney-U test or Kruskal–Wallis test). In cross-tabulations, the chi-square statistics or the McNemar test (linked samples), respectively, were used to analyze the differences between the observed and the expected values. By Cohen's κ-index (29), the degree of agreement of clinical and biophysical parameters and reproducibility were calculated. Correlations between the various clinical, demographical, and biophysical parameters were analyzed using the two-tailed Spearman rank correlation test. The size of estimated effects was judged by the classification of Cohen (30).

An error probability of $<5\%$ was considered statistically significant. For statistical analyses, the statistical software package SPSS^{TM} (version 9.0 D^{TM}, SPSS, Inc., Munich, Germany) was employed.

Results

Cohort

A total of 314 females (median age 27) and 258 males (median age 35) took part (Table 2) in the study. The most frequent profession was "hairdresser" (23%), followed by various "professions in the health sector" (17%), mainly nursing. This explains why the median female age is lower. Male-dominated jobs followed in the third and fourth positions: "metal worker" (7%) and "brick layer" (6%). In 85% of patients, the skin disease was considered to have been induced by the job; overall, the most relevant single factor for the elicitation of the dermatoses had been wet work.

Diagnoses

On investigation, skin lesions were either healed or reduced to minor residuals. Thus, diagnosis had to be made in retrospect. The most frequent primary diagnosis was allergic contact dermatitis ($n = 165$; 28.9%), followed by irritant dermatitis ($n = 158$; 27.6%), and various atopic skin manifestations [e.g., atopic dermatitis; atopic palmar (plantar) eczema]. Owing to the frequent overlap in the pathogenesis of occupational skin diseases in 205 cases, more than one diagnosis was made; most frequently atopic manifestations were diagnosed together with allergic or irritant contact dermatitis. If all the cases in which atopic skin manifestations were diagnosed alone or in combination are taken together, 248 patients (43.4%) were rendered atopics ("atopic skin disposition"). A total of 153 (26.7%) had a history of inhalative atopy (rhinitis or asthma) and this was mostly associated with a history of some kind of atopic skin manifestations.

Pure "irritant contact dermatitis"—without atopic skin manifestations in the history—was $n = 138$ and pure "allergic contact dermatitis" was $n = 130$.

Irritant Patch Testing

During the test period and within a follow-up of at least 24 hours, patients felt no relevant discomfort or pain by the test. Clinical grade 5 ("very marked erythema/vesiculation/edema and/or five or more erosions or necrosis") was never observed. If reactions were positive after 20 minutes, then after 24 hours, some-times, minimal erythema or solitary, small superficial erosions were detected, but no necrosis, scarring, infection, or discoloration. Healing was uneventful in 43.6% of test-positive individuals; skin reactions were completely reversed after 24 hours. Thus, as expected, agreement between 2 × 10-minute- and 24-hour-observation, concerning identifiable skin changes was poor (Cohen's $\kappa = 0.38$). Therefore, test reading after the second 10-minute NaOH provocation phase was considered relevant for clinical outcome. If the result of visual scoring is examined, a good correlation between the degree of clinical reactivity and Δ-TEWL could be demonstrated. Correlation was best after 20-minute NaOH-challenge [$r_s = 0.587$; $P < 0.01$ (Spearman rank correlation)]. Correlation was poor at all measuring intervals for Δ-RSM (20 minutes: $r_s = 0.106$). No signifi-cant correlations could be detected between age or sex and clinical or biophysical findings, or any job-specific effects.

A relevant question was whether biophysical parameters can predict the clinical outcome. In order to answer this question, an ROC analysis was conducted. For the parameter Δ-TEWL after 2 × 10 minute-NaOH, the ROC curve is shown in Figure 3. As a cut point, a Δ-TEWL of $2 \, g/m^2 \, h$ was determined; for this cut point ("critical value"), TEWL has a sensitivity of 76.7% and a specificity of 74.7% ($C = 0.83$), for prediction of the target variable (clinical outcome after 2 × 10-minute NaOH). ROC analysis for Δ-TEWL after 10-minute NaOH for the target variable was not significant ($C = 0.67$). Also for Δ-RSM, at all measuring intervals, there was no relevant ability to significantly discriminate between positive and negative clinical test results.

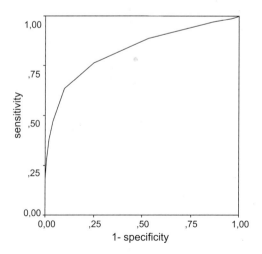

Figure 3 ROC curve for Δ-TEWL after 2 × 10-minute NaOH and clinical outcome after 20 minutes ($n = 572$). X-axis: inverse specificity (equals false-positive classifications). *Abbreviation*: ROC, receiver operating characteristic.

Reproducibility

A total of 14 patients were examined twice in the recruitment phase; the median of the interval between the two separate investigations was two years (range, 1–3 years). In the NaOH-challenge, there were similar clinical findings after 2 × 10-minute NaOH ($\kappa = 0.66$). However, agreement of TEWL values was below significance level [$\kappa = 0.43$; Δ-TEWL dichotomized at cut point (2 g/m^2 h)].

Atopy

If the degree of clinical reactivity after NaOH challenge was analyzed in respect to the presence of "atopic skin disposition," there was a significant negative association with the clinically unresponsive grades "nihil" and "soap effect," and a corresponding positive association with marked clinical reactivity ($\chi_3^2 = 12.17$; $P = 0.007$). This phenomenon is further elucidated by the post hoc comparison of the adjusted, standardized residuals (Table 1).

There was no such association with the other main clinical diagnoses "irritant dermatitis" and "allergic contact dermatitis" (Fig. 4A). Cross-tabulation showed again that distribution was unequal ($\chi_2^2 = 9.65$; $P < 0.01$). By post hoc comparison of the adjusted, standardized residuals, it was obvious that this was only due to the parameter "atopic skin disposition."

There also was a significant positive association of "atopic skin disposition" and the variable Δ-TEWL at all measuring intervals [10-minute NaOH: $z = -2.69$, $P < 0.01$; 20-minute NaOH $z = -3.17$, $P < 0.01$; 24 hours $z = -2.2$, $P = 0.02$ (Mann–Whitney U-test)]. When the association with the other main clinical diagnoses was evaluated, again there were differences detectable for this variable; however, this was significant only after 20-minute NaOH (Fig. 4B): $\chi_2^2 = 10.36$, $P = 0.006$ (Kruskal–Wallis test); in separate

Table 1 Association Between the Clinical Response After 2 × 10-minute NaOH and the Parameter "Atopic Skin Disposition"

			Atopic skin disposition		
			No	Yes	Total
Clinic 20-minute	Nihil/Soap effect	Count	181	104	285
NaOH		Corrected residuals	3.3	−3.3	
	Mild erythema/…	Count	65	58	123
		Corrected residuals	−1.0	1.0	
	Mark eryth./	Count	78	86	164
	edema/vesic.	Corrected residuals	−2.8	2.8	
Total		Count	324	248	572

Note: Clinically unresponsive grades 1 and 2 ("nihil," "soap effect") are included.

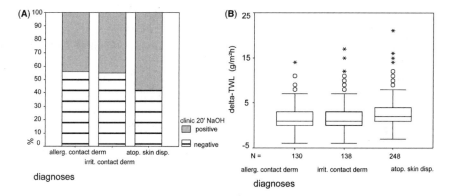

Figure 4 Clinical (**A**) and biophysical (**B**) responses in respect to the three main clinical diagnoses ($n = 516$). (**A**) Percent of positive clinical reactions after 2×10-minute NaOH. (**B**) Boxplot of Δ-TEWL after 2×10-minute NaOH. (○) extremes; (*) outlyers. *Abbreviations*: Δ-TEWL, transepidermal water loss.

Mann–Whitney U-tests, it could be confirmed that differences in distribution were explained only by the parameter "atopic skin disposition." For the variable Δ-RSM, a significant association with clinical diagnoses, single or in combination, was not detectable.

Conclusions

Even in the less rigid modifications (23), Burckhardt's alkali resistance test was shown to induce colliquation necrosis in 1% of the tested individuals (31). The modification with only two 10-minute NaOH challenges did not produce relevant volunteer discomfort when the break-up criteria defined earlier were used. This is a relevant finding when considering that unlike previous studies employing NaOH, where small groups of healthy individuals were studied (18,32), we examined a large cohort of patients with former occupational dermatitis. Even in these patients with a high likelihood of "sensitive skin," the test was well tolerated and yet revealed remarkable individual differences.

Minimal clinical reactions (erythema) were taken as a sufficient sign of positive skin reactivity; clinical findings were objectified by current biophysical techniques. TEWL proved the biophysical variable of relevance, whereas RSM was not useful. The TEWL reading after the second challenge period (2×10-minute NaOH) provided the most relevant results; longer provocations (30 minutes) or late readings (24 hours) did not yield more information, neither clinically nor biophysically. Prediction of clinical outcome by TEWL$_{20\text{-min NaOH}}$ was good; thus, both parameters (clinical grading/TEWL) can serve as internal controls, opening up a kind of stereoscopic view of the test result. If in an individual clinical and biophysical findings are in agreement, measurements are to be considered relevant; if not, especially if there are clinical changes without a corresponding increase of TEWL, the investigation may be repeated. Generally, results should be interpreted, considering the complete range of anamnestic and physical findings in the individual, and the test provides valuable additional information.

In the investigated cohort of 572 clinically thoroughly examined patients with a history of former occupational skin disease, the test seemed helpful to distinguish atopics from non-atopics. The detection of constitutional risks, especially atopy, by irritant patch testing is a controversial issue (3,16,17,33–35). The discrepancies of the investigation results may be explained by the kind and size of cohorts tested, choice of irritants, dose, method, and body site, as irritant reactivity is a complex phenomenon, which is multifactorially influenced, depending on barrier function, inflammatory reactivity, and restitution capacity (1,2,7). These factors are genetically influenced (refer to "Perspectives: Genotyping of Sensitive Skin"). Recent results from a large questionnaire investigation in Denmark show that concordance rate of hand eczema was almost twice as high in homozygotic compared with heterozygotic twins in both sexes (36,37). Also, in earlier studies, reactivity to various irritants such as SLS, benzalkonium chloride, and sapo kalinus showed a significantly higher concordance rate of identical twins as opposed to fraternal twins (38); similar findings were obtained with NaOH (39).

The NaOH test proposed earlier is based on existing procedures, but is less time-consuming, less harmful, and has a better efficacy. The test was found to be reproducible, though further experience has to be gained for confirmation. We called our updated version of Burckhardt's swift modified alkali resistance test (SMART). Table 2 gives an overview on the recommended test protocol on the basis of the obtained findings.

Table 2   Flow Chart of the Swift Modified Alkali Resistance

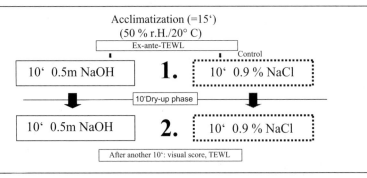

Note: Clinical and biophysical readings are to be conducted 10 minutes after the second provocation phase.
Abbreviation: TEWL, transepidermal water loss.

ACQUIRED SKIN SENSITIVITY ASSESSED WITH SODIUM HYDROXIDE: DIFFERENTIAL IRRITATION TEST

With the aim to distinguish between primary and acquired sensitive skin remaining after previous eczema, we conducted an additional study in another occupational cohort of 554 individuals from risk professions with former eczema. For this purpose, the SMART was applied simultaneously to two different body areas in a comparative fashion (9): one area (back of the hand), which was previously exposed to irritants at the workplace, whereas the other [(mid-)ventral forearm] was not or to a much lesser extent.

Methods

A total of 554 consecutive persons [276 females (median age: 36); 278 males (median age: 42)] from various high-risk professions with former occupational skin diseases, who were seen for medico-legal evaluation in the Osnabrueck University from February 2000 to August 2003, were included in the study. Florid eczematous skin lesions in the hands and forearms had to have healed at least one week before the investigation. Measurements were only performed in clinically healthy skin. SMART was performed as described earlier (refer to "Methods") simultaneously in the two test sites (forearm, back of hand). The back of hand test site was chosen according to chirality (Fig. 5).

The degree of current occupational exposure to wet work/irritants was assessed. For this purpose, the following operational criteria were used—high: three or more hours daily wet work, medium: more than one hour daily wet

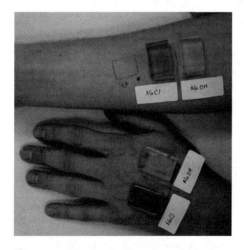

Figure 5 DIT. Back of hand test site is chosen according to chirality. The patient shown is left-handed. *Abbreviation*: DIT, differential irritation test.

work, low: less than one hour daily wet work, none: no wet work. Analogous criteria were used for the assessment of private wet work exposure. Prior to the test, there was no occupational exposure, usually for at least three to five days. Furthermore, to assess possible meteorological effects, the clinical outcome of each patient was related to standardized data on the local ambient temperature and absolute humidity on the day of examination obtained by the German Meteorological Service (9).

Results

In 554 individuals, an NaOH challenge was performed in the forearm and concomitantly in the back of the hand. A total of 212 (38.3%) reacted clinically positive in the forearm and 126 (22.7%) in the back of the hand.

A total of 384 (69.3%) of the cohort were grouped by careful history-taking and thorough clinical examination as atopics (according to the criteria given earlier; refer to "Relevant Variables"). On comparison of positive clinical reactions between the two test sites, stratified for atopic skin disposition, a significant difference in patients with atopic skin disposition ($n = 384$, $P < 0.0001$, exact McNemar test), but not in patients without atopic skin disposition, ($n = 170$, $P = 0.29$) in terms of more positive reactions on the forearm, was observed (Table 3). Atopic skin disposition, as expected, again significantly increased the odds ratio for a positive clinical reaction both at the FA (OR 4.8, 95% CI: 3.0–7.8) and the BOH (OR 3.1, 95% CI: 1.8–5.5).

There was no significant association between the dichotomized clinical test outcome (refer to "Relevant Variables") and the duration of the healing of hand eczema and eczema at other sites, respectively, before the investigation, neither in the back of the hand nor in the forearm ($P > 0.05$, Wilcoxon–Mann–Whitney test). Moreover, there was no significant association with current residual eczema on other parts of the body (present in 17.3% of study patients): OR for back of the hand 1.4 (exact 95% CI: 0.8–2.4) and OR for forearm 1.4 (exact 95% CI: 0.8–2.2).

Table 3 Differential Irritation Test

		Positive atopic skin disposition Forearm		Negative atopic skin disposition Forearm	
		+	−	+	−
Back of hands	+	76	31	1	18
	−	109	168	26	125

Note: Comparison of positive clinical reactions to NaOH between the two test sites stratified for atopic skin disposition. Significant differences in patients with atopic skin disposition ($n = 384, P < 0.0001$, exact McNemar test), but not in patients without atopic skin disposition ($n = 170, P = 0.29$).
Source: Adapted from Ref. 34.

Thirty-nine percent of patients had a high current daily occupational wet work/ irritant exposure; the majority (61%), none to medium (99% had only a low daily *private* wet work/irritant exposure). There was no association between wet workload and NaOH reactivity (BOH and FA: $P > 0.05$; likelihood ratio χ^2-test).

Unlike SLS, NaOH skin challenges seemed robust against seasonal influences in a body area not directly exposed to the environmental factors, such as the forearm. In the back of the hand, however, seasonal effects have been demonstrated, especially, at a temperature $\leq 6°C$ and an absolute humidity ≤ 8 mg/L. Thus, when interpreting NaOH challenges to the back of the hand in very dry and cold weather, it seems helpful to take the ambient meteorological parameters into consideration (9).

IMPLICATIONS FOR CHEMICAL PHENOTYPING OF SENSITIVE SKIN

Primary Sensitive Skin

We have examined two large cohorts of altogether 1126 individuals with former dermatoses in an occupational setting employing NaOH. One might argue that by definition all individuals studied must be "primary skin sensitive;" however, this is not the case. A large questionnaire study in the hairdressing trade has demonstrated that as much as 70% of 4008 hairdresser apprentices described skin lesions in the first year of training (40); further, independent studies with clinical examinations have corroborated very high prevalence rates in hazardous professions (41–43). It is unequivocal from the literature that extensive irritant exposure at the workplace and partial or even complete lack of skin protection can induce skin lesions even in "average" skin sensitivity.

On the other hand, it could be demonstrated that even atopics can almost halve their chances to develop occupational dermatoses, if they use proper skin protection at the workplace (4).

Thus, skin atopy may serve as an approximative marker of primary sensitive skin in our occupational cohorts; certainly, it has to be kept in mind that there is also primary sensitive skin apart from atopy [such as neurosensory stinging, which, so far, has resisted all attempts of objectifying it, e.g., by skin bioengineering (2)]. A high prevalence of skin atopy is to be expected in cohorts with occupational dermatoses (44–46). Accordingly, in both studies, we observed many skin atopics: 43.4% (248 from 572) versus 69.3% (384 from 554), which the test helped to detect. As shown earlier, atopic skin disposition gave an almost fivefold increased chance for a positive reaction in the forearm and still a three-fold increased chance in the back of the hand.

Acquired Sensitive Skin

Some patients with healed irritant contact dermatitis complain of experiencing ongoing increased skin sensitivity. However, in many of these cases, the clinician cannot identify any skin impairment. The differential irritation test (DIT)—comparing NaOH reactivity of the forearm and the back of the hand—is an attempt to objectify such subclinical phenomena. The relatively simple test makes use of two principally known phenomena of skin irritability: (*i*) the back of the hand is physiologically an area of reduced skin irritability and much less responsive than the forearm, but (*ii*) is also the primary site of exposure to occupational irritants and thus of occupational eczema. Comparing the actual irritant-response in the two test sites with the differences, which are physiologically to be expected, allows us to draw conclusions on pathological events—and compensatory mechanisms—in the skin.

In a previous pilot DIT study with 48 patients with completely healed, former occupational eczema (aged 19–68 years; 22 females, 26 males) and 31 healthy volunteers (aged 21–58; 21 females, 10 males) who were not previously exposed to relevant private or occupational skin hazards, we found that in the control group there was reactivity only in the forearm in a minority of (sensitive) individuals, as an indication of constitutionally impaired barrier function. However, there was no reactivity in the dorsum of the hands in any of the controls. Moreover, in the test group with former (healed) dermatitis, a subgroup of four persons (8.3%) was detected where relevant clinical (and biophysical) reactivity to the SMART occurred only in the dorsum of the hands; these patients claimed to have observed remaining increased skin sensitivity. The study is described in detail elsewhere (19). In the present DIT study in a similar but much larger cohort, we again found this unique pattern of skin reactivity and again we could detect a subgroup of a little less than 10%, which seems to be particularly worth looking at from the perspective of a remaining increased skin sensitivity, secondary to former eczema (Table 4).

It has long been known that there are marked regional variations of skin reactivity; they are attributed to differences in keratinization, size and shape of corneocytes, and in the density of epidermal shunts such as hair follicles and sweat ducts (2). Various studies, using different irritants, have convincingly demonstrated that the back of the hand is physiologically a quite robust area, even in skin-sensitive individuals (1,2,19,47). This is corroborated by our data, comparing skin reactivity to the SMART in the forearm and the dorsum of the hand:

1. In this group, most people (52.9%) are non-responsive to the test; we have to expect subjects with normal skin sensitivity and, certainly, also hyposensitive individuals. In the latter group of probably quite a few individuals, the test would not distinguish from the "average" skin sensitivity. This is owing to the well-tolerable test settings, which do not produce necrosis, and to the fact that it is a quick test. Prolonged testing might also reveal hyposensitive subjects.
2. If reactions to the test occur, this happens most likely on the forearm (24.4%); these subjects have an increased likelihood of primary

Table 4 Grouping of Subjects Within the Spectrum of Skin Sensitivity by the Differential Irritation Test

Skin sensitivity	Clinical reaction to NaOH		% of total (n = 554)	% of atopics in respective group
	Forearm	Back of hand		
Normal [and hypo-sensitive/ tolerant]	None	None	52.9 (n = 293)	57.3 (n = 168)
Primary sensitive skin	Positive	None	24.4 (n = 135)	80.7 (n = 109)
	Positive	Positive	13.9 (n = 77)	98.7 (n = 76)
Acquired sensitive skin	None	Positive	8.8 (n = 49)	63.3 (n = 31)

Note: DIT = NaOH-challenge concomitantly to forearm and back of hand.
Abbreviation: DIT, differential irritation test.

sensitive skin in terms of atopy. However, even in many of the atopics, it is evident that they do not react in the back of the hand. Those who react in both locations are almost always atopics (98.7%; Table 4).

3. Only a small proportion of subjects (8.8%) solely reacts in the back of the hand (but not in the forearm); in this group, there is a relatively small proportion of atopics (not much bigger than in the non-responders). This is an a priori paradoxical response pattern, which does not occur in healthy controls who have not previously experienced hand eczema, regardless of whether they are atopics or non-atopics. In this minority of cases, where the physiological hierarchy of skin sensitivity is absent (isolated reactivity in the hands), we claim that this paradoxical constellation provides strong evidence for a remaining acquired hyperirritability. Table 4 outlines the rationale of the concept of comparative (differential) irritation testing in separate body locations in our cohort. Of course, the question "whether the third phenomenon is a persisting one" arises; in our cohort, healing of hand eczema occurred in the subgroup of secondary hyper-reactors between 144 and 1 months (mean 9 months) before the test; further studies will be needed to find out whether it vanishes and when. It may be speculated that the phenomenon may be linked to genetically fixed release and storage of inflammatory cytokines in the keratinocytes in response to irritation.

Assessment of remaining hyperirritability and differentiating between primary and secondary sensitive skin is of great importance for medico-legal evaluations in occupational dermatology (i.e., claims and prognosis). The DIT is a methodical attempt to objectify such subclinical phenomena.

Perspectives: Genotyping of Sensitive Skin

Throughout the last six decades, many scientists have studied sodium hydroxide as an irritant and debated its value, using various test protocols (19). Recently, some epidemiological data from the Swiss metal industry seem to confirm the use of sodium hydroxide for pre-employment screening (48). In the U.S.A., where "alkali resistance" never caught on, two modifications have been proposed recently, one of which only uses skin bioengineering for the assessment of test results obtained with sodium hydroxide (32), whereas the other employs only clinical evaluations (18). Both groups claim high reliability of the respective test procedures. However, results were obtained in small populations and reproducibility has been questioned (49,50).

Unlike the "model irritant" SLS, for which the standardization process is far advanced (20,21), there is no generally accepted test procedure for NaOH. We feel that standardization is needed, as our results confirm that there are pertinent options associated with NaOH-challenges. An interesting aspect, why, in our opinion, NaOH may be a candidate for predictive patch testing for skin sensitivity, especially in the field of occupational dermatology, is that the major cause of occupational dermatoses—"wet work"—inevitably means to alkalinize the skin [dilution and exhausting of buffer systems (51,52)], for which a subset of persons, possibly identifiable by the NaOH test, might be particularly susceptible. This occupational as well as household hazard of alkalinization by wet work may be mimicked by the test. Hachem (22) recently demonstrated the vital importance of a physiological, acidic pH for interacting pH-dependent enzyme systems essential for barrier homeostasis, especially for the formation of the lamellar lipid bilayer system.

As early as 1968, Björnberg (16) showed that one may not necessarily be able to predict the reactivity to one irritant on the basis of the reactivity to another irritant. Generally, the concept of assessing skin sensitivity by a single test rather than by repetitive testing and/or combinations of various irritants is very controversial (7,33,53,54), including the question whether or not by irritant patch testing only a volatile phenomenon is being captured, just reflecting the current state of irritant reactivity rather than an individual trait (2). As yet, the question is open, because presently there is no gold standard to benchmark the various predictive tests. Even prospective cohort studies in risk professions have proven not entirely valid, because other factors such as the individual tendency to use protective measures at the workplace may hide individual risks and successfully prevent disease even in susceptible individuals (4,55).

Nevertheless, it is generally accepted that skin sensitivity to irritants varies interindividually and that this variability is mainly explicable by intrinsic/genetic factors, one of which is atopy [e.g., homozygotic twins show concordant skin reactivity to irritants (36–39)]. However, skin susceptibility also varies intraindividually, dependent mainly on various abundant extrinsic factors such as current irritant influences [e.g., on the workplace, climatic (9)] and modified irritant susceptibility in skin areas, where former eczema occurred ("secondary sensitive skin"). This may explain in partial why results with irritant patch testing are to a relevant extent contradictory. Also, the heterogeneity of human reactivity to irritants, which our data show for NaOH, may be another reason for conflicting results with irritant patch tests, especially when small groups are investigated.

There is recent evidence that skin susceptibility may be related to the presence of certain molecular markers of inflammation (e.g., IL-1a and IL-1RA) in the keratinocytes (56,57). Recently developed techniques allow us to assess the cellular concentrations of these markers non-invasively by tape-stripping (58).

In contrast to contact allergy, the basic inflammatory mechanisms of the response to irritants have been less studied, but recently, new pathogenetic concepts are emerging. For SLS-induced irritation, the role of various inflammatory cytokines, heat-shock proteins, and oxidative stress has been demonstrated (7,59,60). The evidence is growing that in the future we will leave the descriptive level in skin sensitivity research and assess the underlying cascade of pathogenetic events, which seem to be pivotally influenced by multiple genetic polymorphisms (61,62). These findings soon may allow us to explain the—yet enigmatic—great interindividual variability in irritant susceptibility, including the enhanced irritant response in atopics (7).

Eventually, one may speculate we will be able to spare our patients the tortures of irritant patch testing, taking tapes or swabs instead. However, for the time being, clinicians still have to rely on descriptive tests for routine assessment. In this context, the NaOH challenges described above may be helpful.

REFERENCES

1. Agner T. Noninvasive measuring methods for the investigation of irritant patch test reactions. Acta Derm Venereol Suppl 1992; 173:1–26.
2. Frosch PJ, John SM. Clinical aspects of irritant contact dermatitis. In: Frosch P, Menné T, Lepoittevin J, eds. Contact Dermatitis. 4th ed. Berlin/Heidelberg: Springer, 2006:255–294.
3. Frosch PJ. Hautirritation und empfindliche Haut. Berlin: Grosse Verlag, 1985.
4. Uter W. Epidemiologie und Prävention von Handekzemen in Feuchtberufen am Beispiel des Friseurhandwerks. In: Schwanitz HJ, ed. Studien zur Prävention in Allergologie, Berufs- und Umweltdermatologie (ABU 2). Osnabrück: Universitätsverlag Rasch, 1999.
5. Wulfhorst B. Skin hardening in occupational dermatology. In: Kanerva L, Elsner P, Wahlberg J, Maibach H, eds. Handbook of Occupational Dermatology. Berlin, New York: Springer, 2000:115–121.
6. York M, Griffiths HA, Whittle E, Basketter DA. Evaluation of a human patch test for the identification and classification of skin irritation potential. Contact Dermatitis 1996; 34:204–212.

7. Tupker R. Prediction of irritancy in the human skin irritancy model and occupational setting. Contact Dermatitis 2003; 49:61–69.

8. John SM, Schwartz HJ. Functional skin testing: the SMART procedures. In: Chew A-L, Maibach HI, eds. Irritant Dermatitis. Berlin, Heidelberg: Springer, 2006:211–221.

9. John SM, Uter W. Meteorological influence on NaOH irritation varies with body site. Arch Derm Res 2005; 296:320–326.

10. Burckhardt W. Neue Untersuchungen über die Alkaliempfindlichkeit der Haut. Dermatologica 1947; 94:8–96.

11. Burckhardt W. Praktische und theoretische Bedeutung der Alkalineutralisations-und Alkaliresistenzproben. Arch Klin Derm 1964; 219:600–603.

12. Schultheiss E. Eigenuntersuchungen und Alkaliresistenzprobe. Arch klin exp Dermatol 1964; 219:638–648.

13. Wacek A. Weitere Untersuchungen aus dem Gebiet der Alkali- und Säureabwehr der Haut. Dermatologica 1953; 107:369–417.

14. Burckhardt W, Suter H. Kriterien für die Arbeitsfähigkeit nach beruflich ausgelösten Ekzemen. Hautarzt 1969; 20:481–485.

15. Czernielewski A. L'importance pratique du test de résistance de la peau à l'action des alcalis. Symp dermatol Pragae cum participatione internationali de morbis cutaneis professionalibus, Exerpta Lectionum. Prag 1960; 1962:84–85.

16. Björnberg A. Skin Reactions to Primary Irritants in Patients with Hand Eczema. Göteburg: Isaacsons, 1968.

17. Björnberg A. Low alkali resistance and slow alkali neutralization: characteristics of the eczematous subject? Dermatol 1974; 149:90–100.

18. Kolbe L, Kligman AM, Stoudemayer T. The sodium hydroxide erosion assay: a revision of the alkali resistance test. Arch Derm Res 1998; 290:382–387.

19. John SM. Klinische und experimentelle Untersuchungen zur Diagnostik in der Berufsdermatologie. Konzeption einer wissenschaftlich begründeten Qualitätssicherung in der sozialmedizinischen Begutachtung. In: Schwanitz HJ, ed. Studien zur Prävention in Allergologie, Berufs- und Umweltdermatologie (ABU 4). Osnabrück: Universitätsverlag Rasch, 2001.

20. Tupker RA, Willis C, Berardesca E, Lee C, Fartasch M, Agner T, Serup J. Guidelines on sodium lauryl sulfate (SLS) exposure tests: a report from the standardization group of the European society of contact dermatitis. Contact Dermatitis 1997; 37:53–69.

21. Uter W, Geier J, Becker D, Brasch J, Löffler H. The MOAHLFA index of irritant sodium lauryl sulfate reactions: first results of a multicentre study on routine sodium lauryl sulfate patch testing. Contact Dermatitis 2004; 51:259–262.

22. Hachem J, Crumrine D, Fluhr J. pH directly regulates epidermal permeability barrier homeostasis, and stratum corneum integrity/cohesion. J Invest Dermatol 2003; 121:345–353.

23. Locher G. Permeabilitätsprüfung der Haut Ekzemkranker und Hautgesunder für den neuen Indikator Nitrazingelb "Geigy", Modizifierung der Alkaliresistenzprobe, pH-Verlauf in der Tiefe des stratum corneum. Dermatologica 1962; 124:159–182.

24. Pinnagoda J, Tupker RA, Agner T, Serup J. Guidelines for transepidermal water loss (TEWL) measurement. Contact Dermatitis 1990; 22:164–178.

25. Rogiers V, EEMCO Group. EEMCO Guidance for the assessment of transepidermal water loss in cosmetic sciences. Skin Pharmacol Appl Skin Physiol 2001; 14:117–128.

26. Wilson D, Berardesca E, Maibach HI. In vivo transepidermal water loss and skin surface hydration in association of moisturization and soap effects. Int J Cosm Sci 1988; 10:201–211.
27. Green DM, Swets JA. Signal Detection Theory and Psychophysics. New York: Huntington, 1974.
28. Lange N, Weinstock MA. Statistical analysis of sensitivity, specificity, and predictive value of a diagnostic test. In: Serup J, Jemec GBE, eds. Handbook of Non-invasive Methods and the Skin. Boca Raton: CRC Press, 1995:33–41.
29. Cohen J. A coefficient of agreement for nominal scales. Educ Psychol Meas 1960; 20:37–46.
30. Cohen J. Statistical Power Analysis for the Behavioral Sciences. Hillsdale: Erlbaum, 1988.
31. Ummenhofer B. Zur Methodik der Alkaliresistenzprüfung. Dermatosen 1980; 28:104–109.
32. Wilhelm KP, Pasche F, Surber C, Maibach HI. Sodium hydroxide-induced subclinical irritation: a test for evaluating stratum corneum barrier function. Acta Derm Venereol (Stockh) 1990; 70:463–467.
33. Basketter DA, Miettinen J, Lahti A. Acute irritant reactivity to sodium lauryl sulfate in atopics and non-atopics. Contact Derm 1998; 38:253–257.
34. Den Arend JA, De Haan AFJ, Malten KE. Seasonal transepidermal water loss and impedance of forearm skin in atopics and non-atopics. Contact Dermatitis 1988; 19:376–390.
35. Tupker RA, Pinnagoda J, Coenraads PJ, Nater JP. Susceptibility to irritants: role of barrier function, skin dryness and history of atopic dermatitis. Br J Dermatol 1990; 123:199–205.
36. Bryld LE, Agner T, Kyvik KO, Brondsted L, Hindsberger C, Menne T. Hand eczema in twins: a questionnaire investigation. Br J Dermatol 2000; 142:298–305.
37. Bryld LE, Hindsberger C, Kyvik KO, Agner T, Menné T. Risk factors influencing the development of hand eczema in a population-based twin sample. Br J Dermatol 2003; 149:1214–1220.
38. Holst R, Möller H. One hundred twin pairs patch tested with primary irritants. Br J Dermatol 1975; 93:145–149.
39. Gloor M, Schnyder UW. Vererbung funktioneller Eigenschaften der Haut. Hautarzt 1977; 28:231–234.
40. Budde U, Schwanitz HJ. Kontaktdermatitiden bei Auszubildenden des Friseurhandwerks in Niedersachsen. Dermatosen 1991; 39:41–48.
41. John SM, Uter W, Schwanitz HJ. Relevance of multiparametric skin bioengineering in a prospectively followed cohort of junior hairdressers. Contact Derm 2000; 43:161–168.
42. Smit HA, Van Rijssen A, Vandenbrouke JP, Coenrads PJ. Susceptibility to and incidence of hand dermatitis in a cohort of apprentice hairdressers and nurses. Scand J Work Environ Health 1994; 20:113–121.
43. Uter W, Pfahlberg A, Gefeller O, Schwanitz HJ. Prevalence and incidence of hand dermatitis in hairdressing apprentices: results of the POSH study. Int Arch Occup Environ Health 1998; 71:487–492.
44. John SM, Uter W, Richter G, Schwanitz HJ. Unterschiede und Gemeinsamkeiten in der Begutachtung gemäß Berufskrankheiten-Nr. 5101 an zwei berufsdermatologischen Zentren. Dermatol Beruf Umwelt/Occup Environ Dermatol 2002; 50(6):131–218.

45. Shmunes E, Keil J. The role of atopy in occupational dermatoses. Contact Derm 1984; 11:174–178.
46. Uter W, Schwanitz HJ, Pfahlberg A, Gefeller O. Atopic signs and symptoms: assessing the "atopy score" concept. Dermatology 2001; 202:4–8.
47. Schulz D, Korting GW. Zur weiteren Kenntnis der Alkaliresistenz-Probe. Dermatosen 1987; 35:91–94.
48. Berndt U, Hinnen U, Iliev D, Elsner P. Is occupational irritant contact dermatitis predictable by cutaneous bioengineering methods? Results of the Swiss metalworkers' eczema study (PROMETES). Dermatology 1999; 198:351–354.
49. Bangha E, Hinnen U, Elsner P. Irritancy testing in occupational dermatology: comparison between two quick tests and the acute irritation induced by sodium lauryl sulphate. Acta Derm Venereol (Stockh) 1996; 76:450–452.
50. Iliev D, Hinnen U, Elsner P. Reproducibility of a non-invasive skin irritancy test in a cohort of metalworker trainees. Contact Derm 1997; 36:101–103.
51. Batzdorfer L, Schwanitz HJ. Qualität und Qualitätsentwicklung am Beispiel der regelmäßigen Patientenbefragung in einer dermatologischen Heil- und Präventionsmaßnahme. Prävention und Rehabilitation 2000; 12:137–141.
52. Grunewald AM, Gloor M, Gehring W, Kleesz P. Damage to the skin by repetitive washing. Contact Derm 1995; 32:225–232.
53. Koopman D, Kezic S, Verberk M. Skin reaction and recovery: a repeated sodium lauryl sulphate patch test vs. a 24-h patch test and tape stripping. Br J Dermatol 2004; 150:493–499.
54. Smith HR, Rowson M, Basketter DA, McFadden JP. Intra-individual variation of irritant threshold and relationship to transepidermal water loss measurement of skin irritation. Contact Derm 2004; 51:26–29.
55. Löffler H. Der prädiktive Wert von Funktionsprüfungen der Hautirritabilität. JDDG 2003; 1(suppl 1):S138 (abstract).
56. Barland CO, Zettersten E, Brown BS, Ye J, Elias PM, Ghadially R. Imiquimod-induced interleukin-1 alpha stimulation improves barrier homeostasis in aged murine epidermis. J Invest Dermatol 2004; 122:330–336.
57. Spiekstra SW, Toebak MJ, Sampat-Sardjoepersad S, van Beek PJ, Boorsma DM, Stoof TJ, von Blomberg BM, Scheper RJ, Bruynzeel DP, Rustemeyer T, Gibbs S. Induction of cytokine (interleukin-1 alpha and tumor necrosis factor-alpha) and chemokine (CCL20, CCL27, and CXCL8) alarm signals after allergen and irritant exposure. Exp Dermatol 2005; 14:109–116.
58. Perkins MA, Osterhues MA, Farage MA, Robinson MK. A noninvasive method to assess skin irritation and compromised skin conditions using simple tape adsorption of molecular markers of inflammation. Skin Res Technol 2001; 7:227–237.
59. Elias PM, Wood LC, Feingold KR. Epidermal pathogenesis of inflammatory dermatoses. Am J Contact Dermat 1999; 10:119–126.
60. Willis CM. Variability in responsiveness to irritants: thoughts on possible underlying mechanisms. Contact Derm 2002; 47:267–271.
61. Allen M, Wakelin S, Holloway D, Baadsgaard O, Barker J, McFadden J. TNFa and IL-1 receptor antagonist gene polymorphisms in susceptibility to irritant contact dermatitis. Br J Dermatol 1998; 138:735.
62. Allen MH, Wakelin SH, Holloway D, Lisby S, Baadsgaard O, Barker JN, McFadden JP. Association of TNFA gene polymorphism at position -308 with susceptibility to irritant contact dermatitis. Immunogenetics 2000; 51:201–205.

12

Intra- and Inter-Individual Differences in Facial Skin Biophysical Properties

F. Distante, L. Rigano, R. D'Agostino, and A. Bonfigli
Institute of Skin and Product Evaluation, Milan, Italy

Enzo Berardesca
San Gallicano Dermatological Institute, Rome, Italy

INTRODUCTION

Regional differences in skin reactivity to various stimuli according to body site have been widely documented (1–5). Anatomical differences in skin structure and in skin biophysical properties, that is, barrier function, skin permeability, and vascular response to topically applied substances, have been supposed as major factors involved in such skin variability (4,5). Therefore studies on irritation and cosmetic evaluations performed in different body areas cannot be easily compared.

Although cosmetic products are mainly applied on the face, most of the investigative studies by bioengineering methods have been performed on other body sites, that is, the forearm or the trunk, whereas little attention has been paid to investigate regional differences among various facial areas (6–9). Furthermore, many people experience high facial reactivity when exposed to external factors, reporting symptoms such as tightness, burning, itching, and stinging after application of various substances, such as lactic acid, without any objective sign of skin alterations (10). Approximately 40% of the population, when interviewed, suffered from this condition, so that it has been classified as a particular skin type and defined as "sensitive skin" (11–13). However,

149

models to define this condition are not standardized and its boundaries are neither well defined nor extensively investigated, so the term "sensitive skin" can even be misleading (14).

The stinging response after local application of 10% lactic acid (stinging test) is widely used as a marker of skin sensitivity (15). The aim of this study is to objectively investigate and compare facial regional differences in skin barrier function [transepidermal water loss (TEWL)], capacitance, and microcirculation in "sensitive" and "non-sensitive" subjects.

MATERIALS AND METHODS

Study Population

After signing a written informed consent, 20 healthy Caucasian females, aged 19 to 45 years (mean age 36 ± 2; II–IV skin type), 10 of them with sensitive skin and 10 with non-sensitive skin, entered the study. Inclusion criteria for sensitive skin group was a positive stinging response after local application of 10% lactic acid on the naso-labial fold combined with self-reported sensitive skin and perception of at least one of the following symptoms: redness associated with stress/emotion, ingestion of alcohol and spicy food, or rapid temperature change; redness, stinging, tightness after exposure to cold weather or wind; reddening, stinging, burning, itching, scaling after facial application of cosmetics, and contact with water and soap. Subjects suffering from contact dermatitis were excluded from the study. Non-sensitive subjects were defined on the basis of the negative stinging response associated with self-reported normal skin type and the absence of any subjective symptom indicated earlier for the sensitive group.

All subjects, when required, received the same type of make-up removal product and the same facial cream to use for seven days prior to the study entry. Furthermore, they were instructed not to use any cosmetic or soap for at least 12 hours prior to the measurements.

Instrumental Measurements

The following biophysical measurements were performed on 10 selected areas of the face while subjects stayed in lying position: barrier function (TEWL) by an evaporimeter (Tewameter® TM 210 Courage & Khazaka, Germany); hydration by capacitance method (Corneometer® CM 825; Courage & Khazaka, Germany), and skin flux by a laser Doppler (Perimed Periflux PF 4001, Sweden). All measurements were performed after a 30-minute rest period of subjects in an environmentally controlled room ($21–23°C$; RH: $45–55\%$). The sites (2×2 cm^2 size) were selected on 10 anatomically defined facial areas, as reported by Schnetz et al. (9), partially modified (Fig. 1):

> Site 1: the center of the forehead
> Site 2: right forehead superior to the right nerves supraorbital, at the same horizontal level as site 1

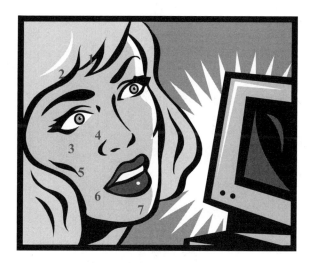

Figure 1   Location of the investigated facial sites.

Site 3: center of the cheekbone (right: site 3R; left: site 3L)
Site 4: cheek, in the infraorbital/paranasal area (right: site 4R; left: site 4L)
Site 5: in the middle of the line that joins the naso-labial fold to the jaw angle (right: site 5R; left: site 5L)
Site 6: 1 cm from the oral commissura (right or left)
Site 7: center of the chin

Statistical Analysis

The data related to each group of subjects (sensitive and non-sensitive) were statistically analyzed by analysis of variance (ANOVA) for repeated measurements and then by Tukey's test for post hoc comparison. The Student's *t*-test was used to compare each facial site between the two groups of subjects.

RESULTS

The results are shown in Table 1 and Figures 2–4.

Transepidermal Water Loss

Intra-Individual Differences

The comparison of all tested facial areas showed a similar pattern of distribution in both groups of subjects: higher TEWL mean values were obtained on the chin (site 7), in the infraorbital sites (sites 4R and 4L), and near the oral commissura (site 6); the lowest values in the lateral part of the cheeks (sites 3R, 3L, 5R, 5L, and 3) and the forehead (sites 1 and 2) (Table 1 and Fig. 2).

Table 1 TEWL, Capacitance, and Laser-Doppler Mean Values and Standard Deviations (in parentheses) in the Tested Facial Sites and the Statistical Comparison Between the Two Groups

Sites	TEWL			Capacitance			Laser-Doppler		
	Sensitive group	Non-sensitive group	P-value (t-test)	Sensitive group	Non-sensitive group	P-value (t-test)	Sensitive group	Non-sensitive group	P-value (t-test)
1	12.86 (4.1)	12.18 (3.4)	n.s.	55.31 (11.7)	56.48 (8.6)	n.s.	43.10 (28.7)	37.52 (19.6)	n.s.
2	12.26 (5.0)	10.91 (3.0)	n.s.	55.41 (14.2)	61.33 (7.7)	n.s.	33.36 (15.5)	37.01 (27.3)	n.s.
3R	12.02 (2.8)	9.34 (2.2)	0.05	66.54 (13.6)	73.42 (7.2)	n.s.	38.15 (21.4)	24.09 (7.9)	n.s.
3L	12.07 (2.9)	9.24 (2.6)	0.03	69.97 (10.8)	75.20 (7.1)	n.s.	34.30 (18.7)	26.45 (9.1)	n.s.
4R	15.79 (3.9)	13.14 (3.0)	n.s.	60.79 (11.7)	70.94 (6.8)	n.s.	72.65 (37.2)	45.09 (17.4)	n.s.
4L	16.11 (4.4)	13.67 (2.9)	n.s.	60.92 (15.2)	67.63 (10.7)	n.s.	73.44 (43.4)	61.18 (22.4)	n.s.
5R	12.24 (3.5)	10.82 (2.4)	n.s.	60.65 (11.5)	62.96 (12.6)	n.s.	50.41 (64.7)	24.32 (9.2)	n.s.
5L	12.94 (3.4)	10.65 (2.9)	n.s.	58.28 (11.8)	62.13 (9.2)	n.s.	32.43 (15.0)	30.87 (6.0)	n.s.
6	14.55 (4.2)	13.85 (2.9)	n.s.	55.76 (15.6)	67.75 (8.5)	n.s.	51.19 (48.6)	46.62 (35.3)	n.s.
7	19.28 (4.7)	17.16 (4.3)	n.s.	61.82 (10.7)	69.56 (10.0)	n.s.	64.77 (36.0)	44.92 (17.1)	n.s.

Abbreviation: TEWL, transepidermal water loss.

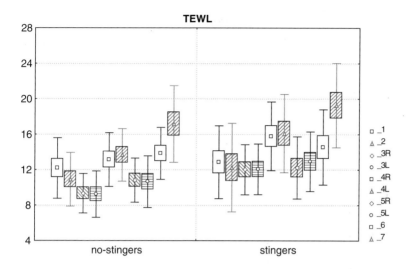

Figure 2 Intra- and inter-individual variations. Distribution of TEWL at different locations in the two groups of subjects (no-stingers = non-sensitive and stingers = sensitive). Data are illustrated as box plots. *Abbreviation*: TEWL, transepidermal water loss.

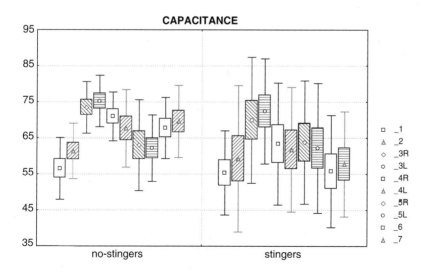

Figure 3 Intra- and inter-individual variations. Distribution of capacitance values at different locations in the two groups of subjects (no-stingers = non-sensitive and stingers = sensitive). Data are illustrated as box plots.

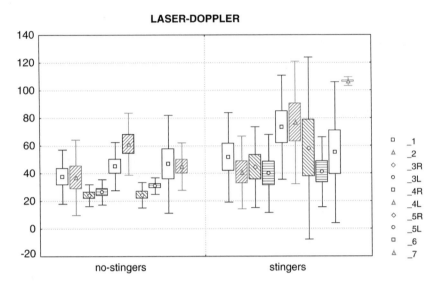

Figure 4 Intra- and inter-individual variations. Distribution of laser Doppler values at different locations in the two groups of subjects (no-stingers = non-sensitive and stingers = sensitive). Data are illustrated as box plots.

Statistically significant differences were found between the chin (site 7) and all the other facial sites ($P < 0.001$), between the paranasal sites (site 4) and the lateral parts of the cheeks (sites 3 and 5), and between the paranasal sites (site 4) and the forehead (sites 1 and 2) ($P < 0.05$ and $P < 0.001$).

Inter-Individual Differences: Sensitive Vs. Non-sensitive Group

The comparison of TEWL values between the two groups showed higher values in all sites in the sensitive skin group compared with the non-sensitive group. Such differences were found statistically significant for the cheekbone and paranasal sites ($P = 0.05$) (Fig. 2).

Capacitance

Intra-Individual Differences

As found for TEWL, the comparison of all tested facial areas showed a similar pattern of distribution in both groups of subjects: higher hydration values were obtained on the chin (site 7) and in the infraorbital and cheekbone sites (sites 3 and 4), the lowest values in the lateral parts of the cheeks (site 5) and the forehead (sites 1 and 2) (Table 1 and Fig. 3). Statistically significant differences were found between the cheekbone areas (site 3) and the forehead (sites 1 and 2) and between the cheekbone sites (site 3) and the lower cheek areas (sites 5 and 6) ($P < 0.05$ and $P < 0.001$). In the non-sensitive group, a statistically significant difference was also found between the chin (site 7) and the forehead sites (sites 1 and 2) ($P = 0.001$).

Inter-Individual Differences: Sensitive Vs. Non-Sensitive Group

The comparison of capacitance values between the two groups showed lower values in all sites in the sensitive group compared with the non-sensitive group (Table 1 and Fig. 3). However, the differences between the two groups were not statistically significant. This result could be due to the small sample size of the study.

Laser Doppler Flowmetry

Intra-Individual Differences

As found for TEWL and capacitance values, the facial profile for skin flux showed higher values in the paranasal sites (site 4) and the chin (site 7) and the lowest in the lateral part of the cheeks (sites 3 and 5) and the forehead (sites 1 and 2) (Table 1 and Fig. 4). In both groups, statistically significant differences were found among the different facial sites: site 4 versus site 3 ($P < 0.05$), site 4 versus site 5 ($P < 0.001$), and site 4 versus site 2 (forehead) ($P < 0.05$).

Inter-Individual Differences: Sensitive Vs. Non-Sensitive Group

The comparison of skin flux values between the two groups showed higher skin flux values in all sites in the skin-sensitive group compared with the non-sensitive group, except for one site on the forehead (site 2). However, the differences between the two groups were not statistically significant (Table 1 and Fig. 4).

DISCUSSION

Contradictory findings about sensitive skin have been reported. The cause may be genetic because racial differences in skin irritability in terms of different reactivity of the water barrier and vascular responses have been documented (12,16–18). The general belief is that hyperreactive people may have a thin permeable stratum corneum with a decreased corneocyte area (19). A heightened neurosensory input could also result in a reduced threshold to irritant stimuli (13).

Regional differences in skin susceptibility to irritants according to body site have been widely reported (1–5). In this study, we investigated the intra-individual and the inter-individual variations of TEWL, capacitance, and microcirculation in 10 different facial areas in subjects with sensitive skin and in subjects with non-sensitive skin. As reported in other works (7), we found regional differences among the investigated facial sites that follow a characteristic profile in both groups of subjects: significantly higher TEWL, higher capacitance, and higher skin flux values were found in the cheekbone, the infraorbital/paranasal sites, and the chin compared with the forehead ($P < 0.05$ and $P < 0.001$). Symmetrical regions on the two cheeks did not show any significant

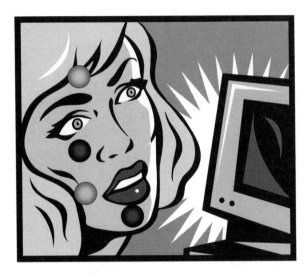

Figure 5 Intra-individual differences: in both groups (sensitive and non-sensitive), the chin and the infraorbital/paranasal facial areas show decreased barrier function (higher TEWL) and increased microcirculation (laser Doppler values) and hydration (capacitance values) compared with the forehead and the lateral facial areas. *Abbreviation*: TEWL, transepidermal water loss.

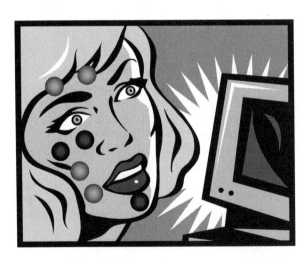

Figure 6 Inter-individual differences: the group with sensitive skin showed higher TEWL, higher skin flux, and lower hydration compared with the non-sensitive group in all the investigated facial sites. *Abbreviation*: TEWL, transepidermal water loss.

differences. The results of this study confirm that intra-regional differences in skin biophysical properties may be behind the variability in skin reactivity among different facial sites. In particular, the decreased barrier function and the increased skin flux found on the chin and the infraorbital–paranasal site could result in a higher permeability of these skin sites, possibly leading to a greater susceptibility to topically applied substances compared with the forehead and the lateral parts of the face (Fig. 5).

These differences were much more marked in the group with sensitive skin, which showed higher TEWL values, higher skin flux, and lower hydration values in all the investigated facial sites compared with the group with non-sensitive skin (TEWL: site 3; $P < 0.05$) (Fig. 6). These findings support the hypothesis that constitutional structural defects in barrier function, stratum corneum structure, and vascular dynamics may induce a higher transcutaneous penetration in subjects with sensitive skin, leading to increased skin hyperreactivity.

REFERENCES

1. Clarys P, Manou I, Barel A. Relationship between anatomical skin site and response to halcinonide and methyl nicotinate studied by bioengineering techniques. Skin Res Technol 1997; 3:161.
2. Henry F, Goffin V, Maibach HI, Pierard GE. Regional differences in stratum corneum reactivity to surfactants. Contact Dermatitis 1997; 37:271.
3. Van der Valk PGM, Maibach HI. Potential for irritation increases from the wrist to the cubital fossa. Br J Dermatol 1989; 121:709.
4. Dupuis D, Rougier A, Lotte C, Wilson D, Maibach HI. In vivo relationship between percutaneous absorption and transepidermal water loss according to anatomical site in man. J Soc Cosmet Chem 1986; 37:351.
5. Pinnagoda J, Tupker RA, Coenraads PJ, Nater JP. Prediction of susceptibility to an irritant response by transepidermal water loss. Contact Dermatitis 1989; 20:108.
6. Le Fur I, Lopez S, Morizot F, Guinot C, Tschachler E. Comparison of cheek and forehead regions by bioengineering methods in women with different self-reported "cosmetic skin types". Skin Res Technol 1999; 5:182.
7. Lopez S, Le Fur I, Morizot F, Heuvin G, Guinot C, Tschachler E. Transepidermal water loss, temperature and sebum levels on women's facial skin follow characteristic patterns Skin Res Technol 2000; 6:31.
8. Le Fur I, Morizot F, Dubourgeat M, Guinot C, Tschauchler E. Comparison of malar and frontal zones by bioengineering methods. In: Second European Symposium of International Society of Bioengineering and Skin, Rome, 2–4 October 1997.
9. Schnetz E, Kuss O, Schmitt J, Diepgen L, Kuhn M, Fartasch M. Intra- and inter-individual variations in transepidermal water loss on the face: facial locations for bioengineering studies. Contact Dermatitis 1999; 40:243.
10. Berardesca E, Cespa M, Farinelli N, Rabbiosi G, Maibach HI. In vivo transcutaneous penetration of nicotinates and sensitive skin. Contact Dermatitis 1991; 25:35.

11. Amin S, Engasser P, Maibach HI. Sensitive skin: what is it? In: Baran R, Maibach HI, eds. Textbook of Cosmetic Dermatology. 2nd ed. London: Martin Dunitz Ltd., 1998:343.
12. Chew A, Maibach HI. Sensitive skin. In: London M, Maibach H, eds. Dry Skin and Moisturizers: Chemistry and Function. CRC Press: Boca Raton, 2000:429.
13. Seidenari S, Francomano M, Mantovani L. Baseline biophysical parameters in subjects with sensitive skin. Contact Dermatitis 1998; 38:311.
14. Berardesca E, Maibach HI. Sensitive and ethnic skin: a need for special skin-care agents? Dermatol Clin 1991; 9(1):89.
15. Frosh PJ, Kligman AM. A method for appraising the stinging capacity of topically applied substances. J Cosmet Chem 1977; 28:197.
16. Berardesca E, Maibach HI. Racial differences in sodium lauryl sulphate induced cutaneous irritation: black and white. Contact Dermatitis 1988; 18:65.
17. Berardesca E, Maibach HI. Sodium-lauryl-sulphate-induced cutaneous irritation: comparison of white and hispanic subjects. Contact Dermatitis 1988; 19:136.
18. Berardesca E, Maibach HI. Cutaneous reactive hyperemia: racial differences induced by corticoid application. Br J Dermatol 1989; 120:787.
19. Hamami I, Marks R. Structural determinants of the response of the skin to chemical irritants. Contact Dermatitis 1988; 18:71.

13

Household Cleaning Products and Sensitive Skin

Gérald E. Piérard, Emmanuelle Xhauflaire-Uhoda, Carole Collard, and Claudine Piérard-Franchimont

Department of Dermatopathology, University Hospital Sart Tilman, Liège, Belgium

INTRODUCTION

Sensitive skin is reported to be increasing in the populations of western countries. In some settings, epidemiological surveys have suggested that one person out of two claims suffering from sensitive skin. However, there are strong cultural differences in the frequency of reporting sensitive skin between different European countries. Overall, complaints relating to consumer products are the most frequent in the U.K., followed by the Netherlands, Belgium, and Germany. When the problem of sensitive skin arises, which the afflicted individual attributes to a consumer product such as cleaning and cleansing formulations, it is often difficult to objectively establish the potential causality. There are genetic, in part ethnic, differences in the susceptibility to react to xenobiotics. Liquid dishwashing detergent ingredients do not escape this rule.

As the business market is large, products intended for individuals with sensitive skin are being increasingly developed by formulators of household cleaning products. However, there is currently no real consensus about the definition and recognition of the biological basis of skin sensitive to detergents. It is likely a multifactorial process leading to skin discomfort that encompasses distinct conditions (1). In a broad sense, sensitive skin means that the skin readily experiences either reduced tolerance or heightened response to external

159

stimuli including physical and/or chemical factors. The perceived adverse reactions may be immediate or delayed, and they begin as a purely sensory phenomenon without any obvious clinical expression (2–5). The discomfort reactions include one or a combination of sensations including tightness, itching, stinging, and burning sensations. Such subjective and subclinical symptoms may be followed by visible effects, including rough- and dry-looking skin, and erythema (4). This common and puzzling condition is often classified in the spectrum of irritant contact dermatitis and thus corresponds to sensory irritation (6).

PHYSIOPATHOLOGY OF SENSORY IRRITATION TO SURFACTANTS

Several targets in the skin may be involved for the abnormal self-perceived sensory response to detergents. It has been suggested that the response of the stratum corneum (SC) to any surfactant threat is impaired in a subset of individuals complaining of sensitive skin (7). Two distinct mechanisms, acting either singly or in combination, are theoretically involved in this process. On the one hand, the surfactant interaction with corneocytes is abnormally pronounced, and consequently, the cells release a variety of mediators including cytokines, prostaglandins, and leukotrienes. In turn, these biomolecules help to release neuromediators from other cells or stimulate nerve endings. On the other hand, the barrier function to surfactants is initially impaired and these compounds directly stimulate sensory nerve endings. According to this hypothesis, enhanced-sensory irritation may be due to subtle variations in the structure of the SC. A thinner SC with or without perturbation of the corneocyte desquamation (8) may be operative. A reduced corneocyte area was also put forward to explain the increased penetration of water-soluble xenobiotics (9,10), including surfactants. Still another possibility involves a lowered threshold reactivity for nerve stimulation. Indeed, free nerve endings and specialized nerve corpuscles receive both excitatory stimuli and antagonist signals. When the latter activity is lowered, the efferent neurosensory input is amplified and perceived as a manifestation of sensitive skin (6–11). As a result, lifestyle including stress and emotions clearly influences this condition.

Some individuals, particularly those complaining of sensitive skin, report unpleasant after-wash tightness. Unlike mild surfactant-based cleansers, harsh cleansers, such as soaps, and some household cleaning products induce skin tightness, about five to ten minutes after washing with a cleanser. The tightness is ascribed to stresses created in the SC by the rapid evaporation of water from the surface. Treatment with harsh surfactants can actually lead to corneocyte hyperhydration and swelling immediately after washing, followed by rapid evaporation of water to equilibrium values that are below the pre-surfactant treatment levels. This hyper-hydration, followed by lower equilibrium hydration levels, creates a higher than normal rate of evaporation. Thus, a differential stress is created in the upper layers of the skin, leading to after-wash tightness. The tendency to cause skin tightness parallels lipid removal, surfactant binding to protein, and change of the overall electrical charge at the surface of the skin.

Controversial Issues about Sensory Irritation to Surfactants

A controversial and blurring issue about sensitive skin to surfactants deals with its putative relationship, if any, with allergic contact dermatitis. Indeed, this disease is characterized by the combination of erythema, serum deposits in the epidermis, scaliness, and pruritus. The latter symptom is almost never encountered in the absence of the clinical signs. Hence, in our opinion, pure sensorial feelings characteristic for sensitive skin are not part of allergic contact dermatitis. However, laypeople often confuse the two conditions. It must be acknowledged that surfactant-based products, as any other irritant xenobiotic, may exacerbate the manifestations of any kind of eczema. Atopic dermatitis is one of the best examples (12,13).

A varied wording is sometimes used to qualify the sensitive skin condition including delicate, damaged, hyperreactive, overreactive, irritated, allergic, hyper-excitable, responsive, and so on. This situation increases confusion about sensory irritation typical for sensitive skin to surfactants. In addition, the consumer perception (14) self-assessment by laypersons is particularly confusing, mixing up specific symptoms and signs of unrelated dermatoses in the broadest non-specific wording of sensitive skin.

The conceptual aspect of sensitive skin, being limited to sensory irritation or expanded to any kind of skin reactivity including allergic contact dermatitis, photodermatitis, or any other dermatitis, is of importance. Quenching sensory irritation due, for instance, to household cleaning products is possible by reducing the irritation potential of this category of products. Much progress has been made in that field by the industry over the past decade. In contrast, the vast majority of cases of allergic contact dermatitis and other unrelated dermatoses are not due to the composition of the household cleaning products. These conditions are not improved by switching the choice of household cleaning products even when they claim hypoallergenicity. Any cleaning product positioned for sensitive skin can realistically only target subjects with sensory irritation to surfactants.

SENSORY IRRITATION TO HOUSEHOLD CLEANING PRODUCTS

In any case of sensory irritation to surfactants, there is a regional variability to the offending agents. Moreover, the nature of the surfactant is of importance because the individual hyperreactivity is often manifest for a limited category of products. The sensory irritation status also varies with the age, gender, and ethnicity of individuals, as well as with environmental and seasonal geoclimatic conditions (5,12,15–22). Women complain more frequently than men from sensitive skin. In the case of household cleaning products, women are indeed more frequently in contact with the triggering agents. As irritation reactivity usually declines with age, it is not surprising that sensory irritation to surfactants appears less frequent in middle-aged and older adults. In general, fair skin is believed to be more susceptible to sensory irritation than darker skin (18,23). The negative geoclimatic influence is manifest when the dew point modifications in winter alter the SC physiology (5,17,18,20,21).

According to these concepts, assessing skin sensitivity to household cleaning products calls for a combined series of tests. The investigative procedure must target sensory irritation, possibly boosted by skin weathering (24). To be clinically relevant, the response of the hands and forearms should be specifically studied. Indeed, one cannot expect salient information by testing facial skin in the context of household cleaning products (25).

Similar test procedures also apply to the evaluation of products such as emollients used to improve sensitive skin. Indeed, vast volumes of emollients are bought every year, but a significant proportion of these products, probably many truckloads worldwide, stays firmly in the tube because of the subjective variation in the tolerance and acceptability of the different preparations by the consumers. Assuming, however, that at least some of the emollients are actually used, the benefit they really provide is often difficult to assess objectively. The effects of emollients and any other protective formulation to sensory irritation can be assessed in two ways, including clinical investigation into their subjective benefits and more rigorous objective assessment (26,27).

The methods for assessing sensitive skin to household cleaning products and those evaluating the efficacy of products aiming to protect against unpleasant sensorial perceptions are numerous. Selected and non-limitative investigative procedures are listed subsequently.

EXPERIMENTAL AND PREDICTIVE METHODS

Subjective self-assessment of sensory irritation is notoriously difficult to interpret. In many instances, it proves to be unreliable. One way to be more confident with the data is to use a blinded device for the subject who positions a cursor on a lath. The back of the device is only seen by the investigator, and the cursor position on a millimetric scale is ranging from 0 (no sensorial stimulation) to 100 (upmost unpleasant sensorial stimulation).

The classical stinging test performed by applying lactic acid to the nasolabial fold may appear irrelevant when assessing sensory irritation of the hands and forearms related to household cleaning products.

Corneosurfametry for Testing SC Reactivity to Surfactants

The ex vivo corneosurfametry test (7,13,25,27–33) can be used for assessing subjects with sensitive skin to household cleaning products, including dishwashing liquids. Human SC is used as a test substrate. The procedure entails the collection of a sheet of SC from the forearms or dorsum of the hands using cyano-acrylate skin surface strippings (CSSSs). Diluted test surfactants are sprayed over the CSSS. Samples are kept for two hours at room temperature in a humid environment. They are then thoroughly rinsed with tap water, dried, and stained for three minutes with a toluidine blue-basic fuschin 30% alcoholic solution. Their color is measured by reflectance colorimetry in the $L^*a^*b^*$ system (Chroma Meter® CR200 Minolta, Osaka, Japan). The L^*- and chroma C^*-values are measured. Their difference L^*-chroma C^* corresponds to the colorimetric index of mildness (CIM). Its value increases with the severity of interaction between corneocytes and surfactants. For a given surfactant-based product, the CIM value is increased in subjects complaining from sensitive skin to surfactants (7). Other types of sensitive skin unrelated to surfactant sensorial irritation do not show similar corneosurfametry changes.

Stinging Response to Electrical Current for Testing Nerve Sensorial Reactivity

Testing skin sensorial perceptions can be performed by electrical stinging stimulations. The skin barrier function has no influence whatsoever on this evaluation. A weak continuous current is delivered by a small device (Herpifix®, C+K Electronic, Cologne). The time for the first perception of stinging is recorded. Some people complaining of sensitive skin detect the stinging sensation after 10 to 20 seconds, which is much shorter than in normal subjects.

Burning Response to Solvents and Corneoxenometry

A chloroform:methanol (20:80) mixture is deposited under occlusion into a chamber test affixed to the skin. The time for the first perception of unequivocal burning is recorded, followed by grading changes in burning sensation over the next five minutes (22). Burning is graded on a nominal scale. This test measures the neurosensory reactivity. It is influenced by the structural integrity of the SC. Occult cracks indeed allow rapid permeation of the solvent mixture.

The corneoxenometry test performed ex vivo gives information correlating with the in vivo test (34). The advantage of corneoxenometry over in vivo tests is the avoidance of discomfort and any other hazards for human volunteers (35) This test is performed and evaluated similar to the corneosurfametry bioassay (27).

Anionic Surfactant-Induced Erythema

The transient erythematous reaction to anionic surfactants such as sodium lauryl sulfate (SLS) can be evaluated by applying 0.75% or less aqueous SLS for 24 hours in a chamber test to the forearms (22,36). Twenty-four hours after removal of the chambers, the reactions can be clinically graded and quantified by reflectance colorimetry. Immersion tests and in-use tests are probably better suited to study sensitive skin to surfactants (37–39). Values of a^* are very informative. A proportion of subjects with sensitive skin to surfactants develop intense erythema without or well before any SC alteration becomes visible. This situation corresponds likely to the rapid release of vasodilation mediators without full-blown irritation with influx of inflammatory cells. This condition is usually unrelated to a defect in the SC barrier function.

Dimethylsulfoxide Wheal and Flare Response

Dimethylsulfoxide (DMSO) is applied for 10 minutes under occlusion. Five minutes after removal, whealing is scored clinically (40,41). The flare surrounding the wheal is also scored on a nominal scale. The whealing response to DMSO is an indirect measure of the permeability of the SC. This test can detect a small proportion of subjects with sensitive skin to surfactants. It is influenced by previous subclinical challenges of the skin by surfactants.

Nicotinates can be used similarly to explore alterations in transcutaneous penetration in subjects with sensitive skin (10).

Corticosteroid Blanching Test

The blanching effect of topical corticosteroids as a measure of SC barrier function can be determined two hours after occlusive film dressing removal (42). Skin colorimetry records the L-value, a measure of skin lightness, and the a^*-value, a measure of skin redness. A controlled amount of topical corticosteroid is applied to both forearms in test chambers affixed to the skin. After 24 hours of occlusion, the chambers are removed, carefully wiping off any residual product, and chromametry is performed again. For a given corticosteroid, the blanching effect is stronger when the SC barrier function is impaired.

Baseline Transepidermal Water Loss

Susceptibility to sensory irritation has been reported, correlated with increased baseline transepidermal water loss (43–45). This characteristic supports the hypothesis according to which skin hyperreactivity to water-soluble irritants is related to increased permeation of the SC to these xenobiotics. Whether this condition is genuine or part of the self-exacerbating loop once irritation is already initiated and the SC damaged is uncertain.

Electrometric Assessments

Skin susceptibility to irritants has been reported to be associated with decreased capacitance (46). In our experience, this change is only present when previous challenges have already damaged the SC (37–39,46,47). It cannot be considered as an initial step of sensitive skin. In contrast, measuring the passive sustainable SC hydration and the SC water-holding capacity (5,47–49) following surfactant challenge might be a tool for discriminating sensitive and non-sensitive skins.

Squamometry and Other Microscopic Assessments of Corneocytes

Sampling corneocytes using self-adhesive clear discs and staining the harvested material by a toluidine blue-basic fuschin dye represent the initial steps of the squamometry test (29,50–53). The color is measured by the chroma C^*-value assessed by reflectance colorimetry. This measurement can be applied for different purposes (53). When it deals specifically with the interaction of surfactants with SC, the method is called squamometry S (53). Indeed, after a subclinical challenge with surfactants, the squamometry index increases (29,51–53). People with sensory irritation to surfactants may show increased reactivity. This finding is likely related to the presence of the so-called immature corneocytes (54).

Surfactants can extract some compounds from the SC, particularly dansyl chloride topically applied on the skin (55,56). This fluorescent dye can be removed more easily from the SC of a subset of subjects claiming to have sensitive skin to surfactants.

Miscellaneous Biometrological Findings

Some authors have reported that susceptibility to irritant xenobiotics was correlated with increased baseline in skin surface pH (36) and skin redness and with decreased sebum excretion (46).

CONCLUSIONS

In the vast majority of cases, sensitive skin to household cleaning products is a manifestation of sensory irritation. Various tricks can be used to assess this common condition. All the available methods only explore a limited aspect of the problem. A multipronged exploration is, therefore, recommended for fully covering the topic.

REFERENCES

1. Simion A, Rau AH. Sensitive skin: what it is and how to formulate it. Cosmet Toiletries 1994; 109:43–50.
2. De Groot AC, Nater JP, Van der Lende R, Ricken B. Adverse effects of cosmetic and toiletries: a retrospective study in the general population. Int J Cosmet Sci 1987; 9:255–259.
3. Kligman AM. The invisible dermatoses. Arch Dermatol 1991; 127:1375–1382.
4. Simion FA, Rhein LD, Morrison BM, Scala DD, Salko DM, Kligman AM. Self-perceived sensory response to soap and synthetic detergent bars correlates with clinical signs of irritation. J Am Acad Dermatol 1995; 32:205–211.
5. Paquet F, Piérard-Franchimont C, Fumal I, Goffin V, Paye M, Piérard GE. Sensitive skin at menopause; dew point and electrometric properties of the stratum corneum. Maturitas 1998; 28:221–227.

6. Lammintausta K, Maibach HI, Wilson D. Mechanisms of subjective (sensory) irritation: propensity to nonimmunologic contact urticaria and objective irritation in stingers. Derm Beruf Umwelt 1988; 36:45–49.
7. Goffin V, Piérard-Franchimont C, Piérard GE. Sensitive skin and stratum corneum reactivity to household cleaning products. Contact Dermatitis 1996; 34:81–85.
8. Piérard GE, Goffin V, Hermanns-Lê T, Piérard-Franchimont C. Corneocyte desquamation. Int J Mol Med 2000; 6:217–221.
9. Hamami I, Marks R. Structural determinants of the response of the skin to chemical irritants. Contact Dermatitis 1988; 18:71–75.
10. Berardesca E, Cespa M, Farinelli N, Rabbiosi G, Maibach H. In vivo transcutaneous penetration of nicotinates and sensitive skin. Contact Dermatitis 1991; 25:35–38.
11. Rietschel RL. Stochastic resonance and angry back syndrome: noisy skin. Am J Contact Dermatitis 1996; 3:152–154.
12. Tupker RA, Coenraads PJ, Fidler V, De Jong MC, Van der Meer JB, De Monchy JG. Irritant susceptibility and wheal and flare reactions to bioactive agents in atopic dermatitis. II. Influence of season. Br J Dermatol 1995; 133:365–370.
13. Goffin V, Piérard GE. Corneosurfametry and the compromised atopic stratum corneum. Arch Dermatol Res 1996; 288:489–491.
14. Paye M, Dalimier Ch, Cartiaux Y, Chabassol C. Consumer perception of sensitive hands: what is behind it? Skin Res Technol 1999; 5:28–32.
15. Coenraads PJ, Bleumink E, Nater JP. Susceptibility to primary irritants. Contact Dermatitis 1975; 1:377–381.
16. Gilchrest BA, Stoff JS, Soter NA. Chronologic aging alters the response to ultraviolet-induced inflammation in human skin. J Invest Dermatol 1982; 79:11–15.
17. Agner T, Serup J. Seasonal variation of skin resistance to irritants. Br J Dermatol 1989; 121:323–328.
18. Maibach HI, Berardesca E. Racial and skin color differences in skin sensitivity: implications for skin care products. Cosmet Toiletries 1990; 105:35–36.
19. Schwindt DA, Wilhem KP, Miller DL, Maibach HI. Cumulative irritation in older and younger skin: a comparison. Acta Derm Venereol 1998; 78:279–283.
20. Uter W, Gefeller O, Schwanitz HI. An epidemiological study of the influence of season (cold and dry air) on the occurrence of irritant skin changes of the hands. Br J Dermatol 1998; 138:266–272.
21. Piérard-Franchimont C, Piérard GE. Beyond a glimpse at seasonal dry skin: a review. Exog Dermatol 2002; 1:3–6.
22. Andersen F, Andersen KH, Kligman AM. Xerotic skin of the elderly: a summer versus winter comparison based on biophysical measurements. Exog Dermatol 2003; 2:190–194.
23. Lammintausta K, Maibach HI, Wilson D. Susceptibility to cumulative and acute irritant dermatitis. Contact Dermatitis 1988; 19:84–90.
24. Piérard GE. Skin weathering: the face at the interface. Dermatology 2003; 207:248–250.
25. Henry F, Goffin V, Maibach H, Piérard GE. Regional differences in stratum corneum reactivity to surfactants: quantitative assessment using the corneosurfametry bioassay. Contact Dermatitis 1997; 37:271–275.
26. Goffin V, Henry F, Piérard-Franchimont C, Piérard GE. Topical retinol and the stratum corneum response to an environmental threat. Skin Pharmacol 1997; 10:85–89.

27. Goffin V, Piérard-Franchimont C, Piérard GE. Shielded corneosurfametry and corneoxenometry: novel bioassays for the assessment of skin barrier products. Dermatology 1998; 196:434–437.
28. Piérard GE, Goffin V, Piérard-Franchimont C. Corneosurfametry: a predictive assessment of the interaction of personal care cleansing products with human stratum corneum. Dermatology 1994; 189:152–156.
29. Piérard GE, Goffin V, Piérard-Franchimont C. Squamometry and corneosurfametry in rating interactions of cleansing products with stratum corneum. J Soc Cosmet Chem 1994; 45:269–277.
30. Goffin V, Paye M, Piérard GE. Comparison of in vitro predictive tests for irritation induced by anionic surfactants. Contact Dermatitis 1995; 33:38–41.
31. Piérard GE, Goffin V, Hermanns-Lê T, Arrese JE, Piérard-Franchimont C. Surfactant induced dermatitis: a comparison of corneosurfametry with predictive testing on human and reconstructed skin. J Am Acad Dermatol 1995; 33:462–469.
32. Goffin V, Piérard-Franchimont C, Piérard GE. Microwave corneosurfametry: a minute assessment of the mildness of surfactant-containing products. Skin Res Technol 1997; 3:242–244.
33. Uhoda E, Goffin V, Piérard GE. Responsive corneosurfametry following in vivo preconditioning. Contact Dermatitis 2003; 49:292–296.
34. Goffin V, Letawe C, Piérard GE. Effect of organic solvents on normal human stratum corneum: evaluation by the corneoxenometry bioassay. Dermatology 1997; 195:321–324.
35. Piel G, Moutard S, Uhoda E, Pilard F, Piérard GE, Perly B, Delattre L, Evrard B. Skin compatibility of cyclodextrins and their derivatives: a comparative assessment using the corneoxenometry bioassay. Eur J Pharm Biopharm 2004; 57:479–482.
36. Wilhelm KP, Maibach HI. Susceptibility to irritant dermatitis induced by sodium lauryl sulfate. J Am Acad Dermatol 1990; 23:122–124.
37. Paye M, Morrison BM, Wilhelm KP. Skin irritancy classification of body cleansing products: comparison of two test methodologies. Skin Res Technol 1995; 1:30–35.
38. Paye M, Gomes G, Zerweg Ch, Piérard GE, Grove GG. A hand immersion test under laboratory-controlled usage conditions: a need for sensitive and controlled assessment methods. Contact Dermatitis 1999; 40:133–138.
39. Paye M, Cartiaux Y, Goffin V, Piérard GE. Hand and forearm skin: comparison of their respective responsiveness to surfactants. Skin Res Technol 2001; 7:78–83.
40. Frosch PJ, Duncan A, Kligman AM. Cutaneous biometrics. I. The response of human skin to dimethyl sulphoxide. Br J Dermatol 1980; 102:263–273.
41. Agner T, Serup J. Quantification of the DMSO-response: a test for assessment of sensitive skin. Clin Exp Dermatol 1989; 14:214–217.
42. Henry F, Fumal I, Piérard GE. Postural skin colour changes during the corticosteroid blanching assay. Skin Pharmacol Appl Skin Physiol 1999; 12:199–210.
43. Muruhata R, Crove DM, Roheim JR. The use of transepidermal water loss to measure and predict the irritation response to surfactants. Int J Cosmet Sci 1986; 8:225–231.
44. Tupker RA, Pinnagoda J, Coenraads PJ, Nater JP. The influence of repeated exposure to surfactants on the human skin as determined by transepidermal water loss and visual scoring. Contact Dermatitis 1989; 20:108–114.
45. Tupker RA, Coenraads PJ, Pinnagoda J, Nater JP. Baseline transepidermal water loss (TEWL) as a prediction of susceptibility to sodium lauryl sulfate. Contact Dermatitis 1989; 20:265–269.

46. Seidenari S, Francomano M, Mantovani L. Baseline biophysical parameters in sub-jects with sensitive skin. Contact Dermatitis 1998; 38:311–315.
47. Goffin V, Piérard-Franchimont C, Piérard GE. Passive sustainable hydration of the stratum corneum following surfactant challenge. Clin Exp Dermatol 1999; 24:308–311.
48. Piérard-Franchimont C, Letawe C, Goffin V, Piérard GE. Skin water-holding capacity and transdermal estrogen therapy for menopause: a pilot study. Maturitas 1995; 22:151–154.
49. Uhoda E, Paye M, Piérard GE. Comparative clinical and electrometric assessments of the impact of surfactants on forearm skin. Exog Dermatol 2003; 2:64–69.
50. Piérard GE, Piérard-Franchimont C, Saint-Léger D, Kligman AM. Squamometry: the assessment of xerosis by colorimetry of D-Squame adhesive discs. J Soc Cosmet Chem 1992; 47:297–305.
51. Charbonnier V, Morrison BM, Paye M, Maibach HI. Open application assay in inves-tigation of subclinical irritant dermatitis induced by sodium lauryl sulfate (SLS) in man: advantage of squamometry. Skin Res Technol 1998; 4:244–250.
52. Paye M, Cartiaux Y. Squamometry: a tool to move from exaggerated to more and more realistic application conditions for comparing the skin compatibility of surfac-tant-based products. Int J Cosmet Sci 1999; 21:9–68.
53. Piérard-Franchimont C, Henry F, Piérard GE. The SACD method and the XLRS squamometry tests revisited. Int J Cosmet Sci 2000; 22:437–446.
54. Hirao T, Denda M, Takahashi M. Identification of immature cornified envelopes in the barrier-impaired epidermis by characterization of their hydrophobicity and and anti-genicities of the components. Exp Dermatol 2001; 10:35–44.
55. Piérard GE. Microscopic evaluation of the dansyl chloride test. Dermatology 1992; 185:37–40.
56. Paye M, Simion A, Piérard GE. Dansyl chloride labelling of stratum corneum: its rapid extraction from skin can predict skin irritation due to surfactants and cleansing products. Contact Dermatitis 1994; 30:91–96.

14

Age and Gender as Influencing Factors in Skin Sensitivity

Michael K. Robinson

Procter & Gamble Company, Cincinnati, Ohio, U.S.A.

INTRODUCTION

Any attempt to assess and thereby to understand skin reactivity differences within and between human subpopulations is complicated by a variety of factors. Perhaps the most important of these is the simple statistical reality of making population-level assertions on the basis of relatively small sample sizes inherent within most comparison studies. This dilemma is illustrated in Figure 1. In Figure 1A, the two samples with very different reactivity profiles are drawn from two relatively non-overlapping parent populations. In Figure 1B, the two samples are of similar reactivity to those in Figure 1A, but are drawn from virtually indistinguishable populations. So, in the first case, measured (and statistically significant) differences between the two sample populations would, in fact, be representative of the actual populations from which the samples were drawn, whereas in the second case, one would only be sampling within the overall range of population variability. The presumption that the sample data truly reflect differences between the populations from which they were drawn would be correct in the first case, but not in the second.

In the case of population differences in skin reactivity, we are uncertain of the nature of the parent populations or the dynamics of those populations over time. So, observations of differences in reactivity among subsets of these populations have to be tempered by this uncertainty. This may also help

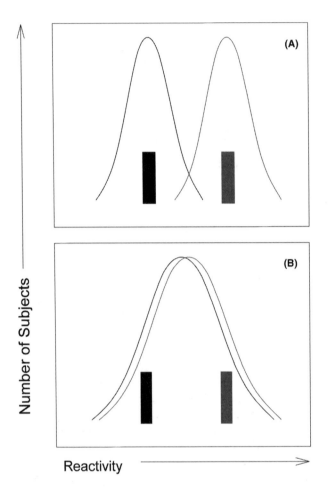

Figure 1   Schematic representation of the two small study populations with different reactivity profiles, but drawn from (**A**) two parent populations with distinctly different profiles or (**B**) two parent populations with virtually identical reactivity profiles.

explain why the literature on population differences in fundamental skin biology or skin responsiveness is so often conflicted (1).

Another critical factor in the effort to understand population differences in skin reactivity relates to the type of responses being evaluated. Some responses are objective in nature and can be measured by instrumental devices or visual grading. However, there are many parameters of skin reactivity, which are purely subjective or symptomatic in nature. These include the self-assessed quality of "sensitive" versus "normal" skin. They also include the various severities (e.g., mild, moderate, and severe) and qualities (e.g., sting, burn, and itch) of skin sensations to physical, chemical, or thermal insult. There are ways to quantify these symptomatic responses, but such measurements must be carefully controlled to avoid artifacts (2). Also, the type of scales used to measure such responses can greatly influence the utility of the data for comparative analyses (2) such as population response patterns or differences.

In the areas of gender- (sex) and age-related skin sensitivity, there have been a small number of studies conducted over the years to determine whether differences within either demographic category affects response profiles in selected test subject populations. Susceptibilities studied have included primary skin irritation, allergic contact sensitization, and self-perceptions of skin sensitivity. Within the context of the provisos stated above, some differences have been noted.

AGE AND GENDER DIFFERENCES IN BASIC SKIN BIOLOGY AND PHYSIOLOGY

Although beyond the scope of this book, it is pertinent to at least briefly consider differences in some of the basic characteristics of skin that may be influenced by gender or age. Characteristics such as skin thickness, barrier function, elasticity, wound repair potential, etc., can certainly influence overall skin reactivity profiles. A selection of published studies and reviews has indicated the following:

1. Reduced forearm skin elasticity with age (comparing pre- and post-menopausal women) (3)
2. Lack of differences in epidermal thickness with age (4)
3. Qualitatively similar wound healing response in elderly versus young subjects, but delayed response in the elderly (5)
4. Literature disparity on effects of aging on wound healing rates (6)
5. Epidermal thickness greater in men than in women (4)
6. Extent of skin barrier disruption (by tape stripping) and poststripping recovery similar in men and women (7)

The variability in results across studies of these types precludes any definitive conclusions.

AGE AND GENDER DIFFERENCES IN OBJECTIVE SKIN IRRITATION RESPONSES

Age Differences

The literature on age-related susceptibility to skin irritation generally shows a reduced sensitivity in older (i.e., >60 years) versus younger adults. A comparison of two widely different age groups (18–25 and 65–84) for reactivity to a strong irritant stimulus [24-hour patch exposure to 5% sodium lauryl sulfate (SLS)] showed greater mean reactivity in the young versus old subjects (4.57 vs. 2.62 on a 0–5 visual grading scale) (8). A similar study using a 20-fold lower SLS concentration gave comparable results (9). The mean response and percent positive responders were greater in young (average age 25.9) versus older (average age 74.6) test subjects. In some areas of the body (e.g., thighs), the response difference was quite dramatic. The lower visual grades in the older subjects were matched by a decrease in the magnitude of SLS-induced changes in barrier function.

Grove et al. (10) studied different types of chemical-induced skin irritation in young and old subjects. Using ammonium-hydroxide-induced blistering responses, they saw a more rapid initiation of blistering in their older (65–75) versus younger (18–30) subjects, but a much slower development of the full blister response. They also examined the response to a variety of irritants (e.g., histamine, DMSO, 48/80, chloroform–methanol, lactic acid, and ethyl nicotinate). In all cases, the visual grades were greater in the younger subjects. Elderly subjects also showed reduced reactivity to ultraviolet irradiation (UV) (11).

Very few studies have shown the opposite effect (increased irritation in the elderly), although some exist (12). Barrier function can also be more susceptible to the compromising effects of UV treatment among older subjects, even though visible skin reactivity is diminished (11).

In a recent survey of acute patch-test reactions to common irritants (13), results from multiple studies conducted over a period of four years were combined. In comparing response profiles across different age clusters, the oldest cohort of study subjects showed significantly reduced reactivity to two strong irritants (Fig. 2). Responses to weaker irritants were directionally, but not significantly, reduced in these subjects (data not shown). Therefore, this larger population analysis supported the conclusions from smaller base size studies that elderly subjects are somewhat less susceptible to common skin irritants.

Gender Differences

There is a longstanding perception that women are more sensitive to skin irritation than men, a finding not necessarily borne out in direct testing (14). In a study of barrier function, no differences were seen between men and women in terms of skin barrier integrity (i.e., loss in barrier function after tape stripping) or time for barrier recovery (7). In terms of irritant reactivity, specific incidences of irritant dermatitis can be either greater in women versus men or about the same, depending on the study (15). In any event, the incidence is almost certainly exposure-related as women are more often exposed to wet work and detergents but less to cutting oils and abrasives. Examination of wheal and flare responses to histamine iontophoresis did show a slight but significant increase in wheal responses in females versus males depending on the body site (16).

Compilation of results from multiple acute skin-irritation patch-test studies again provided an alternative approach to assess gender differences in reactivity versus isolated, smaller base sized studies (13). Each of four response profiles, comparing large cohorts of female and male subjects, showed directional or significantly

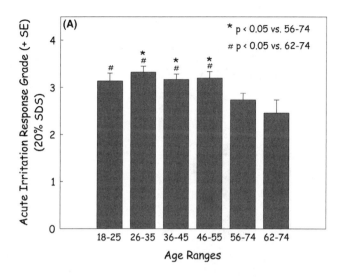

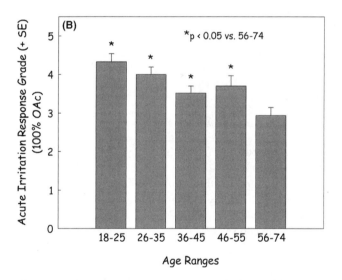

Figure 2 (**A, B**) The mean (±SE) acute irritation response grades for the indicated age group clusters to 20% SDS and 100% OAc, respectively. For SDS, the numbers of test subjects in each age cluster were 18 to 25 years (44), 26 to 35 years (77), 36 to 45 years (118), 46 to 55 years (80), 56 to 74 years (64), and 62 to 74 years (22) (one subject did not have his/her age recorded and was omitted from the analysis). For OAc, the numbers of test subjects in each age cluster were 18 to 25 (21), 26 to 35 (21), 36 to 45 (29), 46 to 55 (30), and 56 to 74 (34). The mean grades for each age cluster were cross-compared by statistical analysis. *Abbreviations*: SDS, sodium dodecyl sulfate; OAc, octanoic acid. *Source*: From Ref. 13.

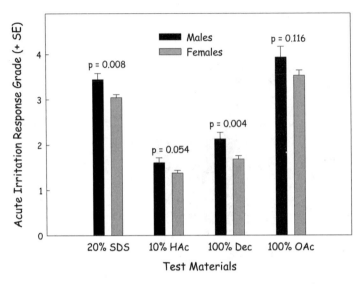

Figure 3 Comparison of acute irritation results for male and female test subjects patch tested with 20% SDS, 100% Dec, 10% HAc, and 100% OAc. The numbers of male and female subjects tested with each chemical were SDS (305 females and 79 males), Dec (203 females and 76 males), HAc (182 females and 77 males), and OAc (106 females and 29 males). The time of response for each subject to each chemical (using graduated 30 minutes to four hours of exposure) was converted to an acute skin irritation response grade. The mean grades ($\pm$SE) were determined and compared by statistical analysis. *Abbreviations*: SDS, sodium dodecyl sulfate; Dec, decanoic acid; HAc, acetic acid; OAc, octanoic acid. *Source*: From Ref. 13.

increased reactivity in the male population, regardless of the overall strength of the chemically induced irritation response (Fig. 3). Although not a definitive statement on gender-related susceptibility in general, these findings clearly did run counter to the common perception of greater reactivity in females. In a similar vein, a recent study has shown that male subjects were more sensitive to UV irradiation than females (lower, minimal erythema dose) (17).

AGE AND GENDER DIFFERENCES IN OBJECTIVE SKIN SENSITIZATION RESPONSES

Skin sensitization differs from skin irritation in its requirement for initial immune recognition of cutaneously encountered low-molecular-weight allergens. However, the dermatitis that is elicited after a secondary exposure to the same allergen can be very similar in appearance to primary irritant dermatitis. The requirement for immune recognition and response introduces an additional factor into the consideration of population differences in reactivity, that is, immune competence.

Age Differences

Age-related studies of skin sensitization are mainly limited to retrospective analysis of elicitation patterns and incidences across patch-testing cohorts. Here, the data are mixed and, because of the nature of the testing approach, it is difficult to separate age-related inherent susceptibility from age-related patterns of exposure. An early study (18) showed no age-related differences in the incidence of allergic patch-test reactions across four common contact allergens (nickel, neomycin, ethylenediamine, and benzocaine). However, other investigators have seen different trends. Goh (19) studied the response incidence to common patch-test tray allergens and saw a general increase in incidence in subjects >40 versus those <40. The trend was even greater when he compared subjects >59 versus those <20. As these totals were cumulative, they may just represent a greater tendency to become sensitized to different allergens as one progresses through life due to possible repetitive exposures. Young et al. (20) looked at the incidence on a per allergen basis and observed different patterns depending on the allergen; cobalt and nickel sensitivity was greater in those <30 versus those >50, but the reverse was true for wood tar. Again, this could be related to the exposure opportunities, but may also be a reflection of some diminution in response in older subjects assuming that they would have had the potential to be sensitized as younger adults.

A study of the elicitation of Rhus reactivity in presensitized young and older subjects showed temporal differences in onset and resolution of skin reactions (8). Young subjects showed a quick onset of reactivity and resolution by 9 to 15 days. Older subjects responded more slowly and the reaction resolved more slowly (12–26 days). Examination of sensitization to standard allergens as a function of age (from birth to >70 years of age) showed similar incidence of response across 0 to 7, 8 to 14, and 20 to 50 age groups, but a reduced incidence in the oldest (>70) age group (21). Kwangsukstith and Maibach (22) have suggested that the incidence of allergic contact dermatitis gradually increases from birth to 14 years of age, then holds steady in overall incidence but greatly varies by allergen on the basis of exposure patterns. The incidence declines with advancing age in terms of both the severity of response (possibly related to similar reduction in irritation responses discussed earlier) and a waning of the allergic response in previously sensitized individuals.

The only way to truly assess allergic sensitivity is to evaluate the induction of allergic contact sensitization in previously naïve subjects. Studies of this type are not generally done today, but studies from the earlier literature do shed some light on age-related susceptibility. Back in the early 1950s, Schwartz (23) studied the induction of sensitization to 2,4-dinitrochlorobenzene (DNCB) in previously naïve subjects of different ages. Approximately half of 174 subjects became sensitized. Among the three age cohorts (21–59, 60–79, and >80), there was no significant difference in the incidence of sensitization. Thus, for very potent sensitizers, there appears to be little age-related difference in allergic sensitivity.

Although focused on the very young, a different result was obtained more recently using DNCB induction and challenge in infants from birth to nine months of age (24). Using a set DNCB dose for induction and one-tenth of that dose for challenge, sensitization rates increased from approximately 7% at birth (up to 15 days of age) to 26% at the end of the first month, to 63% by the third month, and to 91% by the ninth month of life. These results are consistent with the understanding of the fact that the immune system is still maturing in the first months of life.

Gender Differences

Several studies have reviewed the epidemiology of elicited allergic responses to known allergens in men and women. An early study showed that response prevalence among four common allergens was strictly allergen-related (18). Women were far more reactive to nickel and men more reactive to ethylenediamine. Responses to two other allergens (neomycin and benzocaine) were equal. Young et al. (20) reported that women have a higher incidence of responses to cobalt, nickel, and Peru balsam and men have a higher incidence of responses to chromate and carba mix. Goh (19) reported an overall equivalent incidence of positive patch-test reactions among men (51%) and women (47%). Finally, a Finnish study showed a 60/40 preponderance of occupational allergic contact dermatitis among Finnish women versus men. Again, the relative preferential responsiveness was allergen-related. Women showed higher incidences of reactivity to rubber, nickel, and formaldehyde and men showed higher reactivity to epoxy resin, chromate, and colophony (25). As in the age-related studies, the overall findings indicate that exposure is the primary factor in relative incidence of sensitization and that prospective studies are needed to better assess inherent differences in reactivity (22). A compromise between retrospective sensitization rates and controlled exposures was obtained by assessing relative rates of sensitization to a transdermal drug (clonidine) during a clinical trial (26). The sensitization rate for women was twice that for men.

As with age-related studies, there are a few studies from the earlier literature that looked prospectively at the relative sensitivity of men and women to induction of allergic contact sensitization. Jordan and King (27) used the Draize human repeat-insult patch-test method to examine the relative incidences of induced sensitization to common (but not necessarily potent) contact allergens. Of 10 allergens studied, women reacted more frequently to seven. The other three showed equivalent incidences of reactivity. Leyden and Kligman (28) used the human maximization test and studied allergens from each of the five severity classes. Only with the weakest sensitizers (class I) did women react more commonly than men. With the other four classes, the frequencies of response were the same. Rees et al. (29) studied the induction of sensitization to experimental exposures to the strong sensitizer DNCB. They used a single exposure to induce sensitization and then did a dose–response challenge. Women showed a significantly stronger response than men, both in terms of severity of response as well as in the steep slope of the dose–response curve. Thus, from the collective data related to both induced sensitization and frequencies of sensitization in the population, the preponderance of evidence would suggest that women are, at least to a degree, the more sensitive population.

AGE AND GENDER DIFFERENCES IN SENSORY IRRITATION OR PERCEPTIONS OF SKIN SENSITIVITY

Direct testing of sensory irritation involves application of chemical (e.g., lactic acid, capsaicin, and histamine), thermal (heat and cold), or mechanical (tactile) stimuli to various parts of the body and capture of the resulting sensation by symptom grading. Examples include the lactic acid, chloroform/methanol, and capsaicin stinging/burning tests (30–33). Although studies of this type are numerous, few have directly addressed age- or gender-related differences in response profiles. One study of noxious and thermal stimulation of different areas of the face indicated disparate findings on age-related effects, although a slight reduction in response thresholds was observed with increased age (age range 20–89) (34), consistent with results on visible skin irritation described earlier. Although facial sting studies are often conducted in female subjects because of the perception of greater skin sensitivity (14,35), few studies have directly compared gender response patterns. A recent study of facial stinging showed an overall trend toward increased sensitivity among females across multiple test sites; however, individual site comparisons showed no such trend (36). Part of the difficulty in making clear distinctions between gender or age is likely related to the wide variation in response patterns within individual subjects, as a function of test site or chemical stimulant (36,37).

The general perception of sensitive skin is most commonly judged by individual responses to questions about current or past skin conditions (e.g., atopy) and/or sensitivities (e.g., clothing, products, and weather) (38). As with direct sensory response testing, there is a significant literature on the biological assessment of sensitive skin and the comparison with "normal" skin individuals. However, within the self-selected sensitive skin population, however defined, there has been little assessment of age- or gender-related comparisons. One recent study (39) evaluated both parameters. A total of 162 men and 258 women rated, on a scale of 1 (none) to 4 (severe), self-assessed skin sensitivity for a series of questions pertaining to general skin susceptibilities. There was a clear skewing of the response patterns with women assigning significantly greater numbers of moderate, strong, and severe scores. In contrast, the report stated that there was no relationship between response scores and the age of the respondents, although the age range of the respondents was not reported. A similar epidemiology study of sensitive skin (40), conducted via mailed questionnaires, assessed responses provided by 2046 women and 260 men. In sum,

51.4% of women versus 38.2% of men claimed skin sensitivity, with a greater incidence of women responding positively to several questions related to adverse responses to cosmetic or hair-care products. This survey study did not report on any age-related comparisons.

These few studies on direct sensory response testing and sensitive skin surveys tend to support the aforementioned notion that females have greater skin sensitivity than males. However, given the variability in sensory response across different treatments and test sites, even within individual subjects, and the apparent lack of significant gender differences in objective skin irritation responses, much more work is needed to solidify any such conclusion.

SUMMARY

As noted earlier, there is a general caution that needs to be applied to any study reporting differences in skin biology, reactivity, or symptoms. The caution simply relates to the fact that known intra-individual differences in skin reactivity (41) and the potential breadth of reactivity across large population clusters make it difficult to draw definitive conclusions from studies on limited numbers of subjects. With regard to gender-related differences in skin reactivity, there has been a prevailing tendency to regard females as a more sensitive population than males. Objective skin reactivity studies of skin irritation or allergic contact sensitization indicate that this is not necessarily correct, even within limited test populations. However, survey studies on self-assessed skin sensitivity indicate that at least the perception seems to be real. This finding and the gender-specific targeting of many skin-care and cosmetic products perhaps underscore the tendency toward the predominant use of female subjects for clinical skin safety testing and risk assessment (1).

Age-related differences in skin reactivity tend to be more consistent in the response patterns that have emerged from individual studies. The trend toward reduced skin irritation responsiveness in elderly subjects is a fairly common observation. This does not hold for allergic skin responses, where, except for the very young developing immune system, sensitivity is likely more related to exposure history than inherent differences in susceptibility per se. Self-perception of skin sensitivity as a function of age has not been studied well enough to draw conclusions.

The interest in evaluating and understanding inherent patterns of skin reactivity and significant differences in reactivity across populations continues to grow. Much of this is due to the current trend in development of products with improved tolerance profiles for all consumers, especially those with heightened skin sensitivity. It may also reflect the interest in marketing to specifically targeted segments of the population, on the basis of age, race, or gender. Regardless of the driving force, clinical research on this topic is likely to continue and this will only improve our understanding in the years to come.

REFERENCES

1. Robinson MK. Population differences in skin structure and physiology and the susceptibility to irritant and allergic contact dermatitis: implications for skin safety testing and risk assessment. Contact Dermatitis 1999; 41:65.
2. Green BG. Measurement of sensory irritation of the skin. Am J Contact Dermatitis 2000; 11:170.
3. Sumino H, Ichikawa S, Abe M, et al. Effects of aging, menopause, and hormone replacement therapy on forearm skin elasticity in women. J Am Geriatr Soc 2004; 52:945.
4. Sandby-Moller J, Poulsen T, Wulf HC. Epidermal thickness at different body sites: relationship to age, gender, pigmentation, blood content, skin type and smoking habits. Acta Derm Venereol 2003; 83:410.
5. Gosain A, Luisa MD, DiPietro A. Aging and wound healing. World J Surg 2004; 28:321.
6. Norman D. The effects of age-related skin changes on wound healing rates. J Wound Care 2004; 13:199.
7. Reed JT, Ghadially R, Elias PM. Skin type, but neither race nor gender, influence epidermal permeability barrier function. Arch Dermatol 1995; 131:1134.
8. Lejman E, Stoudemayer T, Grove G, et al. Age differences in poison ivy dermatitis. Contact Dermatitis 1984; 11:163.
9. Cua AB, Wilhelm KP, Maibach HI. Cutaneous sodium lauryl sulphate irritation potential: age and regional variability. Br J Dermatol 1990; 123:607.
10. Grove GL, Duncan S, Kligman AM. Effect of ageing on the blistering of human skin with ammonium hydroxide. Br J Dermatol 1982; 107:393.
11. Gilchrest BA, Stoff JS, Soter NA. Chronologic aging alters the response to ultraviolet-induced inflammation in human-skin. J Invest Dermatol 1982; 79:11.
12. Nilzen A, Voss Lagerlund K. Epicutaneous tests with detergents and a number of other common allergens. Dermatologica 1962; 124:42.
13. Robinson MK. Population differences in acute skin irritation responses—race, sex, age, sensitive skin and repeat subject comparisons. Contact Dermatitis 2002; 46:86.
14. Kligman AM. Assessment of mild irritants in humans. In: Drill VA, Lazar P, eds. Current Concepts in Cutaneous Toxicity. New York: Academic Press, 1980:69.
15. Shenefelt PD. Epidemiology of irritant contact dermatitis. In: van der Valk PGM, Maibach HI, eds. The Irritant Contact Dermatitis Syndrome. Boca Raton: CRC Press, 1996:17.
16. Magerl W, Westerman RA, Mohner B, et al. Properties of transdermal histamine iontophoresis—differential effects of season, gender, and body region. J Invest Dermatol 1990; 94:347.
17. Brockmans WMR, Vink AA, Boelsma E, et al. Determinants of skin sensitivity to solar irradiation. Eur J Clin Nutr 2003; 57:1222.
18. Prystowsky SD, Allen AM, Smith RW, et al. Allergic contact hypersensitivity to nickel, neomycin, ethylenediamine, and benzocaine: relationships between age, sex, history of exposure, and reactivity to standard patch tests and use tests in a general population. Arch Dermatol 1979; 115:959.
19. Goh CL. Prevalence of contact allergy by sex, race and age. Contact Dermatitis 1986; 14:237.
20. Young E, van Weelden H, van Osch L. Age and sex distribution of the incidence of contact sensitivity to standard allergens. Contact Dermatitis 1988; 19:307.

21. Wantke F, Hemmer W, Jarisch R, et al. Patch test reactions in children, adults and the elderly—a comparative study in patients with suspected allergic contact dermatitis. Contact Dermatitis 1996; 34:316.
22. Kwangsukstith C, Maibach HI. Effect of age and sex on the induction and elicitation of allergic contact dermatitis. Contact Dermatitis 1995; 33:289.
23. Schwartz M, Eczematous sensitization in various age groups. J Allergy 1952; 24:143.
24. Cassimos C, Kanakoudi-Tsakalidis F, Spyroglou K, et al. Skin sensitization to 2,4-dinitrochlorobenzene (DNCB) in the first months of life. J Clin Lab Immunol 1980; 3:111.
25. Kanerva L, Jolanki R, Toikkanen J. Frequencies of occupational allergic diseases and gender differences in Finland. Int Arch Occup Environ Health 1994; 66:111.
26. Weltfriend S, Bason M, Lammintausta K, et al. Irritant dermatitis (irritation). In: Marzulli FN, Maibach HI, eds. Dermatotoxicology. 5th ed. Washington, DC: Taylor & Francis, 1996:87.
27. Jordan WP Jr, King SE. Delayed hypersensitivity in females: the development of allergic contact dermatitis in females during the comparison of two predictive patch tests. Contact Dermatitis 1977; 3:19.
28. Leyden JJ, Kligman AM. Allergic contact dermatitis: sex differences. Contact Dermatitis 1977; 3:333.
29. Rees JL, Friedmann PS, Matthews JN. Sex differences in susceptibility to development of contact hypersensitivity to dinitrochlorobenzene (DNCB). Br J Dermatol 1989; 120:371.
30. Frosch PJ, Kligman AM. A method for appraising the stinging capacity of topically applied substances. J Soc Cosmet Chem 1977; 28:197.
31. Soschin D, Kligman AM. Adverse subjective responses. In: Kligman AM, Leyden JJ, eds. Safety and Efficacy of Topical Drugs and Cosmetics. New York: Grune & Stratton, 1982:377.
32. Christensen M, Kligman AM. An improved procedure for conducting lactic acid stinging tests on facial skin. J Soc Cosmet Chem 1996; 47:1.
33. Green BG, Bluth J. Measuring the chemosensory irritability of human skin. J Toxicol Cutan Ocul Toxicol 1995; 14:23.
34. Heft MW, Cooper BY, Obrien KK, et al. Aging effects on the perception of noxious and non-noxious thermal stimuli applied to the face. Aging Clin Exp Res 1996; 8:35.
35. Bowman JP, Floyd AK, Znaniecki A, Kligman AM, Stoudemayer T, Mills OH. The use of chemical probes to assess the facial reactivity of women, comparing their self-perception of sensitive skin. J Cosmet Sci 2000; 51:267.
36. Marriott M, Whittle E, Basketter DA. Facial variations in sensory responses. Contact Dermatitis 2003; 49:227.
37. Marriott M, Holmes J, Peters L, Cooper K, Rowson M, Basketter DA. The complex problem of sensitive Skin. Contact Dermatitis 2005; 53:93.
38. Seidenari S, Francomano M, Mantovani L. Baseline biophysical parameters in subjects with sensitive skin. Contact Dermatitis 1998; 38:311.
39. Loffler H, Dickel H, Kuss O, et al. Characteristics of self-estimated enhanced skin susceptibility. Acta Derm Venereol 2001; 81:343.
40. Willis CM, Shaw S, de Lacharriere O, et al. Sensitive skin: an epidemiological study. Br J Dermatol 2001; 145:258.
41. Robinson MK. Intra-individual variations in acute and cumulative skin irritation responses. Contact Dermatitis 2001; 45:75.

15

Sensitive Skin: Epidemiological Approach and Impact on Quality of Life in France

Laurent Misery

CHU Morvan, Service de Dermatologie, Brest, France

Eric Myon and Nicolas Martin

Département Santé Publique, Laboratoires Pierre Fabre, Boulogne, France

Sylvie Consoli

Cabinet Médical, Paris, France

Thérèse Nocera

Laboratoires Avène, Avène, France

Charles Taieb

Département Santé Publique, Laboratoires Pierre Fabre, Boulogne, France

BACKGROUND

Sensitive skin was described by Frosch and Kligman (1) and Thiers (2). Sensitive skin is caused by a combination of nervous and sensory messages from the brain or the central nervous system. Having sensitive skin can be caused by a variety of factors such as a damaged or disrupted skin barrier and a tendency to "overreact" to certain skin-care products. Sensitive skin can be defined as a true skin disease leading to stinging, burning, or tight feeling (possibly associated with pain or itching), which might be caused by the skin's sensitivity to variable climatic conditions (ultraviolet, warm, cold, or wind), "allergic" reactions to certain products (cosmetics, soaps, water, and pollution), psychological (stress), or hormonal actions (menstrual cycles) (3). An erythema is often associated but not always present. Some tests can facilitate the diagnosis and are useful exploratory methods: the stinging, heat sensitivity, and capsaicin tests. Women are more often affected than men, and variations occur during the menstrual cycle. It generally starts in adulthood and ethnic factors are involved. Association with dermatoses (seborrheic, dermatitis, acne rosacea, and atopic dermatitis) is sometimes noted, but the "reactive skin" symptom is generally found in isolation. Reactivity might be induced by cosmetics, especially if they are used incorrectly.

Very few studies have been conducted concerning the physiopathology of reactive skin. Non-allergic, non-immunological mechanisms cause lowering of the skin's tolerance threshold. A change in the skin's barrier function is noted, with insensible water loss that might entrance contact with irritant factors (4). Non-specific inflammation is thought to be associated with the release of IL-1, IL-8, PgE2, PgF2, and TNF-α (5). Histologically, vasodilatation and an inflammatory infiltrate are rarely found. Several arguments plead in favor of the probable role played by the cutaneous nervous system—the influence of psychological factors, abnormal skin sensations, and vasodilatation implies the involvement of the nervous system and the predictive nature of the capsaicin test (6). Neuromediators such as substance P and vasoactive intestinal peptide appear to be sources of neurogenic inflammation, leading to vasodilatation and mast cell degranulation (5).

Cortical factors may also be involved. The activation of certain regions in the brain after the capsaicin test shows that cortical integration occurs. However, the brain might also be the origin of aggravating (triggering?) factors in the case of stress or in certain people who might be in a particular mental state. There are also many cases of spurious sensitive skin: "having sensitive skin is a proclamation of one's sensitivity."

Therefore, it can be mentioned that reactive skin is characterized by abnormal reactivity whose tolerance threshold is lowered. The underlying mechanisms are poorly understood. It seems as if a "storm" of cytokines and neuromediators is unleashed, almost as though reactive skin was "cutaneous asthma."

OBJECTIVES

Despite the significance of sensitive skin, little epidemiological evidence exists with respect to its prevalence (7). Given this lack of epidemiological data on sensitive skin, at least in France, and because we know that skin diseases have a strong impact on the quality of life and psychological well-being of patients (8), we decided to assess its prevalence and consequences in France.

The aims of our study were to assess prevalence of sensitive skin in France and to take into account the patients' feelings and personal experience concerning the idea of sensitive skin and its consequences on their daily life. Moreover, we wanted to see whether seasons had any impact on patients' skin sensitivity, its prevalence, and consequences.

METHODS

Two studies were carried out by IPSOS Santé. The first survey took place in early March 2004 (winter season) and the second at the end of July 2004 (summer season). Samples consisted of, respectively, 1006 and 1001 individuals selected among a national representative sample of the French population over 15 years (omnibus survey). The survey participants were invited stratified by sex, age, profession of the head of family, category of town, and region (quota method).

It was based on the following hypothesis: "If the sample is structurally similar or identical to the reference field, then the results observed by the survey can be extrapolated to this reference population." The method's efficacy in many fields has, of course, been regularly validated by comparing survey data to the reality identified for the general population. The idea is therefore to establish a sample that is structurally comparable to the reference population, based on a certain number of variables for which this structure is known. In general population surveys, the most widely used variables are gender, age, profession, quotas applied in geographical strata (household size X region), and the stratification principle improving the reliability of estimations. Other variables may be individually used as additional quotas. In practice, the objective is therefore to build up a sample whose final structure, at marginal level, will be comparable to that of the reference population. As the global sample is made up of the assembling of all individual samples collected by the interviewers, the latter are frequently given an individual quotas plan, particularly in face-to-face methodology, where analysis of the sample structure can only be performed afterwards.

Questions on how they perceived their skin sensitivity and possible aggravating factors were asked. Quality of life was assessed using the SF-12 (9), a generic measure of health status. Eight concepts are measured through the 12 questions: physical functioning, physical role, bodily pain, general health, energy/ fatigue, social functioning, emotional role, and mental health. The SF-12 is composed of two dimensions, a physical component summary (PCS-12) and a mental component summary (MCS-12). Missing data were not replaced; if a question is left unanswered, then neither the SF-12 mental nor the physical scores can be calculated. The results are standardized on the general U.S. population [mean score of 50 (SD = 10)]; therefore, results can be meaningfully compared to an average and compared to one another. The lower the score, the more the quality of life is affected. Depressive symptomatology was evaluated using a validated scale, the depression subscore of the hospital anxiety and depression (HAD) (10). The depression subscale of the HAD is composed of seven items, allowing calculation of a total score between 0 and 21 and classification of depressive symptomatology into three groups: no symptomatology (total score between 0 and 7), doubtful symptomatology (total score between 8 and 10), and certain symptomatology (total score ≥ 11).

Quantitative data were compared using a Student's t-test (if two mean values were compared) or using analysis of variance (ANOVA) (if more than two mean values were compared). If the required conditions for those tests were not fulfilled, we used non-parametric methods such as Wilcoxon and Kruskal–Wallis tests. Qualitative data were compared with χ^2-test. All statistical analyses were performed using commercial statistical packages such as SAS® software v8.2.

Concerning the epidemiological data, prevalence was compared between the two studies (March and July). Concerning quality of life, results are presented for the two populations grouped for the SF-12 and for the July population for the HAD-depression subscale.

RESULTS

A part of the results from the first survey are already published (11), and some information on the psychological and seasonal impact will be published elsewhere (12). The results presented here are specifically focusing on the epidemiological data of the two surveys' samples and the consequences of sensitive skin on patients' daily life.

Characteristics of both samples were similar in terms of gender, age, profession of the head of family, town category, and region.

Although the survey was performed in two blocks, that is, March ($n = 1006$) and July 2004 ($n = 1001$), we combined both subsamples because no differences in the SF-12 scores were observed (data not shown). Data concerning the epidemiological comparisons are based on the two surveys compared and the HAD-depression subscale was administrated only in July. Both samples could be considered as representative samples of the French population (based on quotas method and therefore compared with the French population).

To make the comparison simpler, in some tables, the first survey concerns wintertime (the March survey) and the second survey summertime (the July survey).

In our population, the sex ratio was the following: men 963 (48%) versus women 1044 (52%). The respondents of the survey were distributed over the five regions of France as following: Ile-de-France (greater Paris) 18.1%, northwest 23.2%, northeast 23.7%, southwest 11%, and southeast 23.9% (Table 1). The largest proportion of respondents lived in municipal communities such as Paris and towns with over 100,000 inhabitants (45.4% together), followed by persons living in rural regions (22.1%). The annual income of the family head (usually father) was well distributed over the five categories, the highest proportion in the category of €13,000 to €23,000 as can be seen in Table 1.

When asked, "Do you have sensitive skin?" 11.9% (wintertime) in the first survey answered "very sensitive," 39.8% "sensitive," 28.5% "slightly sensitive," 19.1% "not sensitive," and 0.6% "gave no answer." For the second survey

Table 1 Demographic Description of the Population Sample of the French Survey

	n	Mean (SD)
Age (years)	2007	45.3 (18.2)

	n	Percent (%)
Region		
Ile-de-France	364	18.1
Northwest	466	23.2
Northeast	476	23.7
Southwest	221	11.0
Southeast	480	23.9
Total	2007	100
Living area/population density		
Rural	504	22.1
Less than 20,000	338	16.8
20,000–100,000	255	12.7
More than 100,000	581	29.0
Paris	329	16.4
Total	2007	100
Family income per year (in Euros)		
Less than 13,720	480	29.6
13,720–23,781	548	33.8
23,782–36,586	342	21.0
More than 36,587	253	15.6
Total	1623	100

(summertime), answers to the same question were different: "very sensitive" 20.7%, "sensitive" 38.2%, "slightly sensitive" 27.5%, "not sensitive" 13.2%, and 0.5% "gave no answer." Therefore, our population reported sensitive skin for 51.7% of the March population and 58.9% of the July one. Globally, the French population reported more skin sensitivity during summertime (Fig. 1).

For both surveys, the level of sensitivity was significantly higher in the female population ($P < 0.0001$). Regarding repartition by gender, comparison between the first and second surveys was significant only for women (Figs. 2 and 3).

Regarding possible seasonal impact on skin sensitivity, summertime favors some factors inducing skin sensitivity among women, such as changes in temperature, air conditioning, and more visible skin redness following exposure to the sun or emotion, whereas wintertime favors skin sensitivity related to cold and wind for men (Table 2). Also, men are more sensitive to pollution.

We also saw that the most reported factors inducing skin sensitivity are changes in temperature, pollution, sun, and tingling due to cosmetics, which are sources of skin sensitivity among, respectively, 57.8%, 54.4%, 53.4%, and 43.9% of the individuals with sensitive and very sensitive skin.

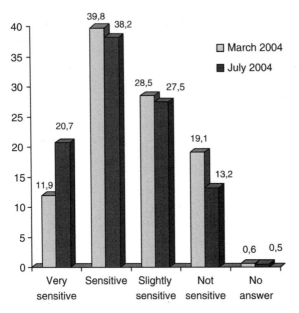

Figure 1 Skin sensitivity according to season (global population)—$P < 0.0001$—March 2004, $n = 1000$ and July 2004, $n = 996$.

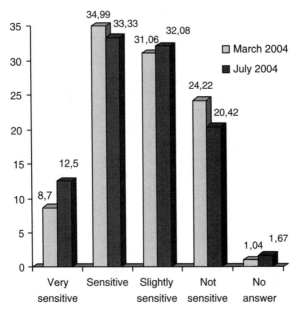

Figure 2 Men skin sensitivity according to season—$P = 0.2116$—March 2004, $n = 478$ and July 2004, $n = 479$.

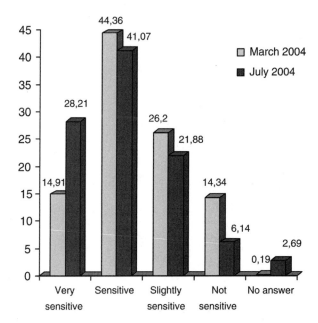

Figure 3 Women skin sensitivity according to season—$P < 0.0001$—March 2004, $n = 522$ and July 2004, $n = 517$.

Concerning sensitive skin and dermatological disorders, 253 persons reported a dermatological disorder (12.6% of the population); 36% were individuals with very sensitive skin, 48.6% had sensitive skin, 11.5% had little sensitive skin, and 4% had non-sensitive skin.

A history of atopic dermatitis or eczema was reported by 18.8% of individuals with sensitive or very sensitive skin.

Regarding dermatologist visits and skin sensitivity, those with sensitive skin were reported to have a dermatologist consultation more frequently when compared with those with non-sensitive skin; for example, if 5.4% of those with very sensitive skin and 9.7% of those with sensitive skin had a dermatologist consultation in the last 12 months, there were only 4.7% among those with little sensitive skin and 1.9% among those with not sensitive skin. For men and women, we demonstrated a more recent visit to the dermatologist during summertime than during wintertime (18.37% of men and 26.15% of women went to the dermatologist in the last 12 months in summertime when compared with 15.45% and 25.54%, respectively, in wintertime, $P = 0.0078$).

Individuals with a dry or oily skin were more numerous to report sensitive skin than the ones with a normal skin (Table 3).

In terms of quality of life, using SF-12, the PCS-12 score (49.87; SD = 8.3; min = 13.6; max = 65.3) was comparable with one of the general U.S. population (50 for the two dimensions).

Table 2 Skin Sensitivity (Percentage Answering Yes) According to Some Possible Factors and According to the Season

	Men			Women		
	First survey	Second survey	P-value	First survey	Second survey	P-value
Dry air	110 (23.31%)	103 (21.55%)	0.5162	211 (41.13%)	181 (35.01%)	0.0431
Skin redness due to sun	176 (36.74%)	194 (40.76%)	0.2031	244 (47.66%)	279 (54.60%)	0.0263
Skin redness due to emotion	197 (41.65%)	215 (45.36%)	0.2496	262 (51.47%)	304 (56.80%)	0.0183
Tingling due to cosmetic at least one time	125 (26.65%)	133 (28.24%)	0.5860	207 (40.04%)	233 (44.98%)	0.1078
Irritations or burns due to cosmetic at least one time	64 (13.62%)	77 (16.24%)	0.2574	131 (25.24%)	146 (28.24%)	0.2755
Changes in temperature	202 (41.82%)	208 (43.61%)	0.5764	272 (52.31%)	308 (59.23%)	0.0246
Pollution	196 (42.24%)	237 (49.79%)	0.0203	247 (49.80%)	278 (53.77%)	0.2058
Air conditioning	151 (32.75%)	181 (38.43%)	0.0705	181 (37.32%)	234 (46.34%)	0.0040
Cold	217 (45.02%)	170 (35.42%)	0.0024	312 (60.23%)	300 (57.80%)	0.4266
Wind	146 (30.48%)	110 (22.96%)	0.0086	252 (48.93%)	220 (42.47%)	0.0371

Table 3 Skin Sensitivity and Skin Characteristics

	Sensitive or very sensitive	Not sensitive or little sensitive	χ^2 *P*-value
Dry skin	521 (69.6%)	228 (30.4%)	94.01 <0.0001
Normal skin	358 (43.2%)	471 (56.8%)	90.33 <0.0001
Oily skin	212 (56.2%)	165 (43.8%)	0.06 0.8116

Concerning the mental dimension, the MCS-12 (46.78; SD = 9.7; min = 12.4; max = 68.7) score was a little bit lower. We observed a significant difference ($P < 0.001$) concerning men and women for the mental and physical dimension scores, the scores being higher for men (Fig. 4).

In addition, comparisons of the various degrees of sensitivity revealed differences, showing that the impairment in the mental dimension was more severe when the skin was more sensitive ($P < 0.005$ for men and women). For the physical dimension, relation between sensitivity and quality of life was not significant (Fig. 5).

Evaluation of depressive symptomatology using the HAD scale, in the July population ($n = 975$), showed that there was no significant link between depressive symptomatology and skin sensitivity: in the group "very sensitive or sensitive," 4.3% of subjects presented a certain depressive symptomatology versus 4.8% in the group "slightly or not sensitive" (Table 4).

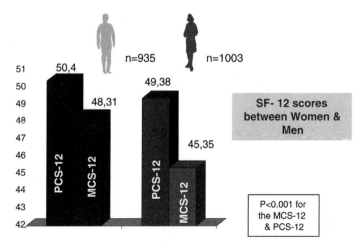

Figure 4 SF-12 scores according to gender.

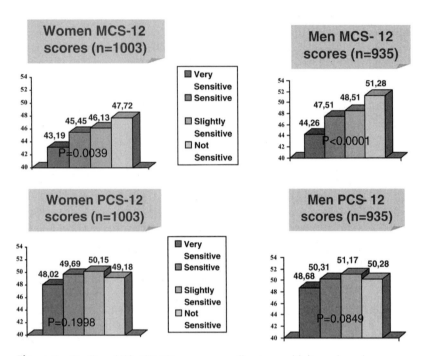

Figure 5   Quality of life (SF-12) scores according to sensitivity and gender.

DISCUSSION

The initial results from our study demonstrate that the idea of "sensitive skin" is perfectly well recognized and accurately rendered by the French men and women. This study is the second one assessing the prevalence of sensitive skin in France (11); the first one compared prevalence during summertime and wintertime. In addition, in the July population, we saw that 58.9% of them considered that their skin was very sensitive or sensitive; the difference in results between both studies suggests greater skin sensitivity during summer.

This study demonstrates a high prevalence of sensitive skin in France, similar to that observed in England (8) (51% of women and 38% of men declare having sensitive skin).

Table 4   HAD-depression Symptomatology According to Skin Sensitivity

	Symptomatology				
	No	Doubtful	Certain	Total	*P*-value
Sensitive or very sensitive	509 (87.9%)	45 (7.8%)	25 (4.3%)	579 (100%)	0.7393
Slightly or not sensitive	351 (88.6%)	26 (6.6%)	19 (4.8%)	396 (100%)	0.7393
Total	860 (88.2%)	71 (7.3%)	44 (4.5%)	975 (100%)	0.7393

Abbreviation: HAD, hospital anxiety and depression.

The phenomenon is very frequent. Although women are more frequently concerned, a high proportion of men suffer from sensitive skin.

Our study measures only subjective feelings of sensitive skin because there was no clinical exam.

As measured by SF-12, the higher the sensitivity, the more the impairment of mental dimension; no significant correlation was shown with the physical dimension.

Concerning the SF-12 scores of our population, they can be compared with the results of the study from Lecha et al. (13) in Spain, where SF-12 mean scores at inclusion for patients ($n = 727$) suffering from mild-to-moderate psoriasis were MCS = 46.6 and PCS = 52.2.

Nevertheless, the HAD-depression scale, which measures depressive symptomatology, did not bring to the fore any relation with skin sensitivity.

An assessment using a specific dermatology QoL scale would be relevant and allows better understanding and comparison of the impact of sensitive skin on patients' daily life.

REFERENCES

1. Frosch PJ, Kligman AM. A method of appraising the stinging capacity of topically applied substances. J Soc Cosmet Chem 1977; 28:197–209.
2. Thiers H. Peau sensible. In: Thiers H, ed. Les Cosmetiques. 2nd ed. Paris: Masson, 1986:266–268.
3. de Lacharriere O. Peaux sensibles, peaux reactives. In: Encycl. Med. Chir. Cosmetologie et Dermatologie Esthetique. Paris: Elsevier, 2002.
4. Seidenari S, Francomano M, Mantavoni L. Baseline biophysical parameters in subjects with sensitive skin. Contact Dermatitis 1998; 38:311–315.
5. Reilly DM, Parslew R, Sharpe GR, Powell S, Green MR. Inflammatory mediators in normal, sensitive and diseased skin types. Acta Derm Venereol 2000; 80:171–174.
6. Misery L. Les nerfs a fleur de peau. Int J Cosmet Sci 2002; 24:111–116.
7. Willis CM, Shaw S, de Lacharriere O, Baverel M, Reiche L, Jourdain R, et al. Sensitive skin: an epidemiological study. Br J Dermatol 2001; 45:258–263.
8. Lewis-Jones S. The psychological impact of skin disease. Nurs Times 2000; 96 (suppl 27):2–4.
9. Ware J, Kosinski M, Keller S. A 12-item short-form health survey. Construction of scales and preliminary tests of reliability and validity. Med Care 1996; 34:220–233.
10. Zigmond AS, Snaith RP. The hospital anxiety and depression scale. Acta Psychiatr Scand 1983; 67:361–370.
11. Misery L, Myon E, Martin N, et al. Peaux sensibles en France: approche epidemiologique. Ann Dermatol Venereol 2005; 132:425–429.
12. Misery L, Myon E, et al. Sensitive skins: psychological impact and seasonal variations. I Invest Dermatol 2005; 125:124.
13. Lecha M et al. Influence of tacalcitol on the quality of life of patients with psoriasis vulgaris in clinical practice. 11th EADV Congress, Prague, 2002.

16

Fabrics and Sensitive Skin

Kathryn L. Hatch

Department of Agricultural and Biosystems Engineering,
College of Agriculture and Life Sciences, University of Arizona,
Tucson, Arizona, U.S.A.

INTRODUCTION

Fabrics—thin, flexible materials composed of fibers, colorants (dyes and pigments), finish chemicals, and sometimes chemical residues acquired during manufacture, use, and cleaning—almost constantly contact human skin because they are made into garments, sheets, pillowcases, blankets, towels, and other household products. As fabric is pressed against the skin and as it moves over the skin surface, there is potential for (*i*) verbal expression of how the fabric feels, (*ii*) physiological responses by nerve endings and other sensory and regulatory mechanisms within the skin structure, (*iii*) mechanical and chemical irritation to the skin, (*iv*) deterioration of the wearers/users' health should the fabric contain allergic contact allergens, toxic, or mutagenic chemicals, and (*v*) transfer of chemicals beneficial to the wearers/users' health.

Ideally, this chapter should concentrate on presenting the results of studies whose objective was to learn why some people are fabric insensitive (have sensitive skin), although most are fabric tolerable (have normal skin sensitivity). Unfortunately, such studies were not found in the literature. Therefore, this chapter concentrates on reviewing research methods and studies that provide the foundation to design and undertake meaningful research into finding the reasons for (causes of) fabric intolerance (fabric sensitivity). Specifically, this chapter (*i*) describes current methods for assessing how the fabric feels against the skin, (*ii*) reviews studies in which changes in neural response, blood capillary flow response, and transepidermal water loss were examined as a result of fabric-to-skin contact, and (*iii*) reviews studies focusing on skin irritation caused by the fabric-to-skin contact. The unique features of this review compared to similar reviews (1–4) are that it includes a review of methods to assess how the fabric feels against the skin and organizes the relevant information differently. This review also adds the latest research papers. Not included in this chapter are discussions about allergic contact dermatitis and potential toxicity due to transfer of textile dyes and chemical-finish compounds from fabric to skin. Readers are referred to recent articles on these topics (5–10).

FABRIC FEEL

When the fabric is held or manipulated in one's hand or when it touches, moves over, or is compressed onto the skin of an individual's legs, arms, torso, neck, etc., it may cause the individual to describe how the fabric feels or responds. A person might use words such as soft, harsh, smooth, rough, prickly, cool, warm, clammy, comfortable, or uncomfortable to describe the sensation. Beginning as early as the 1920s, researchers proposed various sets of terms sometimes defining them, have proposed methods to obtain information from subjects about the intensity of the sensation (how soft and how uncomfortable), and developed procedures (protocols) to help insure the collection of reliable and repeatable data. Such efforts have been expertly reviewed by Cardello et al. (11), Sweeny and Branson (12), Civille and Dus (13), and others.

The purposes of this section of this chapter are to (*i*) describe the two types (classifications) of subjective instruments that have been developed, one for assessing specific sensory attributes (characteristics and perceptions) such as prickliness, softness, smoothness, etc. and one for assessing fabric tactile comfort (an evaluative or affective dimension); (*ii*) make a distinction between studies in which the protocol calls for manipulation of the fabrics in the hand (hand or tactile sensory studies) and those in which the protocol calls for wearing of the fabrics (wear sensory studies); and (*iii*) describe efforts to relate sensory data to fabric characteristics and properties. Readers interested in specific research projects, in which sensory data were collected when subjects wore garments made from different fabrics, are referred to (*i*) a study in which subjects wore garments made from 100% cotton fiber, from a 1.5 denier polyester fiber (14–19), and a 3.5 denier polyester fiber; (*ii*) a study in which subjects wore shirts made from wool or wool blended with other fibers (20); (*iii*) a study in which subjects wore various knit t-shirts (21); (*iv*) a study in which subjects wore sports-wear garments made from different fabrics (22); and (*v*) a study in which subjects wore protective coveralls of various fabrics (23).

Sensory Attribute Instruments

In sensory attribute (perception and characteristic) testing, a listing of possible sensory attribute terms is usually provided to subjects rather than allowing subjects to freely describe sensations, that is, use any word that comes to mind. The listing of the terms provided is often not presented with accompanying definitions. Fabrics may be manipulated in the hands or they may have been made into garments that are worn by the subjects. Such subjective testing can be conducted in a variety of environments with trained or untrained subjects/panelists sitting still, moving about, or following some exercise protocol.

Terms (descriptors) within the sensory attribute lists are thought to describe sensations triggered within the skin's sensory organs with the signals generated being sent to the brain. For example, an expression of prickliness is thought to be the result of the fabric triggering a certain type of nerve fiber, an expression of warmth to triggering of thermal receptors, and an expression of clamminess to the alteration of transepidermal water loss from the skin surface.

Lists of terms tend to be developed for use in hand/tactile studies or for use in wear studies. This makes sense as the types of sensations that might be felt by manipulating fabric in the fingers might not be assessed on other parts of the body and vice versa. One of the earliest and often used wear study sensory attribute lists (24) includes the terms snug, loose, heavy, light-weight, stiff, staticy, sticky, non-absorbent, cold, clammy, damp, clingy, picky, rough, and scratchy. Its intensity scale is partially, mildly, definitely, and totally. In a recently published wear study (20), the attribute terms were warm feeling, sticky feeling, prickle, absorbency, softness, mugginess, and roughness. A 10-point scale was used with descriptive terms at 5-point intervals along the scale. For example, for the term sticky, a subject could select "not at all sticky" associated with the score 0 at one end of the continuum, "slightly sticky" associated with scores of 1, 2, and 3, "sticky" associated with scores of 4, 5, and 6, "very sticky" associated with scores of 7, 8, and 9, or "extremely sticky" at the opposite end of the 10-point continuum.

Distinct from this method is the recently developed handfeel spectrum descriptive analysis (HSDA) (13) used by Cardello et al. (11) in a study about the feel of military fabric. Modeled after the methods used for sensory analysis of consumer products such as foods, perfumes, and skin-care products, the HSDA is said to be free of affective (good/bad) associations and to minimize differences between trained panelist ratings and consumer perceptions. Seventeen sensory attribute terms are included (grainy, gritty, fuzziness, thickness, tensile stretch, hand friction, fabric-to-fabric friction, depression depth, springiness, force to gather, stiffness, force to compress, compression resilience, compression resilience rate, fullness/volume, noise intensity, and noise pitch), each with a definition setting forth an underlying physical dimension. For example, the attribute term springiness is the "perception" of rate at which the sample returns to its original position after the downward force is released. Physical fabric standards are used as reference points along a 15-point intensity scale for each sensory attribute. Thus, the intensity scale for fabric "stiffness" is anchored at the upper end by a cotton organdy standard with a stiffness rating of 14.0 and at the lower end by a 50%/50% polyester/cotton single knit fabric with a stiffness rating of 1.3. Other fabrics define intermediate points on the intensity continuum.

Sensory Comfort Instruments

In contrast to sensory attributes, tactile or sensory comfort is thought not to be associated directly with any single human sense organ. Rather, sensory comfort is an evaluative or affective dimension, analogous to liking. There is no underlying physical dimension of the stimulus that varies continuously and is monotonic. This means that the same stimulus can elicit quite different comfort responses from different individuals. In other words, the subjective perception of fabric sensory comfort is a complex psychological process, involving numerous complex psychological processes, such as clammy, sticky, damp, prickly, and heavy. Each sensation is generated from different signals at the skin surface. By formulating, weighting, combining, and evaluating against past experiences, the brain derives conclusions on sensory comfort. Currently, there are three major methods to obtain a sensory comfort score for a fabric: (*i*) through an individual's subjective judgment of sensory comfort, (*ii*) by using statistical analysis on individual sensory attribute data, and (*iii*) using neural network processes.

Subjective Judgment Method

In this method, untrained subjects/panelists are asked to judge the sensory comfort of a swatch of fabric that they are manipulating in their hand, wearing, or laying upon. Simple scaling methods that require no training are considered to be best.

In a shirt study (20), subjects were to score the fabrics presented for "total comfort" by selecting one of the following expressions of comfort—"extremely uncomfortable" (scored as 0), "uncomfortable" (scored as 1, 2, or 3 depending on where the subject marked the scale line), "slightly uncomfortable" (scored as 4, 5, and 6), "comfortable" (scored as 7, 8, or 9), or "extremely comfortable" (scored as 10). In contrast, in a study about the feel of military fabrics (11), the comfort affective labeled magnitude (CALM) scale was used because the researchers decided that a labeled magnitude scale (sometimes called "semantic" or "category" ratio scales) rather than category scales, labeled category scales, or magnitude estimation methods would result in obtaining the most reliable data for "comfort." Labeled magnitude scales take the form of a visual analog or "line" scale, but are anchored with verbal labels that define a ratio scale of sensory magnitude. Terms along the scale were "greatest imaginable comfort," "extremely comfortable," "very comfortable," "moderately comfortable," "slightly comfortable," "neither comfortable nor uncomfortable," "slightly uncomfortable," "extremely uncomfortable," and "greatest imaginable discomfort."

Statistical Analysis Method

Multiple linear regression, cluster analysis, and factor analysis have been used to determine the contribution of each individual sensory attribute to sensory comfort and to obtain a predicted sensory comfort score (assessment) for a fabric. These methods have been reviewed by Wong et al. (25). Almost without exception, comparison of the predicted comfort scores with subjective comfort scores has resulted in good agreement, indicating that sensory comfort can be predicted using sensory attribute perception data. However, as pointed out by Wong et al. (25), the limitations to this means of establishing the overall sensory comfort of fabric include difficulty with complex non-linear relationships among sensory factors (attributes), lack of self-learning ability, and difficulty in handling the fuzziness of the psychological process.

Neural Network Software Method

Artificial neural networks (ANNs) are computational networks which attempt to simulate, in a gross manner, the networks of nerve cells (neurons) of the biological (human and animal) central nervous system. It is mentioned that defined ANNs are adaptive statistical models based on an analogy with the structure of the brain, because the ANN can learn to estimate the parameters of some populations using a small number of exemplars at a time.

Wong et al. (22,25) hypothesized that human overall comfort perception is determined by a few independent sensory factors (variables) with weights inserted by the brain consciously or unconsciously, which are derived from individual sensory perceptions. So they investigated whether the psychological process could be simulated with the same procedure but with a different methodology, by using statistical models and ANNs. Wong et al. (22) compared the statistical method to the back-propagation neural network approach and found that the neural network is a fast, flexible, predictive tool with a self-learning ability for clothing comfort perceptions. However, the functions and interrelationships of individual sensory perceptions (attributes) and comfort are unknown. Further studies have been completed by Wong et al. (26) and Hui et al. (27).

Sensory Data and Fabric Properties

Fabric/textile scientists have been particularly interested in learning the fabric characteristics (structural features performance properties) that are related to (correlated with) the various sensory attributes and sensory comfort. This information is particularly important in developing fabrics that produce desired sensory attributes and comfort. In turn, such information can be used to recommend certain fabrics to patients who have fabric-intolerant skin.

In this arena of research, considerable work has been directed to develop laboratory instruments that collect data, as the instrument simulates the motion and distortion of fabric using hand manipulation and to a lesser extent the stresses to fabric while worn. Fabric-property data of interest have been (*i*) low-stress mechanical properties such as bending, shear, and tensile deformation and (*ii*) fabric surface data such as smoothness/evenness, roughness, and friction coefficient. The most used instruments are those in the Kawabata evaluation system (KES)-F system (28) and in the fabric assurance by simple testing (FAST) system (29). Yick et al. (30) provide a description and comparison of these systems.

There has been renewed interest in objectively characterizing the surface friction of fabrics (31–33). Of note is Ramkumar's study (32) of changes in surface friction due to treating fabric with enzymes. Swatches of the woven cotton fabric used in the study were treated with cellulose enzymes at six different concentration levels to produce subtle changes in the fabric. A simple sliding friction apparatus was used to obtain data from which *R* (friction factor) was calculated. Those friction factors reflected the subtle differences produced by the finishing treatments. Untreated and finished swatches were also judged for smoothness by a panel of five knowledgeable judges. Findings included a strong correlation between subjective and objective data.

PHYSIOLOGICAL RESPONSES

The skin, composed of three major layers, the dermis, the epidermis, and the stratum corneum (SC), serves as the body's radiator, contains thermal receptors, sensory nerve endings that provide information to the brain about substances/materials that contact it, contains blood-filled capillaries, and controls the passage of transepidermal water through underlying tissues and into the environment at the skin surface. Researchers have investigated how the placement of fabric on the skin alters the skin environment. The purpose of this section is to review those studies.

Neural Response

During the 1980s, research sponsored by the Commonwealth Scientific and Industrial Organization (CSIRO) and undertaken by Garnesworthy et al. (34) focused on understanding the neurological basis for the sensation called prickle, which they defined as "feeling many very gentle pin-pricks." This project also included identifying the construction features of the fabric responsible for this sensation.

The first phase of the work by Garnesworthy et al. involved discovering which nerve fibers in the skin were triggered when fabric/fibers contacted them. Nerve-block experiments were conducted using human subjects and also rabbits. As a result of nerve-block experiments on 12 human volunteers, Garnesworthy et al. thought it was the small diameter nerve fibers of both the thermal and the pain groups that were responsible for the prickle. However, as a result of making recordings of the responses of single nerve fibers in rabbits while they applied fabrics of different prickle intensities to an innervated area of their skin, they noted that only the pain group of receptors responded differently. Thus, it was the pain group of nerves that were triggered by fabrics/fibers. Similar results were achieved from single-fiber recordings conducted with human subjects, demonstrating that pain nerves are involved in prickle sensation.

The second phase of the work involved discovering fabric features that would assist wool-fabric manufacturers in producing fabric free of prickle sensation. These experiments showed that a force of about 100 mgf was required at the end of a 40 μm diameter fiber to trigger a pain receptor. Thus, the stimuli on fabrics that trigger pain receptors to cause prickle are protruding fiber ends capable of supporting loads of about 100 mgf or more without buckling against the skin.

The third phase of the work consisted of psychophysical experiments, in which fabrics of different prickle sensation were pressed onto and slid over different skin areas of human volunteers. CSIRO researchers found that (*i*) prickle results only when the fabric is pressed onto a skin surface, not when the fabric is slid over the skin, and (*ii*) the skin must have hair follicles for the prickle to be felt. So, the prickle can be felt on the forearm but not on the fingers and palms. Further, they discovered that prickle is an elusive sensation and may fluctuate in intensity over a period of seconds. Several seconds usually elapse between the time when the fabric capable of eliciting a prickly sensation is pressed on the skin and when the prickle is felt. They found a pressure of 4 g/cm^2 to be near the upper limit of typical downward pressure at which the prickle is sensed. Other results were that prickle cannot be felt if the skin is uncomfortably cold or the skin contact area is smaller than about 1 cm^2. Moisture on the skin greatly increased the magnitude of the sensation.

It was also found that chemicals are released at or near the nerve endings, which dilate surface blood capillaries. Reddening first occurred in the vicinity of activated pain nerve endings and then diffused over larger areas. Inflammation may appear within one hour or more slowly after several hours of skin contact. It usually subsides rapidly after the removal of the irritant from the skin unless the skin/fabric contact over several days has produced a severe inflammation. Fabrics that are abrasive or poke the skin may produce this irritant response.

LaMotte (35) studied cutaneous receptor response due to sliding fabrics and a bare metal plate over a monkey's hand. An electromechanical device displaced the monkey's skin. The response of the nerve fibers to fabric was always greater than the response to the smooth, uncovered metal plate. The intensity of response of the mechano-receptive nerve fibers to the fabrics depended on the amount of skin displacement, the weave of the fabric, the density of the fabric, and the rate of movement of the fabric. Precise relationships between nerve response and fabric construction were not obtained.

Gwosdow et al. (36) studied the degree of unpleasantness experienced by eight male volunteers when six different fabrics were slid across their forearms. Force required to pull each fabric over the skin increased as the skin became wetter. As force and skin wetness increased, subjects rated all fabrics as feeling rougher and less pleasant. The researchers concluded that "moisture on the skin surface increases skin friction, which enhances perception of roughness..."

Capillary Blood Flow

Wester et al. (37) were interested in whether the insulative nature of certain fabrics altered human capillary blood flow. Capillary blood flow was measured using laser Doppler velocimetry, a non-invasive low-power laser-light optical technique. Two fabrics that differed significantly in thermal conductivity, a fourfold difference as determined by the guarded hot-plate method, were placed on the upper arm of 10 female volunteers. Blood flow was significantly higher under the fabric with lower thermal conductivity.

Wester et al. (37) investigated whether the abrasive nature and/or prickliness of certain fabrics might alter capillary blood flow. Two fabrics were selected that differed substantially in contact sensation; one was soft and the other coarse. The thermal effect was controlled by layering of the fabrics before they were worn under a tricot top on the upper back. On one side of the upper back, the coarse fabric contacted the skin; on the other side, the soft fabric contacted the skin. Skin blood flow increased from zero to three hours, but there was not statistically significant difference between the fabrics. However, six of the nine volunteers showed higher blood flow when the coarser fabric was next to the skin than when the softer fabric was next to the skin. The researchers concluded that fabric influences skin blood flow, but that it is not known whether the prickling of or abrasive action on the skin by fibers in the fabric altered the blood flow or whether any flow alteration was undetectable due to instrumentation and methodological limitations.

Transepidermal Water Loss

Placing fabric over the skin surface without any downward or lateral movement of the fabric relative to the skin may cause changes in the skin. One of the primary ones is hydration of the SC because (*i*) the fabric usually acts as a barrier to the loss of transepidermal water evaporated at the skin surface or (*ii*) the fabric is a source of water that may contribute to the SC hydration. The primary change, an increase in the SC hydration, may lead to other events such as increased susceptibility to microbial growth, abrasive damage, and absorption of chemicals, and altered pH with inflammation of the skin as a final outcome or manifestation (38).

Two main types of assessments have been used to determine the effect of fabric on moisture in or on the skin. The first type involves the use of instruments that measure the water content of the SC or measure the rate of evaporative water loss as an indication of the SC water content. Hydration due to fabric covering the skin is the difference between measurements taken after covering the skin with fabric and those taken on uncovered skin. The second type involves the use of rating scales by which subjects indicate skin wetness, procedures described in the "Fabric Feel" section of this chapter.

Studies in which the effect on the skin of diaper and incontinence materials/products while dry, wetted with water, and soiled during use have been reviewed by Cottenden et al. (39) and by Hatch and Maibach (3). In general, researchers have found that wearing diapers, incontinence pads, or patches cut from these products does elevate skin wetness as determined instrumentally. This is not surprising in that these products are designed to hold urine (liquid water). The inner layers absorb the urine and the outer materials are usually water resistant (waterproof) and not water vapor permeable. The products fit tightly to the skin allowing little opportunity for ventilation. The SC hydration differs depending on the materials used in the product. In general, products containing super-absorbent polymers keep the skin driest. A notable exception occurred in the study by Dallas and Wilson (40) in which no significant differences in skin wetness were found for disposable incontinence pads containing super-absorbent and not containing super-absorbent and reusable pads. However, there were several significant differences within the groups.

Cottenden et al. (39) focused on discovering the pad characteristics (absorption capacity, strike-through time, and rewet property) that resulted in the best-wet comfort. To do so, they used experimental pads composed of different combinations of materials, but the same design (hourglass-shaped). Twenty lightly incontinent women used the range of experimental pads. In the first phase, the women used a random mix of three of the six pad variants, they logged the time at which they put on and took off each pad, and scored it for leakage performance, wet comfort, and absorbance using a 3-point scale (good, ok, and poor). Used pads were weighed and the pad performance studied as a function of urine weight, wear time, and put-on time. In the second phase, the women were asked to compare the overall performance and leakage performance of different pairs of pad variants after a week of use. Pads with high absorption capacity and low rewet were rated the best. However, they concluded that "differences are smaller than conventional wisdom would have predicted and often failed to reach statistical significance."

Hatch et al. (15,18,19) and Cameron et al. (41) assessed the SC hydration when garments made by commonly used fabrics were worn by subjects. In an initial study by Hatch et al. (42), subjects wore patches of dress-weight woven fabrics composed of triacetate and polyester. The longer the patches were in place, the higher the SC hydration became. The SC hydration was higher when a water vapor impermeable film was placed over the swatches than when it was absent. The SC hydration differed depending on the moisture-absorbing properties of the fabrics when the water vapor impermeable film was in place, but did not differ when the impermeable film was not used. This initial study was followed by a series of studies in which the same set of three jersey knit fabrics (the first of all cotton fibers, the second of all 1.5-denier polyester fibers, and the third of all 3.5 polyester fibers) was used. In the first phase of the study, subjects exercised while wearing garments made from the three fabrics. At intervals during the exercise protocol, subjects reported sensory attribute and comfort sensations and the research team instrumentally determined the SC water content and the rate of evaporative water loss. There were no significant differences in water evaporation or the SC water content because of the type of fabric, a result that was not expected due to significant differences in water absorption capability of the fabrics. Further, subjects did not indicate differences between fabrics for wetness sensation. Because the fabrics did not lie on the skin where the SC assessments were made, the next phase of the study involved placing swatches of the fabrics with different amounts of moisture in them on the volar forearm of sedentary volunteer subjects. These swatches were covered with a water vapor impermeable film. Under these conditions, the trend was that the wetter the fabric applied to the skin, the higher the SC hydration at its removal.

In the study by Cameron et al. (41), placement of dry fabrics on the skin with a water vapor impermeable cover did not significantly affect the hydration level of the SC, though all dry fabrics did increase the hydration level slightly. Wet wool and cotton fabrics significantly hydrated the SC when the levels were compared with either uncovered skin or skin covered by dry fabrics. Of the seven synthetic-fiber fabrics tested in a wetted state, three (acrylic, PTFE, and spun nylon) significantly increased the SC hydration level. These three fabrics and the natural fabrics had comparable wetted moisture content.

SKIN IRRITATION

This section considers studies in which fabric was rubbed on the skin, sometimes on pre-irritated skin. Assessment focused on changes to the structure, coloration, or functional properties of the skin. The subsection on mechanical irritation focuses on those studies in which fabrics differing in softness were rubbed on the skin. The subsection on chemical irritation focuses on studies in which the fabrics being rubbed contained substances that might cause chemical as well as mechanical irritation. Studies are in chronological order in both subsections.

Mechanical

Piérard et al. (43) studied the effects of gently rubbing swatches of cotton terrycloth fabric on the forearm skin. Two sets of swatches were prepared: one set was cut from terrycloth that had been laundered with detergent only and the others cut from terrycloth softened with a fabric softener product following laundering in detergent. Fifteen volunteers who (*i*) had "sensitive" skin according to dermatological and their own assessment, (*ii*) had "dry" forearm skin, and (*iii*) were free of any pre-existing allergic sensitivity to materials were selected. Three days before the testing, skin areas on each forearm were treated with 0.2 mL of a 2% solution of sodium lauryl sulfate under plastic occlusion to produce pre-irritated skin areas. Other skin areas were wetted with water to produce control areas. During the testing, dry swatches of softened and unsoftened terry-cloth were rubbed gently on the prepared skin areas of one forearm and wet swatches on the prepared areas of the other forearm. Skin effects were determined by visual grading (redness, dryness, and smoothness), by non-invasive skin stripping and measuring of chroma C^* (squamometry), and by instrumental measurements (capacitance, transepidermal water loss, and colorimetry).

No deleterious effects on control or pre-irritated skin were induced by softened or unsoftened terrycloth (wet or dry). A mild beneficial effect was observed with the softened terrycloth particularly on pre-irritated skin. The authors state that "the study findings suggest that softened fabrics may exert a reduced frictional effect on the skin."

Hermanns et al. (44) undertook a study to confirm the safety of atopic skin exposure to fabrics softened during laundering with a fabric softener product and to determine whether softened fabric offers a skin benefit relative to fabric not softened during laundering. The fabric was a 100% cotton terrycloth washed five times with a powder detergent to remove any chemical finishes. Half of the terrycloth was laundered again with the same detergent in a normal cycle at 60°C and line dried. The other half of the fabric was identically washed and dried, but liquid fabric softener was added during the rinse cycle.

Twenty volunteers with atopic skin were selected. The experimental design was the same as for the Píerard et al. (43) study, except the concentration of sodium lauryl sulfate for each volunteer was determined in a dose–range study to induce a similar slight-to-moderate erythema. Data were analyzed for differences between softened and unsoftened terrycloth.

The findings were that rubbing of atopic skin with terrycloth generally resulted in discrete-to-moderate alterations of the structure of the SC. Both for control and for pre-irritated skin, all measured parameters indicated that softened terrycloth was less aggressive to the skin than unsoftened terrycloth. In the case of pre-irritated skin, the recovery of the skin was significantly faster when rubbed with softened rather than unsoftened fabric. The researchers concluded that "softened fabrics help mitigate the skin condition in atopic patients."

Farage et al. (45) sought to improve upon two standard tests—the semi-occluded patch on the upper arm (46) and the wrist-band test, six-hour exposures daily for four days (46), to increase the reliability of selecting fabrics that would not irritate human skin as they repeatedly moved over the skin surface.

In their study, the two fabrics used—a satin fabric (a smooth-surfaced fabric) and a burlap fabric (a rough-surfaced fabric)—represented a non-irritating fabric and a highly irritating fabric because they wanted two fabrics that should produce significantly different results. If they did not, then it would not be reasonable to expect their procedures to differentiate among/between other materials. Subjects were females 18 to 65 years old with no skin irritation. Swatches from the irritant and non-irritant fabrics were secured to the back of the knee using an Ace elastic bandage, to the axilla using a snug-fitting garment, and to the wrist using an athletic band. These methods of application were thought to provide continuous skin contact between fabric and skin while allowing movement of the fabric over the skin surface. Exposure regimens were (*i*) six hours daily for four days, (*ii*) 24 hours daily for three days, and (*iii*) 24 hours daily for four days. Irritation on the test sites was scored on a 9-point visual scale prior to initial application and 30 to 60 minutes after removal of the fabrics each day.

Mean differences between scores of the irritant and non-irritant fabrics were calculated. The regimen that resulted in the greatest mean difference with the smallest variability (as a function of the standard deviation) was considered to be the most likely to detect small differences in intermediate levels of irritation. Quantitative measures of these abilities were used to rank the overall effectiveness of various test protocols as a model for mechanical irritation. The result was that attaching the test fabric to the back of the knee for six hours daily for four days, led to the most effective test system for evaluating mechanical irritation of the fabric to the skin.

Farage et al. (47) also wanted to find the best method to differentiate the irritation potential of fabrics having intermediate ability to cause mechanical irritation. So, they had the following three objectives in the follow-up study to the one reported earlier.

1. Validate the test model using a variety of conditions, including those that mimic the conditions that exist during normal product use.
2. Determine the most cost-effective protocol to use for screening different product executions for potential irritant effects.
3. Evaluate sensory responses that consumers often associate with irritation to determine whether any of these sensations correlated with objective measures of irritation.

In this experiment, the test materials were products intended to be worn for prolonged periods of time on body sites that include the mucous membrane and non-keratinized epithelium in addition to normal squamous cell epithelium. More specifically, the products were catemenial pads. These pads were applied daily to the area behind the knee and held in place for six hours by an elastic knee band. Irritation was graded 30 to 60 minutes after test product removal and the following morning before application of the next sample. Two products were compared using four different protocol variations: dry product on intact skin, dry product on tape-stripped (compromised) skin, wet product (product loaded with 8 mL of saline) on intact skin, and wet product on compromised skin. An additional study compared the two products using two protocol variations (intact skin/dry product vs. compromised skin/wet product). In addition, a study (#5) was conducted to compare a third product applied wet on intact versus compromised skin. In the final two studies, information was collected from the panelists on subjective sensations of irritation. Words used were burning, sticking, pain, and any complaint.

Findings were that all four protocol variations were capable of detecting significant differences between the products. Product differences were directionally similar to those provided in subjective consumer comment data. In addition, a higher number of certain perceived sensory effects were reported for the more irritating product.

Chemical Irritation

Detergent Residue

Matthies (48) provides a recent, comprehensive review of the literature pertaining to the role of detergents in textiles in causing irritant dermatitis. His review includes detergent left in fabric as it enters the consumer marketplace and detergent left in fabric after home and/or commercial laundering of soiled fabric as well as irritation to hands when textiles are hand-washed. The reader is referred to this excellent review for specifics. The conclusion Matthies reached is as follows:

"The main intended contact between detergents and textiles is laundering of clothes in household or in professional laundries. There is little evidence that usual procedures of cleaning might lead to a health risk for the consumers. Residues of detergents on fibres are present at an amount which is typical for the respective type of textile. Repeated evaluations of residue analysis, especially surfactants, showed a significantly higher capacity of adsorption of cotton compared to synthetic fibres (e.g., polyester). However, even the highest measured amounts of residues on textile probes were unable to induce irritation to the skin of volunteers. This holds true for open as well as for fully occluded application."

This conclusion was also reached in those few studies not cited in the Matthies review (48) and those studies published after the Matthies review was completed. For example, Bannan et al. (49) studied whether the introduction of enzymes into detergent formulations (in liquid, powdered, or concentrated packets) introduced irritant effects to fabrics laundered with these products. The exposures used for each of the 17 treatments were a wrist-band test (simulates a tight-fitting garment), a men's briefs test (also simulates a tight-fitting garment), a men's t-shirt test, an infant wear and cloth-diaper test, and extended home-usage tests. These test conditions simulated tight-fitting garments— situations in which there is close contact of the fabric with the skin. Subjects were volunteers. Only the 150 volunteers for the men's t-shirt test claimed to have a history of sensitive skin. The results under all the conditions of test were that "the presence of enzymes in laundry detergents does not introduce irritant properties of fabrics." Dermal irritation grades (medical and subjective) were not always zero—no irritation. Also, a number of itch/rash comments were received from volunteers in the t-shirt-irritation test and the three-month laundry product home-usage test.

In 2003, Kiriyama et al. (50) investigated whether residual washing detergent in cotton clothes plays a role in the winter deterioration of atopic dry skin because they noticed that skin areas covered with clothes tended to be drier than exposed areas. They knew through experimentation that (i) the common practice of washing cotton garments in cold water (10°C) using an anionic detergent followed by rinsing in cold water led to concentrations of residual detergent of 125 mg in 100 g of cotton fabric and (ii) cold water washing of cotton garments in non-ionic detergent resulted in one-third of the residue left by cold water washing with anionic detergent. They were also aware that dryness of the skin was most prominent around the shoulders of atopic patients; an area where there was the most movement of fabric across the skin.

In their experiment, photographs were taken to record the distribution of dry skin on the trunks of 148 of their patients with atopic dermatitis. Of these, 115 (76%) had widespread or localized dry skin on the trunk with 95 of these patients having prominent dry skin around the shoulders and 33 (22%) did not have clinically recognizable dry skin on the trunk. All 115 patients were asked to stop washing their clothes with common anionic, additive-enriched detergents and to use a non-ionic additive-reduced detergent for two weeks. Cold water washing and rinsing continued. Change in the severity of dry skin was assessed comparing skin dryness in the before photos with the after photos. Visual assessment was markedly improved, moderately improved, slightly improved, unchanged, and worsened. Patients were also asked whether the severity of dryness on their trunk has attenuated, unchanged, or worsened.

Eighty-seven of the 115 patients showed marked or moderate improvement of dry skin after the two-week use of the non-ionic, additive-reduced detergent. No patient had a worsening of dry skin. The researchers concluded that residues of common washing detergents in cotton underclothes play an important role in the winter deterioration of dry skin in patients with atopic dermatitis who use cold tap water for washing their clothes.

Belsito et al. (51) undertook a study of allergic contact dermatitis to detergents, a skin condition that is clearly not the focus of this manuscript, but that study needs to be referred to here because this team concluded that previously reported "incidence rate for detergent-induced allergy of 0.7% of dermatitic patients may be too high, possibly because of false-positive irritant reactions." They invited 3120 eligible patients to enroll in their study. Of these, 738 volunteered. Patch testing of these 738 patients led to five (0.7%) positive patch tests.

Laundry-Applied Fabric Softeners

Matthies (48) reviewed the literature pertaining to fabric softeners and irritant dermatitis. He concluded that "the use of after-treatments and functional treatments seems to be an area of special attention. While typical after-treatment like softeners were seen as helpful and safe even in atopic and in children's skin, functional treatments for antibacterial or antifungal efficacy may cause problems when applied under stress conditions. New clothes therefore should be rinsed carefully before wearing. Unspecified skin symptoms like itching, redness, folliculitis, etc., may be connected with indirect influences. This means changes in the surface electrical charge, change in the permeability against vaporizing sweat, but also contaminations with materials from occupational or accidental contact. Last but not least, it should be remembered that simple mechanical alterations may lead to friction, tension, and abrasion with subsequent skin symptoms."

Matthies (48) also says that "it becomes clear that diagnosing . . . dermatitis from textiles and detergents is a complex and meaningful procedure. There are . . . factors that . . . contribute to a better state of the skin [such as] softeners for diapers or wool treatments, [in] which the amount of residue of detergents should normally be too low to cause direct reactions. On the other hand, changes in the surface of textiles may lead to discomfort if microclimate and vaporization is worsened. This will be an interesting and wide field for research in the future."

Hygiene Products

Ehretsmann et al. (52) conducted a three-part study to confirm the safety and cutaneous tolerability of a new brand of baby wet wipes. The three clinical study methods and results were as follows:

Study A was a double-blind in-use design involving 102 infants over a period of two weeks to compare skin tolerance of the wipes versus water and a cleansing material. Skin condition was assessed visually for the presence and severity of erythema and diaper dermatitis. The overall skin condition was not different in the group using wipes and in the group using only water and a cleansing material, indicating comparable skin mildness for both regimes.

Study B was a chamber scarification test on adults to assess the skin-irritation potential of the baby wipe. This study confirmed that the lotion contained in the wipe had a very low-irritation potential, lower than that of a currently marketed baby wipe and comparable to that of water under occlusive patch-test conditions.

Study C was a four-week clinical in-use study in 60 babies with atopic dermatitis, to confirm the safety and skin tolerability in a sensitive-skin subpopulation. The good skin tolerance of the wipes in study B was supported by the observations of a dermatologist in this study.

Ehretsmann et al. (52) concluded that "these data strongly support the suitability of the baby wipes tested for daily cleansing of the diapered area, even for infants with sensitive skin."

Farage et al. (53) conducted a study to (*i*) optimize the current arm patch-test method, so they might detect more effectively the problems with products designed to be inherently non-irritating (feminine-hygiene products), (*ii*) reduce the cost of product chemical irritation studies by shortening the protocol, and (*iii*) increase the understanding of the contribution of mechanical irritation to any skin effects produced by "non-irritating" products. They were also interested in furthering their understanding of the relationship of sensory effects to objective measures of irritation.

To accomplish their objectives, swatches were prepared from three feminine-protection pads, currently sold in the consumer marketplace. Some forearm sites were tape stripped prior to the initial patch application to create compromised skin. Wet and dry swatches were applied to the upper arm on the intact and compromised test sites using the standard 24-hour patch test producing four protocol variations (intact skin/dry swatches, compromised skin/dry swatches, intact skin/wet samples, and compromised skin/wet swatches). Applications were repeated daily for four consecutive days. Test sites were scored for irritation prior to the first patch application, and 30 to 60 minutes after patch removal. In one experiment, panelists were asked to keep a daily diary describing any sensory skin effects noticed at each test site.

Similar results were obtained for the four protocol variations for the products tested. When compared to the behind-the-knee test method, the standard upper-arm patch test gave consistently lower levels of irritation when the test sites were scored shortly after swatch removal, even though the sample application was longer (24 vs. 6 hours) in the standard patch test. The higher level of irritation in the behind-the-knee method was likely due to mechanical irritation. The sensory skin effects did not appear to be related to a particular test product or a particular protocol variation. However, the mean irritation scores at those sites where a sensory effect was reported were higher than the mean irritation score at those sites where no sensory effects were reported.

Six well-stated conclusions are provided by Farage et al. (53). First, all four protocol variations of the standard upper-arm patch test can be used to assess the inherent chemical irritation properties of feminine-protection products. Secondly, for these products, which are inherently non-irritating, tape stripping and/or applying wet samples do not increase the sensitivity of the patch-test method. Thirdly, differences in irritation potential were apparent after one to three 24-hour applications. Therefore, the standard patch-test protocol can be shortened to three applications without compromising our ability to detect differences in the chemical irritation produced by the test materials. Next, the patch test can be used to evaluate effectively the inherent chemical irritation potential of these types of products. However, this method is not suitable for testing the mechanical irritation due to friction that occurs during product use. Further, there is no relationship between specific text conditions, that is, compromised skin and/or testing wet samples and reports of perceived sensory reactions. Finally, there seems to be a clear relationship between sensory reactions and objective irritation scores.

DISCUSSION

The significance of this chapter is that it brings together the information the researchers need to design and carry out research projects that focus on discovering differences (if these exist) between people who express intolerance to fabrics and those who do not. This chapter presented information about methods to subjectively assess the feel of fabric, to objectively assess the feel of fabric, reviewed studies in which researchers discovered which nerve fibers were involved when prickly fabrics were pressed on the skin surface, reviewed studies in which bioengineering instrumentation was used to assess changes in capillary blood flow and in rates at which transepidermal water loss occurred when the fabric covered the skin surface, and reviewed studies on mechanical and chemical irritation to fabric-covered skin.

Methods to subjectively study the feel of fabric on skin were presented first, because the current basis for saying a sensitive-skin fabric syndrome exists is based on verbal reports of intolerance to fabrics by "skin sensitive" individuals. Although research to date using subjective instruments has concentrated on dis-covering differences between fabrics, these subjective sensory instruments should prove valuable in discovering differences among people in their judgment of the feel of fabric. Are there certain sensory attributes that separate fabric-tolerant and fabric-intolerant people? Or, do fabric-intolerant people report greater intensity for each sensory attribute? Might it be possible to place individuals on a fabric-sensitivity scale on the basis of the data from and analysis of subjective sensory study results? A key element in such studies will be the set of fabrics presented to the subjects/panelists. The capability to objectively measure fabric properties, such as surface friction, allows appropriate sets of fabrics to be selected. Guidelines for the design of fabric-feel (tolerance) studies might parallel those established for non-textile products (e.g., cosmetics).

Interestingly, the sensory attribute called prickle has been the sole sensory attribute linked to a specific neural receptor in the skin. It was usually 100% wool or wool-blend fabrics that were used in these studies. Researchers were able to discover how to change the composition and structure of wool fabrics to eliminate the unacceptable prickliness of the fabrics. Researchers might use this fabric prickle model to investigate which neural receptors are linked to other sensory attributes (such as stiff, picky, and scratchy).

Studies involving bioengineering instrumentation to study change in capillary blood flow and transepidermal water loss from the skin surface due to placing fabric over the skin have focused on finding differences due to fabric type (fiber composition, thickness, etc.) and sometimes to relating the physiological information collected to sensory attribute and sensory-comfort data collected. The question to ask in the context of studying sensitive-skin syndrome is "might the use of these instruments and procedural methods worked out for collecting the physiological data lead to discover differences in physiological response for fabric-intolerant subjects and fabric-tolerant subjects?" In this case, the emphasis is on finding subject-group differences, not on discovering fabric differences.

The significance of studies reported in the "Mechanical Irritation" section of this chapter is discovering that methods have been established for rubbing fabrics on the skin surface, for pre-irritating skin sites, and for measuring skin redness and other skin characteristics that may change due to mechanical (rubbing) action. Might not these methods and procedures be used in conjunction with fabric-feel (sensory) methods to determine how the subjects would subjectively rate fabric feel under various degrees of mechanically abraded skin? Might not the fabrics used in these tests be objectively analyzed for surface friction and other fabric properties? Might not these methods and procedures be used to discover differences in response within fabric-tolerant and fabric-intolerant populations?

The last section of this chapter, chemical irritation to skin by fabric, establishes that chemical irritation to skin is the least likely of all factors reviewed in this chapter to explain skin intolerance to fabric. This statement is based on the fact that studies to date on chemical irritation have found that fabrics containing detergent residues, and laundry-applied fabric softeners, do not cause chemical irritation to the skin, at least not to the skin of the subjects used in these studies.

Much remains to be known about the relationship of fabric to skin and to sensitive skin, in particular. Research on discovering the causes of fabric intolerance will advance as research teams composed of scientists from the medical, biotechnology, and textile science fields are formed. The medical community will bring expertise about the grading of skin, skin structure, and skin function; the biotechnology community will develop the required instrumentation; and textile scientists will bring knowledge about methods for assessing the feel of fabric on skin as well as characterizing the structure and properties of fabrics. Investigating the causes of fabric-sensitivity syndrome is bound to expand rapidly in the future with the marvelous foundation built by those scientists listed in the reference section of this chapter.

REFERENCES

1. Hatch KL, Markee NL, Maibach HI. Skin response to fabric, a review of studies and assessment methods. Cloth Text Res J 1992; 10(4):54.
2. Hatch KL, Maibach HI. Fiber. In: Maibach HI, ed. Toxicology of Skin. Chapter 79. Philadelphia, PA: Taylor & Francis, 2001:207–234.
3. Hatch KL, Maibach HI. Assessing the effects of fiber-based materials on skin using bioengineering instrumentation. In: Agache P, Humbert P, eds. Measuring the Skin: Non-invasive Investigations. Chapter 56. New York: Springer-Verlag, 2004:565–582.
4. Elsner P, Hatch KL, Wigger-Alberti W. Textiles and the Skin. Basel: Karger, 2003.
5. Hatch KL. Textile dyes as allergic contact allergens. Curr Probl Dermatol 2003; 31:139.
6. Hatch KL, Motschi H, Maibach HI. Disperse dyes in fabrics of patients patch-test positive to disperse dyes. Am J Contact Dermat 2003; 14(4):205.
7. Hatch KL, Motschi H, Maibach HI. Identifying the source of textile–dye allergic contact dermatitis, a guideline. Exog Dermatol 2003; 2(5):240.
8. Platzek T. Introduction to the problem of clothing textiles. BGVV textile working group report, http://www.bfr.bund.de/cms/detail.php?template = internet_en_index_js, 2002-08-01.

9. Schneider K, Hafner C, Jäger I. Mutagenicity of textile dye products. J Appl Toxicol 2004; 24:83.
10. Knittel D, Beermann K, Schollmeyer E. Surface of textiles and the human skin. Part 2: testing methods for skin compatibility of textiles, textile ingredients and textile auxiliaries. Exog Dermatol 2003; 2:17.
11. Cardello AV, Winterhalter C, Schutz HG. Predicting the handle and comfort of military clothing fabrics from sensory and instrumental data: development and application of new psychological methods. Text Res J 2003; 73(3):221.
12. Sweeny MM, Branson DH. Sensorial comfort. Part I: a psychophysical method for assessing moisture sensation in clothing. Text Res J 1990; 60:371.
13. Civille GV, Dus CA. Development of terminology to describe the handfeel properties of paper and fabrics. J Sens Stud 1990; 5:19.
14. Hatch KL, et al. In vivo cutaneous and perceived comfort response to fabric. Part I: thermophysiological comfort determinations for three experimental knit fabrics. Text Res J 1990; 60:406.
15. Barker R, Radhakrishnaiah P, Woo SS, Hatch KL, Markee NL, Maibach HI. In vivo cutaneous and perceived comfort response to fabric. Part II: mechanical and surface related comfort property determinations for three experimental knit fabrics. Text Res J 1990; 60:490.
16. Barker R, Hatch KL, Markee NL, Maibach HI, Woo SS, Radhakrishnaiah P. In vivo cutaneous and perceived comfort response to fabric. Part III: water content and blood flow in human skin under garments worn by exercising subjects in a hot, humid environment. Text Res J 1990; 60:510.
17. Barker R, Markee NL, Hatch KL, Maiback HI, Radhakrishnaiah P, Woo SS. In vivo cutaneous and perceived comfort response to fabric. Part IV: perceived sensations to three experimental garments worn by subjects exercising in a hot, humid environment. Text Res J 1990; 60:561.
18. Hatch KL, Markee NL, Prato H, et al. In vivo cutaneous response to fabric. Part V: the effect of fiber type and fabric moisture content on the hydration state of human stratum corneum. Text Res J 1992; 66:638.
19. Hatch KL, Prato HH, Zeronian SH, Maibach HI. In vivo cutaneous and perceived comfort response to fabric. Part VI: the effect of moist fabrics on stratum corneum hydration. Text Res J 1997; 67:926.
20. Wang G, Zhang W, Postle R, Phillips D. Evaluating wool shirt comfort with wear trials and the forearm test. Text Res J 2003; 73(2):113.
21. Fuzek JF. Some factors affecting the comfort assessment of knit T-shirts. Ind Eng Chem Prod Dev 1981; 20:254.
22. Wong ASW, et al. Neural network predictions of human psychological perceptions of clothing sensory comfort. Text Res J 2003; 73(1):31.
23. Laing RM, Ingham PE. The effectiveness of specimen tactile evaluation as a predictor of garment tactile acceptability for garments as a whole and on a regional basis. Cloth Text Res J 1983–1984; 2:58.
24. Hollies NRS. Visual and tactile perceptions of textile quality. J Text Inst 1989; 80(1):1.
25. Wong ASW, et al. Statistical simulation of psychological perception of clothing sensory comfort. J Text Inst. In press.
26. Wong ASW, Li Y, Yeung PKW. Predicting clothing sensory comfort with artificial intelligence hybrid models. Text Res J 2004; 74(1):13.

27. Hui CL, Lau TW, Ng SF, et al. Neural network prediction of human psychological perceptions of fabric hand. Text Res J 2004; 74(5):375.
28. Kawabata S. Standardization and Analysis of Hand Evaluation. 2nd ed. Osaka: The Textile Machinery Society of Japan, 1980.
29. CSIRO Division of Wool Technology. The FAST System for the objective measurement of fabric properties—operation, interpretation and applications, 1989.
30. Yick KL, Cheng KPS, Dhingra RC, How YL. Comparison of mechanical properties of shirting materials measured on the KES-F and Fast instruments. Text Res J 1996; 66(10):622.
31. Bueno M-A, Durand B, Renner M. A non-contact measurement of the roughness of textile fabrics. Exp Tech 2000; 24(2):23.
32. Ramkumar SS. Frictional characterization of enzyme-treated fabrics. AATCC Rev 2002; 2(11):24.
33. Chinnasami SK, Ramkumar SS. Development of an automated fabric friction factor calculator. AATCC Rev 2003; 3(11):20.
34. Garnesworthy RK, Gully RL, Kandiah RP, et al. Understanding the causes of prickle and itch from the skin contact of fabrics (Report No. G64). Belmont, Australia: CSIRO Division of Wool Technology, 1988.
35. LaMotte RH. Psychophysical and neurophysical studies of tactile sensibility. In: Hollies NRS, Goldman RF, eds. Clothing Comfort. Ann Arbor, MI: Ann Arbor Science, 1977:83–106.
36. Gwosdow AR, Stevens JC, Berglund LG, Stolwijk JAJ. Skin friction and fabric sensations in neutral and warm environments. Text Res J 1986; 54:574.
37. Wester RC, Hatch KL, Maibach HI. Blood flow changes in fabric-contacted human skin. Bioeng Skin 1982; 3:276.
38. Zha IH, Maibach HI. Skin occlusion and irritant and allergic contact dermatitis: an overview. Contact Dermatitis 2001; 44:201.
39. Cottenden AM, Thornbur PH, Dean GE, Fader MJ. Wet comfort of small disposable incontinence pads. Text Res J 1998; 68:479.
40. Dallas MJ, Wilson PA. Adult incontinence products: performance evaluation on healthy skin. INDA J Nonwovens Res 1992; 4(2):26.
41. Cameron BA, Dallas MJ, Brandt B, Brown D. Effect of natural and synthetic fibers and film and moisture content on stratum corneum hydration in an occlusive system. Text Res J 1987; 67:585.
42. Hatch KL, Wilson D, Maibach HI. Fabric-caused changes in human skin: in vivo water content and water evaporation. Text Res J 1987; 57:583.
43. Piérard GE, et al. Effects of softened and unsoftened fabrics on sensitive skin. Contact Dermatitis 1994; 30:286.
44. Hermanns J-F, et al. Beneficial effects of softened fabrics on atopic skin. Dermatology 2001; 202:167.
45. Farage MA, Gilpin DA, Enane NA, Baldwin S. Development of a new test for mechanical irritation: behind the knee as a test site. Skin Res Technol 2001; 7(3):193.
46. Farage MA. Development of a new mechanical irritation test. Toxicologist 2000; 54:203.
47. Farage MA, Meyer S, Walter D. Development of a sensitive test method to evaluate mechanical irritation potential on mucosal skin. Skin Res Technol 2004; 10(2):85.
48. Matthies W. Irritant dermatitis to detergents in textiles. Curr Probl Dermatol 2003; 31:123.

49. Bannan EA, et al. Skin testing of laundered fabrics in the dermal safety assessment of enzyme-containing detergents. J Toxicol Cutan Ocular Toxicol 1992; 11:327.
50. Kiriyama T, Sugiura H, Uehara M. Residual washing detergent in cotton clothes: a factor of winter deterioration of dry skin in atopic dermatitis. J Dermatol 2003; 30(10):708.
51. Belsito DV, et al. Allergic contact dermatitis to detergents: a multicenter study to assess prevalence. J Am Acad Dermatol 2002; 46(2):200.
52. Ehretsmann C, Schaefer P, Adam R. Cutaneous tolerance of baby wipes by infants with atopic dermatitis, and comparison of the mildness of baby wipe and water in infant skin. J Eur Acad Dermatol Venereol 2001; 15(1):16.
53. Farage MA, Meyer S, Walter D. Evaluation of modifications of the traditional patch test in assessing the chemical irritation potential of feminine hygiene products. Skin Res Technol 2004; 10(2):73.

17

Contact Urticaria Syndrome and Sensitive Skin: Clinical Approach

Marina Goldovsky and Howard I. Maibach

Department of Dermatology, University of California, San Francisco, California, U.S.A.

Patients with sensitive skin may have one or more mechanisms as triggers. Contact urticaria syndrome (CUS) [non-immunologic (NICU) and immunologic (ICU)] may be readily missed by the patient, consumer, and health care worker, as the signs and symptoms are transient (minutes to an hour or so) and not always morphologically overt, especially on damaged skin of the face. Thus, when the symptom is transient burn, sting, or itch (BSI), contact urticaria of the NICU and ICU type should be ruled out (Table 1, Fig. 1).

CUS comprises an inflammatory reaction that usually appears within minutes after cutaneous or mucosal contact with the eliciting agent (2). Subdivided into two categories, NICU and ICU are distinct processes, as the former requires no presensitization of the patient's immune system to an allergen, whereas the latter does. Even though these processes are different, patients' symptoms can overlap at presentation, making diagnosis more challenging for a clinician. Therefore, careful history taking is essential (Table 2).

The mechanisms underlying contact reactions comprised two types: immunologic [immunoglobulin E (IgE)-mediated] and non-immunologic immediate contact reaction (4). However, many unknowns remain about substances causing immediate contact reactions (immunologic or not).

Immediate contact reactions appear on normal or eczematous skin within minutes to an hour after inducing-substances have contacted the skin. The reaction

Table 1 Definitions and Terms

Immediate contact reaction	Immunologic (allergic) or non-immunologic (irritant), urticarial or non-urticarial reaction
Contact urticaria	Allergic and non-allergic urticarial reactions
Non-immunologic contact urticaria	The most common type of immediate contact reaction, that occurs without previous sensitization in most patients. Reaction remains localized; no spread; no systemic symptoms
Immunologic contact urticaria	Immediate allergic reaction in patients previously sensitized to the causative agent (refer to Table 4 for the list of agents)
Immediate-type irritancy	Non-allergic urticarial or non-urticarial reactions
Protein contact dermatitis	Allergic or nonallergic eczematous reactions caused by proteinaceous material
Contact urticaria syndrome	Local reactions in the skin and systemic symptoms in other organs, usually allergic. Reaction usually extends beyond the contact site, causing generalized urticaria or targeting other organs (e.g., rhinitis, conjunctivitis, asthma attack, and anaphylaxis in rare cases)

Source: From Ref. 1.

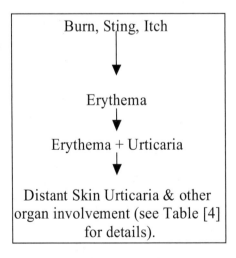

Figure 1 Signs and Symptoms of CUS. (*i*) NICU: The skin response is dose-related. (*ii*) ICU: The skin response is dose-, host-, and sensitivity-related. *Abbreviations*: CUS, contact urticaria syndrome; NICU, non-immunologic contact urticaria; ICU, immunologic contact urticaria.

Table 2   Essential Details in Patient's History to Narrow Down Many Agents Capable of Causing CUS

Contact urticaria reactions appear within minutes to an hour after exposure of the urticariant to the skin.

Patient may complain of a local burning sensation, tingling, or itching. Swelling and redness may be seen (wheal-and-flare).

Patient may be able to associate the symptoms to exposure to a specific substance. In some cases, this exposure may include the application of cosmetic products, especially to the face (cosmetic intolerance syndrome).

Details of the patient's employment provide insight into possible causes in the workplace, especially if the symptoms are temporally related to work.

Patient may be able to identify what he or she was doing at the onset of symptoms, again allowing the physician to narrow down the possible causes.

Presence and extent of extracutaneous involvement (asthma, rhinitis, conjunctivitis, and gastrointestinal upset) should be ascertained.

History of previous anaphylaxis should be sought, as should a personal or family history of atopy.

Abbreviation: CUS, contact urticaria syndrome.
Source: From Ref. 3.

disappears within 24 hours, usually within a few hours. The symptoms include itching, tingling, or burning accompanied by erythema. Local wheal-and-flare is the prototype reaction of contact urticaria. Contact urticaria can be allergic (immunologic) or irritant (NICU).

NICU is the most common immediate contact reaction and occurs without presensitization in most exposed patients. This reaction can also be called a form of immediate-onset irritancy. The mechanism of NICU is not completely understood. Previously, histamine was thought to be released from mast cells in response to exposure to an eliciting substance. NICU may be mediated by prostaglandins (3).

Some commonly reported causes of NICU include balsam of Peru, benzoic acid, cinnamic alcohol, cinnamic aldehyde, sorbic acid, and dimethylsulfoxide (5). In some patients, NICU may account for cosmetic intolerance syndrome.

The intensity of the reaction depends on the concentration, the vehicle, the skin area exposed, the mode of exposure, and the substance itself. Itching, tingling, or burning with erythema are the weakest types of reactions seen. As shown in Table 3, CUS can be staged according to symptomatology. Sometimes local sensations are not accompanied by any visible skin changes. The erythema is follicular at presentation, followed by spreading over application site. Generalized urticaria after contact with NICU agents is rare but has been reported more often after contact with agents eliciting immunologic IgE-mediated contact urticaria.

Repeated applications of ICU agents may cause eczematous reactions. Immediately appearing microvesicles are frequently described after contact with food products in protein contact dermatitis, which can be caused by

Table 3 CUS: Staging by Symptomatology

Stage 1	Localized urticaria
	Dermatitis
	Non-specific symptoms (itching, tingling, burning, etc.)
Stage 2	Generalized urticaria
	Cutaneous and extracutaneous reactions
Stage 3	Rhinoconjunctivitis
	Orolaryngeal symptoms
	Bronchial asthma
	Gastrointestinal symptoms
Stage 4	Anaphylactic symptoms

Note: This table reflects the variety of clinical manifestations that can be found in a patient suffering from this syndrome. The severity of reactions to a causative agent can be categorized by stages. Stage 1 is the least severe and localized, whereas Stage 4 is the most severe and spread.
Abbreviation: CUS, contact urticaria syndrome.
Source: From Ref. 4.

immunologic (allergic) mechanisms. The symptoms are usually limited to the contact area in NICU reactions.

ICU is less frequently encountered in clinical practice than NICU. ICU is a type 1 hypersensitivity reaction mediated by IgE antibodies in the patient's serum made against the specific eliciting substance. IgE molecules react with IgE receptors on the mast cells, basophils, eosinophils, Langerhans' cells, and other cells. Allergen penetrates through the skin or mucosal membrane to react with adjacent IgE molecules bound to mast cells. Within minutes, histamine, neutral proteases, and proteoglycans are released from the mast cells, leading to the immediate skin reaction. In addition, the mast cells release chemotactic factors attracting eosinophils and T cells from vascular system into the dermis. This mechanism requires that the patient has previously been exposed to the causative agent and has become "sensitized" (i.e., has produced specific IgE antibodies). Foods, drugs, and inhalants, among other substances, can interact as antigens with membrane-bound IgE, causing degranulation of mast cells. Sensitization can be at the cutaneous level (natural latex and some foods), but it may also be via the mucous membranes, such as in the respiratory or gastrointestinal tracts.

Generally, individuals with atopic dermatitis may be more predisposed to ICU. This is thought to be secondary to the presence of IgE antibodies on epidermal Langerhans' cells in these patients. This could explain the high frequency of positive patch-test reactions to inhalant allergens, such as house dust mites, birch and grass pollen, and animal danders in such patients.

ICU reactions may spread beyond the site of contact and progress to generalized urticaria (Table 3). When more severe, ICU may lead to anaphylactic shock. One such example is ICU from natural rubber latex (6). Typically, latex gloves cause a wheal-and-flare reaction at the site of contact. This reaction can affect either the person wearing the gloves or the person being touched by the person wearing the gloves. In addition to direct skin contact, allergy may be caused by airborne natural rubber latex. Thus, sensitized, yet undiagnosed, individuals are at risk when in contact with airborne ICU allergens.

In skin challenge, the molecules of a contact reactant penetrate the epidermis and react with specific IgE antibodies attached to mast cell membranes. Skin symptoms and signs, such as pruritis, erythema, and edema, are elicited by histamine and other vasoactive substances released from mast cells. ICU reactions have also been reported to result from cross allergy. The patient could be sensitized to a specific protein, but also react to other proteins that possess a similar antigenic molecular site. In the example of latex allergy, patients may experience symptoms from banana, chestnut, and avocado, as well as a number of other fruits, vegetables, and nuts. This phenomenon places patients with ICU at further risk.

Table 4 Agents Producing ICU

Food	Sunflower seed
Dairy	Meats
Cheese	Beef
Egg	Chicken
Milk	Lamb
Fruits	Liver
Apple	Turkey
Appricot	Seafood
Banana	Fish
Kiwi	Prawns
Mango	Shrimp
Orange	Vegetables
Peach	Beans
Plum	Cabbage
Grains	Carrot
Buckwheat	Celery
Maize	Chives
Malt	Cucumber
Rice	Endive
Wheat	Lettuce
Wheat bran	Onion
Honey/Nuts/Seeds	Parsley
Peanut	Parsnip
Sesame seed	Potato

(Continued)

Table 4   Agents Producing ICU (*Continued*)

Rutabaga
Tomato
Soybean

Fragrances and flavorings
Balsam of Peru
Menthol
Vanilin

Medications
Acetylsalicylic acid
Antibiotics
Amoxicillin, Ampicillin
Bacitracin
Cephalosporins (Cefotiam
 dihydrochloride, Cephalotin)
Chloramphenicol
Cloxacillin
Gentamycin
Iodochlorhydroxyquin
Mezlocillin
Neomycin
Nifuroxim
Penicillin
Rifampin
Rifamycin
Streptomycin
Virginiamycin
Benzocaine
Benzoyl peroxide
Clobetasol 17-propionate
Dinitrochlorbenzene
Etophenamate
Fumaric acid derivatives
Mechlorethamine
Pentamidine
Phenothiazines
Chlorpromazine
Levomepromazin
Promethazine
Pyrazolones
Aminophenazone
Methamizole
Propylphenazone
Tocopherol

Metals
Cobalt
Gold
Mercury
Zinc
Copper
Nickel
Platinum
Rhodium
Palladium
Iridium
Rutherium

Plant products
Abietic acid
Algae
Birch
Camomile
Castor bean
Chrysanthemum
Cinchona
Colophony
Corn starch
Emetin
Fennel
Garlic
Grevillea juniperina
Hakea suaveolens
Hawthorn, *Crataegus monogyna*
Henna
Latex rubber
Lichens
Lily
Lime
Limonium tataricum
Mahogany
Mustard
Papain
Perfumes
Pickles
Rose
Rouge
Spices
Strawberry

(*Continued*)

Table 4 Agents Producing ICU (*Continued*)

Teak	Ammonia
Tobacco	Ammonium persulfate
Tulip	Aminothazole
Winged bean	Benzophenone
Preservatives and disinfectants	Carbonless copy paper
Benzoic acid	Chlorothanil
Benzyl alcohol	Cu(II)-acetyl acetonate
Butylated hydroxytoluene	Denatonium benzoate
Chlorhexidine	Diethyltoluamide
Chloramine	Epozyresin
Chlorocresol	Lanolin alcohols
1,3-Diiodo-2-hydroxypropane	Lindane
Formaldehyde	Methyl–ethyl ketone
Gentian violet	Monoamylamine
Hexantriol	Naphtha
para-Hydroxybenzoic acid	Naphthylacetic acid
Parabens	Nylon
Phenylmercuric propionate	Oleylamide
ortho-Phenylphenate	Paraphenylenediamine
Polysorbates	Patent blue dye
Sodium hypochlorite	Perlon
Sorbitan monolaurate	Phosphorus sesquisulfide
Tropicamide	Plastic
Enzymes	Polypropylene
alpha-Amylase	Polyethylene glycol
Cellulases	Potassium ferricyanide
Xylanases	Seminal fluid
Miscellaneous	Sodium silicate
Acetyl acetone	Sodium sulfide
Acrylic monomer	Sulfur dioxide
Alcohols (amyl, butyl, ethyl,	Terpinyl acetate
isopropyl)	Textile finish
Aliphatic polyamide	Vinyl pyridine
	Zinc diethyldithiocarbamate

Abbreviation: ICU, immunologic contact urticaria.

Reported causes of ICU include natural rubber latex, many antibiotics, some metals (e.g., platinum and nickel), acrylic monomers, short-chain alcohols, benzoic and salicylic acids, parabens, polyethylene glycol, polysorbate, and other miscellaneous chemicals. Table 4 describes different agents capable of producing ICU. Prick testing is an investigation tool used to trace etiological factors responsible for ICU (4).

Although immediate readings of all epidermal tests are rarely possible in clinical practice, one should try to perform testing on selected substances as

A. Epidermal application

1) Open application to:

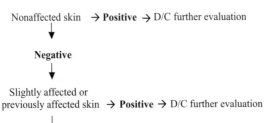

2) Occlusive application (patch or chamber) to:

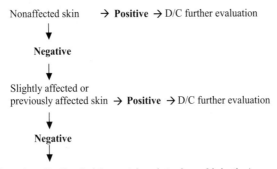

B. Intradermal application (prick, scratch or intradermal injection)

When it comes to diseased skin, one should test only the slightly affected areas to insure
clear interpretation and most accurate results.

Figure 2   Algorithm for Contact Urticaria Testing. *Source*: From Ref. 5.

guided by the patient's history Table 2. The above testing outline (Fig. 2) can be
used as a guideline for clinicians taking care of CUS suspected patients, listing
test procedures for evaluation of immediate responses; order as recommended.
Tests should first be performed on non-diseased skin; if negative, repeat the
test on the involved or previously affected areas.

REFERENCES

1. Lahti A. Non-immunologic contact urticaria. In: Amin S, Lahti A, Maibach HI, eds.
   Contact Urticaria Syndrome. Chapter 3. CRC Press, 1997.
2. Amin S, Maibach HI. Immunologic contact urticaria—definition. In: Amin S, Lahti A,
   Maibach HI, eds. Contact Urticaria Syndrome. Chapter 2. CRC Press, 1997.
3. Bashir S, Maibach HI. Urticaria, contact syndrome. eMedicine 2004.
4. Lachapelle JM, Maibach HI. Patch Testing and Prick Testing. Berlin: Springer, 2003.
5. von Krogh G, Maibach HI. The contact urticaria syndrome—1982. Semin Dermatol
   1982; 1:59–66.

6. Jaeger D, Kleinhans D, Czuppon AB, Baur X. Latex-specific proteins causing immediate-type cutaneous, nasal, bronchial, and systemic reactions. J Allergy Clin Immunol 1992; 89(3):759–768.
7. Elpern DJ. The syndrome of immediate reactivities (contact urticaria syndrome): a historical study from a dermatology practice. II. The atopic diathesis and drug reactions. Hawaii Med J 1985; 44(12):466–468.
8. Hannuksela M. Mechanisms in contact urticaria. Clin Dermatol 1997; 15(4):619–622.
9. Kanerva L, Toikkanen J, Jolanki R, Estlander T. Statistical data on occupational contact urticaria. Contact Dermatitis 1996; 35(4):229–223.
10. Kanerva L, Jolanki R, Toikkanen J, Estlander T. Statistics on occupational contact urticaria. In: Amin S, Lahti A, Maibach HI, eds. Contact Urticaria Syndrome. CRC Press, 1997:57–70.
11. Maibach HI, Johnson HL. Contact urticaria syndrome: contact urticaria to diethyltoluamide (immediate type hypersensitivity). Arch Dermatol 1975; 111:726–730.

18

Contact Allergy and Sensitive Skin

Harald Löffler

Department of Dermatology, Philipp University of Marburg, Marburg, Germany

The interrelation between contact allergies and sensitive skin is multiple and can be investigated from various angles: Do individuals with contact allergies have a higher skin sensitivity? Do individuals with sensitive skin have more allergies or a higher risk to develop allergies? Which are the mechanisms of interaction between contact allergies and sensitive skin?

In this book, the various manifestations of sensitive skin are discussed in detail. Regarding the interaction between contact allergies and sensitive skin, highly irritable skin (as one manifestation of a sensitive skin) is the focus of attention. It appears obvious that individuals with a contact allergy, especially when acute eczemas are present, do have a higher skin sensitivity. The eczematous skin of allergic contact dermatitis is more susceptible to various environmental influences, for example, chemical or mechanical irritation, climatic conditions, and skin-care products. On the other side, irritated skin might imply a risk concerning sensitization. However, this mechanism is rather complex and will be discussed in detail.

Because irritant and allergic dermatitis are two completely different diseases, one would expect that the immunopathological features of both are completely different. The first investigations seemed to support this expectation: some cytokines (especially, IL-1-beta and IL-6) were thought to be specific for the allergic contact dermatitis (1–6). However, further investigations revealed that mostly every cytokine that has been found in the course of allergic contact dermatitis can also be found in the course of irritant contact dermatitis.

The differences in the expression of some cytokines were mostly dependent on the concentration and types of the allergen or irritant applied (7–11). In addition, histological, immunohistochemical, and electron microscopical investigations could not detect any relevant differences between these two different types of contact dermatitis (12–14).

CONTACT ALLERGY: THE INFLUENCE OF IRRITATION ON TYPE-IV ALLERGY

In immunology, the decision between "self" and "non-self" is of highest relevance. One unspecific signal that is responsible for the decision of "non-self" is irritation and leads to an activation of the immune system. This activation can be induced by irritants. For efficient vaccination strategies, the immunological activation is used, for example, by the application of Freund's adjuvant for BCG vaccination. An irritation induces multiple changes in the chemical, physical, and biological structure of the skin, which are responsible for enhancing the skin reaction even to allergens by multiple mechanisms.

Disturbance of the Cutaneous Barrier

Patients with leg ulcer have a high risk to get multiple sensitization against, for example, compounds of external therapeutics (15,16). It was recognized early that the underlying stasis dermatitis was a risk factor for sensitization, and the impaired skin barrier was thought to be responsible for this problem. The idea is simple and convincing: the limit of a molecular size that can penetrate the stratum corneum easily is about 500 Dalton (17). When the normal skin barrier is disturbed (due to a stasis dermatitis, due to an irritant dermatitis, or experimentally by tape stripping), molecules with a size much higher than 500 Dalton can penetrate the skin. This 500 Dalton rule is used for therapeutic purposes when the atopic dermatitis is treated with topical tacrolimus because only when the skin barrier is disturbed can the active component penetrate the skin. However, from an allergological point of view, it is essential that proteins reacting as a full antigen penetrate such eczematous skin. Smaller molecules (haptens) may also penetrate in a higher amount into the skin. Hence, the amount of allergens in the skin that may induce allergic contact dermatitis is higher than that in normal skin (17). It is known that the sensitization and elicitation of allergic contact dermatitis is easier when the concentration of the allergen is higher (no. 1 in Fig. 1) (18,19).

Modification of Allergens

By the various attempts to sensitize mice against the common allergen nickel, it is known that a simple injection or application of $Ni(II)Cl_2$ does not induce sensitization (20). However, when applied together with an irritant, the

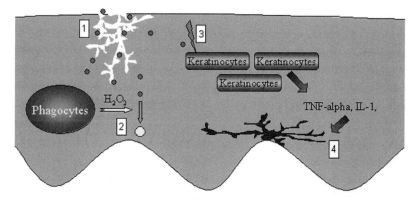

Figure 1 Model of the influence of irritation on type-IV-allergy: (1) Disturbance of the cutaneous barrier leads to a higher amount of haptens in the skin. (2) Inflammation leads to a modification of allergens. (3) The irritant property of the hapten (or an additional irritant) induces cytokine expression from keratinocytes. (4) Cytokines activate Langerhans cells. *Abbreviations*: H_2O_2, hydogen peroxide; TNF-alpha, tumor necrosis factor-alpha; IL-1, interleukin-1.

experimental sensitization to $Ni(II)Cl_2$ can be successful (21). A possible explanation for this observation is that the Ni ion is altered in inflamed skin. Phagocytes that are activated by irritants produce oxidants such as hypochloride (OCl^-) and hydrogen peroxide (H_2O_2), which are able to generate Ni(III) and Ni (IV) from Ni(II) (22,23). In this higher oxidation state, nickel contains a far higher chemical reactivity. Besides this higher chemical reactivity, Artik et al. (21) proved that Ni(III) and Ni(IV) were able to sensitize naive T cells. Hence, the inflammation induced by an irritant does alter the nickel hapten so that a sensitization is possible. The same mechanism can be found for gold. When gold(I)—a weak sensitizer—is oxidized to gold(III), the sensitization capacity is raised enormously (24,25). These two metals cannot be compared completely because the inability of Ni(II) to induce sensitization is due to an inadequate provision of signal 2, whereas the inability of gold(I) to induce sensitization is most likely due to its lack to induce signal 1 (21). However, the mechanism to alter these metals to an oxidation state in which they are potent sensitizers is the same. The impact on oxidation to the sensitizing capacity of allergens is generally known. Especially, the dramatic effect of air oxidation to various allergens (terpenes, fragrances, and ethoxylated surfactants) has been investigated over the past years (26–28). However, we are more and more aware that acute or chronic inflammation can also provide the environment (29,30) in which an alteration of allergens can take place, so that the probability of a sensitization against formerly harmless molecules rises (no. 2 in Fig. 1). Beyond it, irritants may most likely change the haptens directly in a way that sensitization becomes more likely.

"Danger" Model and Sensitization

In earlier years, there was the impression that allergic contact dermatitis could be caused by minimal doses of allergens. However, it has been shown that, not only in the elicitation but also in the sensitization process, the concentration of the allergen per area is a crucial point. White et al. (31) have shown that the sensitization to dinitrochlorobenzene (DNCB), a potent sensitizer, only occurs when a defined concentration threshold is reached. The explanation for this phenomenon was seen in the irritant feature of DNCB. Only if DNCB was applied in a concentration that a distinct irritant reaction was achieved, the sensitization process could take place. This irritation is, therefore, accepted as the "danger" signal necessary for each sensitization (30,32). Mostly, the hapten itself can induce this "danger" signal (no. 3 in Fig. 1) because we know that almost every known relevant allergen is also an irritant. But if the hapten has a very low irritability, high concentrations are necessary for the sensitization. If lower concentrations are applied, the "danger" signal can be induced by additional substances. Experimentally, it has been shown that the vehicle of the hapten can induce this "danger" signal, so that the hapten itself does not necessarily have an irritant activity (33). The co-administration of sodium lauryl sulfate (SLS), a model irritant, with a hapten increases the chances of successful sensitization (34,35). Furthermore, when DNCB in a very low concentration is applied for sensitization, the accumulation of Langerhans' cells in the draining lymph node and the proliferative response by draining lymph node cells can be increased by co-administration of the irritant SLS. This raised immunological activity can be compared with the one induced by DNCB alone in higher concentrations (35). It can be assumed that in these higher concentrations, the irritant feature of DNCB is sufficient to induce a strong immunological reaction.

What happens when the hapten penetrates the skin? What is the "danger" signal? Which cells are responsible for its initiation? Today, keratinocytes are the focus of attention. It has been shown that after stimulation by irritants (such as SLS, DMSO, croton oil, and phorbol myristate acetate), keratinocytes produce a number of cytokines, for example, tumor necrosis factor-alpha (TNF-alpha), IL-1-beta, and IL-8 (9,36–39). Even the irritant property of nickel is sufficient to induce such a cytokine release by keratinocytes (40). TNF-alpha does, of course, induce an unspecific proinflammatory response by the activation of T-cells, macrophages, and granulocytes; it activates the expression of cellular adhesion molecules and the release of further cytokines (41). More important in our context is the ability to activate Langerhans' cells. TNF-alpha down-regulates E cadherin and induces the production of type-IV collagenase (MMP-9) so that the Langerhans' cells can migrate more easily in the local lymph node (42,43). Moreover, TNF-alpha induces the up-regulation of MHC class I and II molecules, thus increasing the possibility of presentation of an allergen. As a consequence, TNF receptor p75 knockout mice are hardly sensitizable (44), and anti-TNF-alpha antibodies or recombinant soluble receptors were able to block the sensitization (45,46). Besides the known IL-1-beta production (which is also induced by irritants), the TNF-alpha production by keratinocytes seems to be a crucial point in the activation of the Langerhans' cells and, therefore, in the concept of a "danger" signal (nos. 3 and 4 in Fig. 1). An interesting theory is that in the absence of such a "danger" signal, the contact of the allergen with immunologic competent cells might induce tolerance (30,32,47,48). This absence can be achieved by a very low dose of the allergen, so that the irritancy of the allergen is too small to induce any unspecific reaction, although the immunologic (allergenic) effect is still present. At this moment, the immunologic reaction might lead to tolerance. Experimentally, this was shown in mice by various groups (49–52); the confirmation in humans is still missing.

"Danger" Model and Elicitation

In principle, the same danger signal may be necessary for elicitation and for sensitization. Even the cytokine profile is very similar to that at sensitization: TNF-alpha and IL-1 are of highest relevance (53). Often, the irritant property of the allergen may be sufficient to induce this danger signal. But if the allergen is applied on non-irritated skin in a concentration that no irritant reaction is induced, no allergic reaction takes place. The elicitation of an allergic response can then be achieved by co-administration of an irritant (54). For example, in humans, the allergic reaction to very low concentrations of allergens such as iso-eugenol, nickel, or dimethylaminopropylamine was markedly enhanced by the administration of irritants such as SLS (55,56). For the clinical practice, it is of highest relevance that in irritated skin, the danger signal is already present. This means that a hapten does not have to induce the "danger" signal in the skin, and therefore, even a much lower concentration of the hapten is necessary for the sensitization and elicitation of allergic dermatitis. Hence, especially patients with irritant or atopic dermatitis have a much higher risk of developing a further skin sensitization and additional allergic contact dermatitis. This association was assumed by epidemiological studies (57,58).

During the course of an allergic skin reaction, once reaction is induced, the "danger" signal is present due to the persistent inflammation. Further contact to the allergen may maintain this reaction, even when the concentration of the relevant allergen is below the concentration that would normally be needed for the elicitation of the reaction (below the concentration which induces an unspecific irritant reaction).

CONTACT ALLERGY AND UNSPECIFIC IRRITABILITY

When the danger signal is of such a high relevance for induction and elicitation of a cutaneous hypersensitivity reaction, it may be postulated that individuals with a higher skin sensitivity, in a narrower sense individuals who react more often and more intense to irritation, do have more sensitizations. In addition, a sufficient elicitation might also be achieved more easily. In a first study, the correlation between sensitization against colophony and irritation threshold against the irritant SLS was investigated by Smith et al. (59). They compared a group with an allergy against colophony with a control group and found that the group sensitized against colophony had a lower irritation threshold to the irritant SLS. Therefore, it might be possible that in individuals with a lower irritation threshold, sensitization and elicitation do occur more easily. However, when comparing the SLS reactivity to the amount and degree of sensitization in a patch test for contact allergens, Geier et al. (60,61) and (in a large multicenter study) our own group found that mostly irritant and doubtful reactions to the allergens are enhanced in the group with a positive SLS test. This can be explained by higher skin sensitivity at the time of testing, so that the irritant property of an allergen might be sufficient to induce an unspecific (irritant or doubtful) skin reaction. Therefore, the visible reaction in the patch test is rather an artificial reaction without any clinical relevance. The fact that also weak positive test reactions to several allergens were increased in SLS-positive individuals may be due to a false positive reading. In this case, the individual is not sensitized against the allergen. However, it may also be assumed that in the SLS-positive group, more real sensitizations are found in the patch test with contact allergens because the irritant property of the hapten may be sufficient to induce the "danger" signal necessary for the elicitation. In this case, the individual is sensitized against the allergen. Which of these two hypotheses is mostly relevant cannot be answered at this time.

CONTACT ALLERGY TO TYPE-1-ALLERGENS AND UNSPECIFIC IRRITABILITY

As mentioned above, the interrelation between contact allergy and irritation has been shown for multiple type-IV-allergens. Especially, the co-administration of an allergen and an irritant leads to an enhanced allergic reaction because of the "danger" signal of the irritant. This mechanism was investigated also for type-I-allergens. The administration of type-I-allergens does induce an atopic/allergic contact dermatitis in sensitized atopic patients (62). The barrier disruption seems to be an important condition for the development of a skin reaction to type-I-allergens. The question arises whether an irritation is also necessary for such a skin reaction or whether this reaction to an allergen is at least supported and enhanced by the co-administration of an irritant. Many type-I-allergens do induce proinflammatory reactions in keratinocytes (63,64); therefore, they also seem to have the ability to induce a "danger" signal on their own. In an experimental design, it has been shown that the tandem application of SLS and a type-I-allergen does lead to a much stronger skin reaction compared with SLS or the type-I-allergen alone (65). These findings confirm the hypothesis that the co-administration of an irritant does enhance the skin reaction to type-I-allergens in atopics comparable with the findings to type-IV-allergens. In daily life, taking showers or bathing in a tub during the pollen season may exert a calamitous effect on the skin of atopic individuals, as this provides an adverse association of aeroallergen and irritant exposure. Especially, individuals with a higher skin susceptibility to irritants may, therefore, also have a higher risk of developing skin reaction due to type-I-allergens.

CONTACT ALLERGY AND SELF-ESTIMATED SKIN SUSCEPTIBILITY

The difficult distinction between an objective estimate of skin susceptibility and a self-estimated skin susceptibility is the subject of discussion in various parts of this book. In a recent study, individuals with known nickel allergy stated that their skin had a higher unspecific susceptibility than those without nickel sensitization (66). However, the question whether the higher skin susceptibility was due to the sensitization to nickel (and the cutaneous problems following this sensitization) or the sensitization to nickel was due to the higher skin susceptibility (with e.g., an impaired barrier function of the skin) could not be answered. It is interesting to note that the estimated skin susceptibility in this work did not correlate with a subsequently performed irritant patch test with SLS, indicating that a self-estimated skin susceptibility is not the same as the one evaluated by testing with an irritant (66). Hence, although the hypothesis regarding an association between an increased skin susceptibility to irritants and contact allergy is mostly accepted, the association between a self-estimated enhanced skin susceptibility and contact allergy cannot be seen at the moment.

REFERENCES

1. Enk AH, Angeloni VL, Udey MC, et al. An essential role for Langerhans cell-derived IL-1 beta in the initiation of primary immune responses in skin. J Immunol 1993; 150:3698.
2. Enk AH, Katz SI. Identification and induction of keratinocyte-derived IL-10. J Immunol 1992; 149:92.
3. Dearman RJ, Kimber I. Cytokine production and the local lymph node assay. In: Rougier A, Goldber AM, Maibach HI, eds. In Vitro Skin Toxicology. New York: Liebert, 1994:367.
4. Müller G, Knop J, Enk AH. Is cytokine expression responsible for differences between allergens and irritants? Am J Contact Dermat 1996; 7:177.
5. Enk AH, Katz SI. Early molecular events in the induction phase of contact sensitivity. Proc Natl Acad Sci USA 1992; 89:1398.
6. Katz SI, Aiba S, Cavani A, et al. Early events in contact sensitivity. Adv Exp Med Biol 1995; 378:497.
7. Effendy I, Löffler H, Maibach HI. Epidermal cytokines in murine cutaneous irritant responses. J Appl Toxicol 2000; 20:335.

8. Wilmer JL, Burlesón FG, Kayama F, et al. Cytokine induction in human epidermal keratinocytes exposed to contact irritants and its relation to chemical-induced inflammation in mouse skin. J Invest Dermatol 1994; 102:915.
9. Lisby S, Muller KM, Jongeneel CV, et al. Nickel and skin irritants up-regulate tumor necrosis factor-alpha mRNA in keratinocytes by different but potentially synergistic mechanisms. Int Immunol 1995; 7:343.
10. Kondo S, Pastore S, Shivji GM, et al. Characterization of epidermal cytokine profiles in sensitization and elicitation phases of allergic contact dermatitis as well as irritant contact dermatitis in mouse skin. Lymphokine Cytokine Res 1994; 13:367.
11. Corsini E, Galli CL. Epidermal cytokines in experimental contact dermatitis. Toxicology 2000; 142:203.
12. Willis CM, Young E, Brandon DR, et al. Immunopathological and ultrastructural findings in human allergic and irritant contact dermatitis. Br J Dermatol 1986; 115:305.
13. Vestergaard L, Clemmensen OJ, Sorensen FB, et al. Histological distinction between early allergic and irritant patch test reactions: follicular spongiosis may be characteristic of early allergic contact dermatitis. Contact Dermatitis 1999; 41:207.
14. Nater JP, Hoedemaeker PJ. Histological differences between irritant and allergic patch test reactions in man. Contact Dermatitis 1976; 2:247.
15. Marasovic D, Vuksic I. Allergic contact dermatitis in patients with leg ulcers. Contact Dermatitis 1999; 41:107.
16. Tavadia S, Bianchi J, Dawe RS, et al. Allergic contact dermatitis in venous leg ulcer patients. Contact Dermatitis 2003; 48:261.
17. Bos JD, Meinardi MM. The 500 Dalton rule for the skin penetration of chemical compounds and drugs. Exp Dermatol 2000; 9:165.
18. Boukhman MP, Maibach HI. Thresholds in contact sensitization: immunologic mechanisms and experimental evidence in humans—an overview. Food Chem Toxicol 2001; 39:1125.
19. Basketter DA, Angelini G, Ingber A, et al. Nickel, chromium and cobalt in consumer products: revisiting safe levels in the new millennium. Contact Dermatitis 2003; 49:1.
20. Mandervelt C, Clottens FL, Demedts M, et al. Assessment of the sensitization potential of five metal salts in the murine local lymph node assay. Toxicology 1997; 120:65.
21. Artik S, von Vultee C, Gleichmann E, et al. Nickel allergy in mice: enhanced sensitization capacity of nickel at higher oxidation states. J Immunol 1999; 163:1143.
22. Naskalski JW. Oxidative modification of protein structures under the action of myeloperoxidase and the hydrogen peroxide and chloride system. Ann Biol Clin (Paris) 1994; 52:451.
23. Testa A, Serrone M, Foti C, et al. Neutrophil activation in nickel sensitized subjects. Cytobios 1996; 86:193.
24. Goebel C, Kubicka-Muranyi M, Tonn T, et al. Phagocytes render chemicals immunogenic: oxidation of gold(I) to the T cell-sensitizing gold(III) metabolite generated by mononuclear phagocytes. Arch Toxicol 1995; 69:450.
25. Griem P, Panthel K, Kalbacher H, et al. Alteration of a model antigen by Au(III) leads to T cell sensitization to cryptic peptides. Eur J Immunol 1996; 26:279.
26. Karlberg AT, Bodin A, Matura M. Allergenic activity of an air-oxidized ethoxylated surfactant. Contact Dermatitis 2003; 49:241.

27. Bergh M, Shao LP, Hagelthorn G, et al. Contact allergens from surfactants. Atmospheric oxidation of polyoxyethylene alcohols, formation of ethoxylated aldehydes, and their allergenic activity. J Pharm Sci 1998; 87:276.
28. Matura M, Goossens A, Bordalo O, et al. Oxidized citrus oil (R-limonene): a frequent skin sensitizer in Europe. J Am Acad Dermatol 2002; 47:709.
29. Dahl MV. Chronic, irritant contact dermatitis: mechanisms, variables, and differentiation from other forms of contact dermatitis. Adv Dermatol 1988; 3:261.
30. McFadden JP, Basketter DA. Contact allergy, irritancy and "danger". Contact Dermatitis 2000; 42:123.
31. White SI, Friedmann PS, Moss C, et al. The effect of altering area of application and dose per unit area on sensitization by DNCB. Br J Dermatol 1986; 115:663.
32. Smith HR, Basketter DA, McFadden JP. Irritant dermatitis, irritancy and its role in allergic contact dermatitis. Clin Exp Dermatol 2002; 27:138.
33. Heylings JR, Clowes HM, Cumberbatch M, et al. Sensitization to 2,4-dinitrochlorobenzene: influence of vehicle on absorption and lymph node activation. Toxicology 1996; 109:57.
34. Kligman AM. The identification of contact allergens by human assay. II. Factors influencing the induction and measurement of allergic contact dermatitis. J Invest Dermatol 1966; 47:375.
35. Cumberbatch M, Scott RC, Basketter DA, et al. Influence of sodium lauryl sulphate on 2,4-dinitrochlorobenzene-induced lymph node activation. Toxicology 1993; 77:181.
36. Muller Decker K, Furstenberger G, Marks F. Keratinocyte-derived proinflammatory key mediators and cell viability as in vitro parameters of irritancy: a possible alternative to the Draize skin irritation test. Toxicol Appl Pharmacol 1994; 127:99.
37. Corsini E, Marinovich M, Galli CL. In vitro keratinocytes responses to chemical allergens. Boll Chim Farm 1995; 134:569.
38. Hunziker T, Brand CU, Kapp A, et al. Increased levels of inflammatory cytokines in human skin lymph derived from sodium lauryl sulphate-induced contact dermatitis. Br J Dermatol 1992; 127:254.
39. Grangsjo A, Leijon-Kuligowski A, Torma H, et al. Different pathways in irritant contact eczema? Early differences in the epidermal elemental content and expression of cytokines after application of 2 different irritants. Contact Dermatitis 1996; 35:355.
40. Barker JN, Mitra RS, Griffiths CE, et al. Keratinocytes as initiators of inflammation. Lancet 1991; 337:211.
41. Groves RW, Allen MH, Ross EL, et al. Tumour necrosis factor alpha is pro-inflammatory in normal human skin and modulates cutaneous adhesion molecule expression. Br J Dermatol 1995; 132:345.
42. Kobayashi Y, Matsumoto M, Kotani M, et al. Possible involvement of matrix metalloproteinase-9 in Langerhans cell migration and maturation. J Immunol 1999; 163:5989.
43. Kobayashi Y. Langerhans' cells produce type IV collagenase (MMP-9) following epicutaneous stimulation with haptens. Immunology 1997; 90:496.
44. Wang B, Fujisawa H, Zhuang L, et al. Depressed Langerhans cell migration and reduced contact hypersensitivity response in mice lacking TNF receptor p75. J Immunol 1997; 159:6148.

45. Cumberbatch M, Dearman RJ, Kimber I. Langerhans cells require signals from both tumour necrosis factor-alpha and interleukin-1 beta for migration. Immunology 1997; 92:388.
46. Piguet PF, Grau GE, Hauser C, et al. Tumor necrosis factor is a critical mediator in hapten induced irritant and contact hypersensitivity reactions. J Exp Med 1991; 173:673.
47. Matzinger P. The danger model: a renewed sense of self. Science 2002; 296:301.
48. Matzinger P. Tolerance, danger, and the extended family. Annu Rev Immunol 1994; 12:991.
49. Steinbrink K, Sorg C, Macher E. Low zone tolerance to contact allergens in mice: a functional role for CD8+ T helper type 2 cells. J Exp Med 1996; 183:759.
50. Lowney ED. Topical hyposensitization of allergic contact sensitivity in the guinea pig. J Invest Dermatol 1964; 43:487.
51. Lowney ED. Simultaneous development of unresponsiveness and of sensitivity following topical exposure to contact sensitizers. J Invest Dermatol 1967; 48:391.
52. Lowney ED. Immunologic unresponsiveness appearing after topical application of contact sensitizers to the guinea pig. J Immunol 1965; 95:397.
53. Grabbe S, Schwarz T. Immunoregulatory mechanisms involved in elicitation of allergic contact hypersensitivity. Am J Contact Dermat 1996; 7:238.
54. Grabbe S, Steinert M, Mahnke K, et al. Dissection of antigenic and irritative effects of epicutaneously applied haptens in mice: evidence that not the antigenic component but nonspecific proinflammatory effects of haptens determine the concentration-dependent elicitation of allergic contact dermatitis. J Clin Invest 1996; 98:1158.
55. Angelini G, Rigano L, Foti C, et al. Contact allergy to impurities in surfactants: amount, chemical structure and carrier effect in reactions to 3-dimethylamino-propylamine. Contact Dermatitis 1996; 34:248.
56. Allenby CF, Basketter DA. An arm immersion model of compromised skin (II). Influence on minimal eliciting patch test concentrations of nickel. Contact Dermatitis 1993; 28:129.
57. Uter W, Gefeller O, Schwanitz HJ. Occupational dermatitis in hairdressing apprentices. Early-onset irritant skin damage. Curr Probl Dermatol 1995; 23:49.
58. Uter W, Pfahlberg A, Gefeller O, et al. Preventing skin damage in beauticians. Gesundheitswesen 2001; 63(suppl 1):S32.
59. Smith HR, Holloway D, Armstrong DK, et al. Irritant thresholds in subjects with colophony allergy. Contact Dermatitis 2000; 42:95.
60. Löffler H, Becker D, Brasch J, et al. Simultaneous sodium lauryl sulfate testing improves the diagnostic validity of allergic patch tests. Br J Dermatol 2005; 152:709.
61. Geier J, Uter W, Pirker C, et al. Patch testing with the irritant sodium lauryl sulfate (SLS) is useful in interpreting weak reactions to contact allergens as allergic or irritant. Contact Dermatitis 2003; 48:99.
62. Darsow U, Vieluf D, Ring J. Evaluating the relevance of aeroallergen sensitization in atopic eczema with the atopy patch test: a randomized, double-blind multicenter study. Atopy Patch Test Study Group. J Am Acad Dermatol 1999; 40:187.
63. Hewitt CR, Foster S, Phillips C, et al. Mite allergens: significance of enzymatic activity. Allergy 1998; 53:60.

64. Ghaemmaghami AM, Gough L, Sewell HF, et al. The proteolytic activity of the major dust mite allergen Der p 1 conditions dendritic cells to produce less interleukin-12: allergen-induced Th2 bias determined at the dendritic cell level. Clin Exp Allergy 2002; 32:1468.
65. Löffler H, Steffes A, Happle R, et al. Allergy and irritation: an adverse association in patients with atopic eczema. Acta Derm Venereol 2003; 83:328.
66. Löffler H, Dickel H, Kuss O, et al. Characteristics of self-estimated enhanced skin susceptibility. Acta Derm Venereol 2001; 81:343.

19

Photobiology and Sensitive Skin

Giovanni Leone and Alessia Pacifico

Phototherapy Unit, San Gallicano Dermatologic Institute, IRCCS, Rome, Italy

INTRODUCTION

Topically and systemically administered chemical substances have the capability to access the skin. Some of these chemicals may absorb ultraviolet or visible light and are, therefore, potential photosensitizers.

Chemical photosensitivity is a term used to describe skin disease caused by the interaction of light and exogenously acquired chemical agents. In all such reactions, both the chemical substance and radiation are necessary for the response to be produced. The mechanism of the response can be either irritant or allergic.

Chemical photosensitivities may be classified into two distinct entities: photoirritant contact dermatitis (PICD) and photoallergic contact dermatitis (PACD). In the case of topically applied chemicals, it is quite easy to distinguish the mechanism of action (irritant vs. allergic) on the basis of clinical history and morphology. In fact, the reaction occurs on the first exposure to the chemical agent and light in PICD, whereas there is sensitization delay for PACD (1).

The timing of response to testing or in the clinical history of the eruption is delayed in PACD, as it is in allergic contact dermatitis. In PICD, the timing of the response varies depending on the chemical involved. For example, tars usually induce a quick response that occurs as the patient is being exposed to radiation, whereas psoralens, whether from natural or synthetic material, produce in skin a response ranging from 48 to 72 hours after exposure to sunlight.

Photopatch testing to the chemical-inducing PACD reveals positive responses only in sensitized subjects and negative responses in the general population, whereas the majority of the population will develop positive reactions to photopatch testing to a phototoxic agent (PICD).

On clinical and histological examinations, PACD presents as an eczematous reaction, whereas PICD appears clinically with erythematous, edematous, and bollous lesions. Moreover, histological examination of biopsies from skin specimens reveals PICD necrosis of keratinocytes (2).

The dose of both chemical and radiation necessary to induce the response is usually considered to be critical, especially to the production of PICD when compared with PACD, but such factors may also play a role in PACD. Photopatch testing in PICD patients is usually contraindicated because a positive response might be severe (3).

PACD is a classic T-cell-mediated or delayed-type hypersensitivity reaction of the skin in response to a photoallergen or photoantigen in a subject who has previously been sensitized to the same or a cross-reacting chemical. When a complete antigen is formed, the pathogenesis of a photocontact dermatitis is identical to that of allergic contact dermatitis: epidermal Langerhans' cells process the antigen and present it in the draining lymph nodes to antigen-specific T-lymphocytes. Cutaneous lesions will develop when activated T-cells circulate to the exposed areas of the skin and recognize the photoallergen (4).

The action spectrum, which is the quality of the radiation that induces photocontact dermatitis, both toxic and allergic, falls almost always in the ultraviolet A (UVA) longwave (320–400 nm) and in the visible range (400–800 nm); some photoallergens elicit reactions in both UVA and UVB ranges as is the case with diphenhydramine hydrochloride and non-steroidal, anti-inflammatory agents (NSAIDS) (5). When photopatch testing is performed, therefore, it is necessary to use a UVA source for the testing.

Often in the clinic, diagnostic difficulties center around whether a patient has phototoxicity or photoallergy. Photoallergy as a type IV hypersensitivity reaction usually presents as a dermatitis. Phototoxicity, on the other hand, is considered to have an exaggerated sunburn appearance, an oversimplification complicated by the fact that repeat episodes can produce a dermatitis, both clinically and histologically.

Although there is a lack of information, it is generally accepted that photoallergy is a relatively uncommon event that follows exposure of the skin to a topical photoallergen such as a non-steroidal, anti-inflammatory cream that sets off a type IV hypersensitivity contact allergic reaction following irradiation within the skin with ultraviolet. Phototoxicity can follow exposure to topical drugs, but more often is seen following drug ingestion or injection.

PHOTOIRRITANT CONTACT DERMATITIS

The real incidence of PICD in the general population is unknown. Review of large studies of patients being evaluated for photosensitivity reveals a low incidence of this diagnosis. This may be because the diagnosis is made clinically.

For this reason, patients with PICD would not undergo testing and would not appear in statistics. It is probably more common than PACD in the general population (6).

Several agents may commonly induce PICD; among them there are tar-related products and furocoumarins. Every subject with an eruption in photo-distribution should be suspected of having PICD, and a careful history of exposure to photosensitizers at home or at the workplace should be taken.

Clinical features are characterized by an erythematous and edematous eruption in the absence of eczematous lesions in most individuals. In more severe cases, bullae are also present. Frequently, the lesions of PICD heal with pigmentation, especially when resulting from furocoumarin sensitizers. In fact, the majority of patients present with only hyperpigmentation without a history of preceding inflammation.

TAR PRODUCTS

Tar and related products produce a particular photosensitive reaction known as "tar or pitch smarts" (7). Patients experience burning and stinging almost immediately when exposed to the sun. Roofers with exposure to pitch and coal tar are most susceptible, and direct skin contact is not necessary because aerosolized contact is sufficient to produce the reaction. Associated ophthalmologic involvement may also occur. The sensitizers in coal tar include acridine, anthracene, benzopyrene, and fluoranthene.

FUROCOUMARINS

Furocoumarins are photosynthesizing chemicals which occur naturally in wild and in cultivated plants, and have also been synthesized for its many uses, for example, as fragrances and therapeutic agents.

The most common agents used therapeutically, 8-methoxypsoralen and 5-methoxypsoralen, are also the ones present in plant extracts, which are potent photosensitizers. After irradiation, maybe the most striking and best documented reaction pattern is seen with psoralens where phototoxicity is used therapeutically for the treatment of psoriasis and other conditions (photo-chemotherapy-PUVA). This family of naturally occurring drugs is used predominantly in a systemic form although they may be applied also as a topical emulsion or in a bath routinely producing a phototoxic rather than photoallergic reaction type.

When an individual develops PICD to a fragrance product, it usually appears as a hyperpigmented macule at the site of application. This has been called "berloque dermatitis" (2). Because most fragrance agents containing photosensitizers have been removed from products used in the U.S.A. and Europe, these reactions are currently relatively rare.

Common reactions are those that occur to plant and plant products, which are referred to as "phytophotodermatitis." Unlike reaction to tar products, reaction to furocoumarins is delayed. Healing is often accompanied with hyperpigmentation. The plant most often reported to induce phytophotodermatitis is lime. This reaction usually occurs in a recreational setting and small quantities of UVA radiation may then elicit a response.

PHOTOALLERGIC CONTACT DERMATITIS

The incidence of PACD is unknown. The available incidence data are based on positive photopatch test results in groups of patients with presumed photosensitivity (8).

Although PACD has been considered to be uncommon, several substances cited in the literature such as sunscreens, antibacterial agents, fragrances, and therapeutic agents give these reactions (9).

The clinical symptoms of PACD are those of an eczematous reaction, with histopathologic features identical to other forms of allergic contact dermatitis. It may be acute, subacute, or chronic. There are many similarities to phototoxic reactions, and clinical and histopathologic features may help to differentiate between these two entities.

PACD generally affects well-demarcated areas of the light-exposed areas: the face, neck, V-area of the upper chest, the backs of the hands and forearms, and sometimes the legs.

Peculiar clinical features may sometimes occur, such as an erythema multiform-like eruption, leukomelanoderma, and a lichenoid-photosensitive eruption. Systemic reactions including fever, rigors, diarrhea, and abnormalities of liver function have been reported in association with photocontact dermatitis (10).

Patients may have an underlying idiopathic type of photosensitivity such as polymorphous light eruption (PLE) or chronic actinic dermatitis and have a secondary PACD from using sunscreens to treat the original type of photosensitivity.

SUNSCREENS

Despite the enormous increase in sunscreen use, PACD reactions to ultraviolet filters are considered rare.

UV filters can be classified into two major types: chemical and physical. The physical UV filters, zinc oxide and titanium dioxide, reflect and scatter UV radiation and are not sensitizers, whereas chemical UV filters reduce the amount of UV radiation reaching the stratum corneum by absorption and can therefore cause sensitization. The chemical UVB filters include *p*-aminobenzoic acid (PABA), its ester derivatives octyl dimethyl PABA and amyl dimethyl PABA, and cinnamate derivatives. Chemicals absorbing UVB and some UVA radiation include the benzophenones (11). Butyl methoxydibenzoylmethane predominantly absorbs UVA radiation. Microfine titanium dioxide can, however, reflect and absorb UV radiation. As the chemical UV filters are used in relatively rare concentrations, it has been postulated that sensitization may occur fairly readily.

ANTIBACTERIAL AGENTS

Antibacterial agents used in soap, such as halogenated salicylanilides and chlorinated phenols, for example, fentichlor, were found to be potent photoallergens in the 1960s and 1970s and are now seldom used (12).

FRAGRANCES

Probably the best known photoallergen, the fragrance musk ambrette, was long ago removed from the marketplace, although it remains in the photopatch test series, as it can still be found in products from Asia and may cause prolonged photosensitivity reactions (13).

THERAPEUTIC AGENTS

Several drug families have the ability to change a patient's sensitivity to artificial or solar irradiation. They act by having a radiation absorbance characteristic, which after interaction with normally harmless doses of radiation, particularly in the UVA (315–430 nm) and sometimes in the visible region, will produce a photochemical effect with damage to cellular components within the skin, resulting in the clinical presentation (14).

The two systemic drugs that most frequently produce photosensitivity are the two phenotiazines, chlorpromazine hydrochloride and promethazine (15).

Ketoprofen, an NSAID used topically in Europe and other parts of the world, has been shown to be a photoallergen and has been recently included in the North American Contact Dermatitis Group Photopatch Test Series. It has been shown to cross-react with the benzophenone sunscreens and two other systemic agents, tiaprofenic acid, another NSAID, and fenofibrate, a cholesterol-lowering agent (16).

PERSISTENT LIGHT REACTION

This term describes the continuing state of eczematous photosensitivity following an initial photoallergic episode. It is supposed that despite avoidance of the original photoallergen, photosensitivity of a type-IV-delayed hypersensitivity is induced following UVB/A exposure. For many authors, the term is used synonymously with chronic actinic dermatitis (17).

PHOTOPATCH TESTING

In May 2002, a panel representing contact dermatology, photobiology, photophysics, with a special interest in photopatch testing, on behalf of the European

Society of Contact Dermatitis and European Photodermatology Society, met to establish a consensus methodology, a list of recommended test agents, and interpretation guidelines for photopatch testing. It is believed that photopatch testing, which is the clinical investigation of choice for suspected photocontact dermatitis and photoallergies, is significantly underused in Europe and its methodology varies greatly throughout the world (18).

As with the technique of patch testing, this investigation should not be undertaken when the skin test area is active. Furthermore, the use of the mid-upper-back skin, avoiding the paravertebral groove area, is recommended with photoallergen application in a duplicate set. At 24 hours, both patch applications are removed and one set carefully irradiated with UVA, followed by readings over the next 72 hours. In order to reduce unspecific test reactions, the suggested UVA dose has recently been reduced from 10 to $5 \, \text{J/cm}^2$. Only in the case of chronic actinic dermatitis with a minimal erythema dose $<5 \, \text{J/cm}^2$ UVA, suberythematous doses of UVA are allowed (19).

As with conventional patch testing, a range of reaction types from mild irritant to strong allergic, with the addition of a photoaggravated response may be seen. There is a move away from chemicals known historically to cause photoallergy but no longer in routine use. On this basis, revised series need to be produced and kept updated (20,21).

Review of the relevant allergens for photopatch testing shows that all positive photopatch tests in recent years are because of sunscreen ingredients. In fact, sunscreen chemicals are the most common photoallergens, although the incidence of photoallergy is low. Sunscreen photoallergy has been reported in patients with PLE and may be difficult to distinguish. Previous photoallergens such as 6-methyl coumarin, musk ambrette, and related molecules have been discontinued by the perfume industry in Europe because of previous relatively frequent sensitization. Testing perfume ingredients and plant materials and drugs such as promethazine, chlorpromazine, and non-steroidal, anti-inflammatory drugs leads to such a number of false-positive phototoxic reactions, hence better to omit these agents.

Reading of photopatch testing should be recorded using the International Contact Dermatitis Research Group (ICDRG) scoring system, pre-irradiation, immediately postirradiation, and 48-hour postirradiation. Further readings at 72 and 96 hours postirradiation may enable increasing or decreasing scoring patterns, suggesting allergic and non-allergic mechanisms, respectively (22,23).

REFERENCES

1. Murphy GM. Investigation of photosensitive disorders. Photodermatol Photoimmunol Photomed 2004; 20:305–311.
2. DeLeo VA, Harber LC. Contact photodermatitis. In: Fisher AA, ed. Contact Dermatitis. 3rd ed. Philadelphia: Lea & Febiger, 1986.

3. Marks JG, Elsner P, DeLeo VA. Contact and Occupational Dermatology. 3rd ed. Chicago: Mosby Yearbook, 2002:217–258.
4. Mang R, Krutmann J. Mechanisms of phototoxic and photoallergic reactions. In: Rycroft RJG, Mennè T, Frosch PJ, Lepoittevin J-P, eds. Textbook of Contact Dermatitis. 3rd ed. Berlin: Springer, 2001:134–143.
5. Adamski H, Benkalfate L, Delaval Y, et al. Photodermatitis from non-steroidal anti-inflammatory drugs. Contact Dermatitis 1998; 38:171–174.
6. Thune P, Jansen C, Wennersten G, et al. The Scandinavian multicenter photo-patch study: 1980–1985 final report. Photodermatology 1988; 5:261–269.
7. Emmett EA. Cutaneous and ocular hazards of roofers. Occup Med 1986; 1:307–322.
8. Ferguson J. Photosensitivity due to drugs. Photodermatol Photoimmunol Photomed 2002; 18:262–269.
9. Daevay A, White IR, Rycroft RJG, Jones AB, Hawk JLM, McFadden JP. Photo-allergic contact dermatitis is uncommon. Br J Dermatol 2001; 145:597–601.
10. White I. Phototoxic and photoallergic reactions. In: Rycroft RJG, Mennè T, Frosch PJ, Lepoittevin J-P, eds. Textbook of Contact Dermatitis. 3rd ed. Berlin: Springer, 2001:134–143.
11. Thune P. Contact and photocontact allergy to sunscreens. Photodermatology 1984; 1:5–9.
12. Wilkinson DS. Photodermatitis due to tetrachlorosalicylanilide. Br J Dermatol 1961; 73:213–219.
13. Cronin E. Photoallergic reactions to musk ambrette. Contact Dermatitis 1984; 11:88–92.
14. Johnson BE, Ferguson J. Drug and chemical photosensitivity. Semin Dermatol 1990; 9:39–46.
15. Llunggren B, Moller H. Phenotiazine phototoxicity: an experimental study on chlor-promazine and its metabolites. J Invest Dermatol 1977; 68:313–317.
16. Ophaswonge S, Maibach H. Topical nonsteroidal anti-inflammatory drugs: allergic and photoallergic contact dermatitis and phototoxicity. Contact Dermatitis 1993; 29:57–64.
17. Schauder S, Schroder W, Geier J. Olaquindox-induced airborn photoallergic dermati-tis followed by transient or persistent light reactions in 15 pig breeders. Contact Dermatitis 1996; 35:344–354.
18. The European Taskforce for Photopatch Testing. Photopatch testing: a consensus methodology for Europe. J Eur Acad Dermatol 2004; 18:679–682.
19. Neumann NJ, Holzle E, Plewig G, et al. Photopatch testing: the 12 year experience of the German, Austrian and Swiss photopatch test group. J Am Acad Dermatol 2000; 42:183–192.
20. Neumann NJ, Lehmann P. The photopatch test procedure of the German, Austrian and Swiss photopatch test group. Photodermatol Photoimmunol Photomed 2003; 19:8–10.
21. Beattie PE, Traynor NJ, Woods JA, Dawe RS, Ferguson J, Ibbotson SH. Can a posi-tive photopatch test be elicited by subclinical irritancy or allergy plus suberythemal UV exposure? Contact Dermatitis 2004; 51:235–240.
22. British Photodermatology Group. Workshop report: photopatch testing—methods and indications. Br J Dermatol 1997; 136:371–376.
23. Neumann NJ, Holzle E, Lehman P, et al. Pattern analysis of photopatch test reactions. Photodermatol Photoimmunol Photomed 1994; 10:65–73.

20

Treatments for Sensitive Skin: An Update

Zoe Diana Draelos

Department of Dermatology, Wake Forest University School of Medicine, Winston-Salem, North Carolina, and Dermatology Consulting Services, High Point, North Carolina, U.S.A.

Treating sensitive skin can indeed present a challenge to the physician because formulations that are typically not problematic for the general population cause intense stinging, burning, and redness in individuals with sensitive skin. Patients with sensitive skin can present with either skin that appears normal to the eye or overt skin disease. This chapter discusses methods of treating both invisible and visible sensitive skin from the standpoint of prescription medications, over-the-counter actives, and final cosmetic formulations. It will also present guidelines for patients to self-test products for skin sensitivity and a list of basic recommendations that may help the patient with sensitive skin find methods to minimize the signs and symptoms of their condition.

TREATING VISIBLE SENSITIVE SKIN

Visible sensitive skin is the easiest condition to diagnose because the outward manifestations of erythema, desquamation, lichenification, and inflammation identify the presence of a severe barrier defect. Any patient with a barrier defect will possess the signs and symptoms of sensitive skin until complete healing occurs. The three most common causes of barrier defect–induced facial sensitive skin are eczema, atopic dermatitis, and rosacea. These three diseases nicely illustrate the three components of sensitive skin, which include barrier disruption, immune hyperreactivity, and heightened neurosensory response.

Eczema

Eczema is characterized by barrier disruption, which is the most common cause of sensitive skin. The barrier can be disrupted chemically through the use of cleansers and cosmetics that remove intercellular lipids or physically through the use of abrasive substances that induce stratum corneum exfoliation. In some cases, the barrier may be defective due to insufficient sebum production, inadequate intercellular lipids, abnormal keratinocyte organization, etc. The end result is the induction of the inflammatory cascade accompanied by erythema, desquamation, itching, stinging, burning, and possibly pain. The immediate goal of treatment is to stop the inflammation through the use of topical, oral, or injectable corticosteroids, depending on the severity of the eczema and the percent body surface area involved. In dermatology, topical corticosteroids are most frequently employed with low-potency corticosteroids (desonide) used on the face and intertrigenous areas, medium-potency corticosteroids (triamcinolone) on the upper chest and arms, high-potency corticosteroids (fluocinonide) on the legs and back, and ultra-high-potency corticosteroids (clobetasol) used on the hands and feet. Newer topical options for the treatment of eczema-induced sensitive skin include the calcineurin inhibitors, pimecolimus, and tracrolimus.

However, the resolution of the inflammation is not sufficient for the treatment of eczema. Proper skin care must also be instituted to minimize the return of the conditions that led to the onset of eczema. This includes the selection of maintenance skin-care products, such as cleansers and moisturizers, a topic discussed later in the chapter. Thus, the care of sensitive skin involves not only the treatment of the acute skin disease, but also the prevention of recurrence through proper skin-care maintenance.

Atopic Dermatitis

Sensitive skin due to eczema is predicated only on physical barrier disruption, whereas the sensitive skin associated with atopic dermatitis is predicated both on a barrier defect and an immune hyperreactivity, as manifested by the association of asthma and hay fever. Patients with atopic dermatitis not only have sensitive skin on the exterior of the body, but also have sensitive mucosa lining the eyes, nose, and lungs. Thus, the treatment of sensitive skin in the atopic population involves topical and systemic considerations. There is also a prominent link between the worsening of hay fever and the onset of skin symptoms, requiring broader treatment considerations.

All of the treatments previously described for eczema also apply to atopic dermatitis, but additional therapy is required to minimize the immune hyperreactivity. Although this may take the form of oral or injectable corticosteroids, antihistamines (hydroxyzine, cetirizine hydrochloride, diphenhydramine, fexofenadine hydrochloride, etc.) are typically added to decrease cutaneous and ocular itching. Antihistamines also improve the symptoms of hay fever and may prevent a flare if the patient is exposed to pollens or other inhaled allergens. The avoidance of sensitive skin in the atopic patient is largely predicated on avoidance of inciting substances. This means creating an allergy-free environment by removing old carpet, non-washable drapes, items likely to collect dust, feather pillows and bedding, stuffed animal toys, heavy pollinating trees and plants, live pets, etc. The prevention of the release of histamine is the key to control the sensitive skin of atopic dermatitis.

Rosacea

Rosacea is an example of the third component of sensitive skin, which is heightened neurosensory response. This means that patients with rosacea experience stinging and burning more frequently than the general population to minor irritants. For example, I demonstrated that 62.5% of randomly selected rosacea patients showed a positive lactic acid sting test for sensitive skin (1). Furthermore, rapid prolonged facial flushing is one of the main diagnostic criteria for rosacea. Whether this sensitive skin is due to nerve alterations from chronic photodamage, vasomotor instability, altered systemic effects to ingested histamine, or central facial lymphedema is unclear.

The treatments for rosacea-induced sensitive skin are much different than those for eczema or atopic dermatitis. Anti-inflammatories in the form of oral and topical antibiotics form the therapeutic armamentarium. Antibiotics of the tetracycline family are most commonly used orally, whereas azelaic acid, metronidazole, sulfur, and sodium sulfacetamide are the most popular topical agents. However, the effect of the anti-inflammatory antibiotic can be enhanced through the use of complementary skin-care products that enhance barrier function. This statement was validated through a clinical study I conducted evaluating the effect of both a 15% azelaic acid gel and a gluconolactone-containing cleanser and moisturizer in the treatment of 66 subjects with moderate rosacea for 12 weeks.

Subjects entered the study with an average of 11.82 facial inflammatory lesions that were reduced to 4.61 facial inflammatory lesions after 12 weeks of treatment with 15% azelaic acid gel ($P < 0.0001$). The addition of a gluconolactone-containing cleanser and moisturizer to the 15% azelaic acid gel resulted in a statistically significant reduction in erythema ($P = 0.001$) over the 15% azelaic acid gel and patient self-selected skin-care products (2). This is due to the ability of gluconolactone to function as a humectant by enhancing the water-binding capabilities of the stratum corneum, which can strengthen the resiliency of the skin barrier to insult (3). This nicely demonstrates the importance of skin-care product selection in the treatment of sensitive skin associated with rosacea.

TREATING INVISIBLE SENSITIVE SKIN

Eczema, atopic dermatitis, and rosacea are in some ways the easiest forms of sensitive skin to treat. The skin disease is easily seen and treatment success can be monitored visibly. If the skin looks more normal, generally the symptoms of itching, stinging, burning, and pain will also be improved. Unfortunately, there are some patients who present with sensitive skin and no clinical findings. These patients typically present with a bag full of skin-care products they claim cannot be used because they cause facial acne, rashes, and/or discomfort. This situation presents a challenge for the physician, as it is unclear how to proceed.

Several treatment ideas are worth considering. The patient may have subclinical barrier disruption. For this reason, treatment with an appropriate strength topical corticosteroid for two weeks may be advisable. If symptoms improve, then the answer is clear. The patient may have subclinical eczematous disease. If the symptoms do not improve, it is then worthwhile to examine the next most common cause of invisible sensitive skin, which is contact dermatitis. This is accomplished by considering the ideas presented in Table 1 (4). Sometimes, a more regimented approach to contact dermatitis is required. This is the next topic of discussion.

ALGORITHM FOR EVALUATING INVISIBLE SENSITIVE SKIN

If the prior treatment recommendations have failed, a systemic approach must be undertaken to further elucidate the nature of the invisible sensitive skin. I would say that this algorithm is based more on the art of medicine than science, but it provides a systemic approach to treat the patient with sensitive skin. The algorithm is discussed subsequently.

Table 1   Considerations for the Minimization of Contact Dermatitis from Skin Care Products and Cosmetics

---

Eliminate common allergens and irritants or reduce their concentration

Select products from a reputable manufacturer who uses high-quality pure ingredients free of contaminants

Products should be well preserved to prevent the formation of auto-oxidation byproducts

Paraben preservatives have proven to be the least problematic

Avoid solvents, volatile vehicles, vasodilatory substances, and sensory stimulators in all products

Minimize the use of surfactants and select minimally irritating emulsifier systems

---

1. Discontinue all topical cosmetics, over-the-counter treatment products, cleansers, moisturizers, and fragrances. Use only a lipid-free cleanser and a bland moisturizing cream for two weeks.
2. Discontinue all topical prescription medications for two weeks. Especially avoid medications containing retinoids, benzoyl peroxide, glycolic acid, and propylene glycol.
3. Eliminate all sources of skin friction by selecting loose, soft clothing.
4. Discontinue any physical activities that involve skin friction, such as weight lifting, running, horse-back riding, etc.
5. Evaluate the patient at two weeks to determine whether any improvement has occurred or any visible dermatoses are present. If an underlying dermatosis, such as seborrheic dermatitis, psoriasis, eczema, atopic dermatitis, acne, rosacea, or perioral dermatitis is present, treat as appropriate until two weeks after all visible signs of skin disease have disappeared.
6. Patch and photopatch test patient to elicit any allergens with the standard dermatologic patch-test substances. Determine which of these allergens are clinically relevant and make avoidance recommendations.
7. Test for contact urticaria.
8. Perform facial sting testing with 10% lactic acid to one nasolabial fold and normal saline to the opposite nasolabial fold.
9. Evaluate the patient's mental status, especially noting signs of depression, menopause, or psychiatric disease.
10. Allow the female patient to add one facial cosmetic of low allergenic potential, following the guidelines in Table 1, in the following order: lipstick, face powder, and blush.
11. Use test cosmetics by applying them to a 2-cm area lateral to the eye for at least five consecutive nights. Cosmetics should be tested in the following order: mascara, eye-liner, eyebrow pencil, eye shadow, facial foundation, blush, facial powder, and any other colored facial cosmetic.
12. Use test leave-on skin-care products on the face individually as previously outlined with one product applied to a 2-cm area lateral to the eye for at least five consecutive nights.
13. Use test rinse-off skin-care products for five consecutive nights in the manner specified by the manufacturer.
14. Evaluate all positive and negative data and develop a list of products and ingredients that the patient should use or avoid to minimize the symptoms of sensitive skin.

This is indeed a time-consuming undertaking, but it is a thorough approach to determine the possible cause or causes of invisible sensitive skin.

BOTANICAL TREATMENT CONSIDERATIONS FOR SENSITIVE SKIN

The chapter began with an overview of the prescription treatments for the three components of sensitive skin to include barrier disruption, immune hyperreactivity, and heightened neurosensory responsiveness. Each of these components activates the inflammatory cascade, which is the final common pathway for all skin diseases, including sensitive skin. In addition to prescription therapies, a variety of cosmeceutical botanicals have been studied, which may be helpful in the maintenance phase of sensitive-skin treatment. These botanical anti-inflammatories include ginkgo biloba, green tea, aloe vera, and allantoin. They are most relevant to the sensitive-skin patient in the form of topical moisturizers, which may help reduce the symptoms of sensitive skin.

Ginkgo Biloba

Ginkgo biloba is a plant with numerous purported benefits and is a common part of homeopathic medicine in the Orient. The plant leaves contain unique polyphenols such as terpenoids (ginkgolides and bilobalides), flavonoids, and flavonol glycosides that have anti-inflammatory effects. These anti-inflammatory effects have been linked to antiradical and antilipoperoxidant effects in experimental fibroblast models (5). Another aspect of ginkgo in relation to sensitive skin is its ability to modify skin microcirculation. Vascular alterations induced in the skin include a blood-flow decrease at the capillary level and a vasomotor change in the arterioles of the subpapillary skin plexus. These changes may lead to decreased skin redness, sometimes a concern of patients with sensitive skin (6).

Green Tea

Green tea, also known as *Camellia sinensis*, is another botanical anti-inflammatory containing polyphenols, such as epicatechin, epicatechin-3-gallate, epigallocatechin, and epigallocatechin-3-gallate (7). The term "green tea" refers to the manufacture of the botanical extract from fresh leaves of the tea plant by steaming and drying them at elevated temperatures, being careful to avoid oxidation and polymerization of the polyphenolic components. A study by Katiyar et al. (8) demonstrated the anti-inflammatory effects of topical green tea application on C3H mice. A topically applied green tea extract containing GTP [(−)-epigallocatechin-3-gallate] was found to reduce UV-B-induced inflammation as measured by double skin-fold swelling. Green tea containing moisturizers may be valuable in the sensitive skin patient.

Aloe Vera

The most widely used cutaneous botanical anti-inflammatory is aloe vera. The mucilage is released from the plant leaves as a colorless gel and contains 99.5% water and a complex mixture of mucopolysaccharides, amino acids, hydroxyquinone glycosides, and minerals. Compounds isolated from aloe vera juice include aloin, aloe emodin, aletinic acid, choline, and choline salicylate (9). The reported cutaneous effects of aloe vera include increased blood flow, reduced inflammation, decreased skin bacterial colonization, and enhanced wound healing (10). The anti-inflammatory effects of aloe vera may result from its ability to inhibit cyclooxygenase as part of the arachidonic acid pathway through the choline salicylate component of the juice. However, the aloe vera final concentration in any moisturizer must be at least 10% to achieve a cosmeceutical effect.

Allantoin

Allantoin is the commonly added anti-inflammatory ingredient in moisturizers labeled as designed for sensitive skin. It is naturally found in the comfrey root, but synthesized in a large quantity by the alkaline oxidation of uric acid in a cold environment. It is a white crystalline powder that is readily soluble in hot water, making it easy to formulate in cream and lotion moisturizers designed for sensitive skin.

SENSITIVE SKIN PRODUCT GUIDELINES

In many cases, it is impossible to determine the exact cause of the sensitive skin. No obvious skin disease is present, yet the patient notes intense stinging and burning whenever skin-care products or cosmetics are applied to the skin. Frequently, patch testing reveals no obvious source of irritant or allergic contact dermatitis. This then leaves the physician to use empiric methods to make product recommendations to the patient. Products must be carefully selected on the basis of the use of ingredients that are least likely to damage the skin barrier, elicit a noxious sensory response, or alter the skin structure. Products with botanical anti-inflammatories may be helpful, but most patients want specific suggestions on how to select skin-care products and cosmetics. This section discusses the approach I use in my practice for product selection in the sensitive-skin patient who has not responded to any of the previously outlined treatment modalities.

Even patients with sensitive skin require basic hygiene. The face and body must be cleansed. There is no doubt that the synthetic detergent cleansers, also known as syndets, provide the best skin cleansing while minimizing barrier damage. Bars based on sodium cocyl isethionate appear to perform the best. However, there are some patients who only require the use of a facial syndet cleanser occasionally, because sebum production and physical activity are minimal. For these patients, a lipid-free cleanser is preferable because it can be used without water and wiped away. These products may contain water, glycerin, cetyl alcohol, stearyl alcohol, sodium lauryl sulfate, and occasionally propylene glycol. They leave behind a thin moisturizing film and can be used effectively in persons with excessively dry, sensitive, or dermatitic skin. However, they do not

Table 2   Draelos Cosmetic Selection Criteria in Sensitive-Skin Patients

Powder cosmetics should be selected
Cosmetics should be water removable
Old cosmetics should be discarded
Eyeliner and mascara should be black
Pencil formulations should be used for eyeliner and eyebrow cosmetics
Eye shadows should be earth toned (tan, beige, light pink, and cream)
Avoid chemical sunscreens in cosmetic formulations
Select cosmetic formulations with as few ingredients as possible
Avoid nail polishes
Select cream/powder facial foundations, or if liquid, silicone-based formulations

have strong antibacterial properties and may not remove odor from the armpit or groin. Lipid-free cleansers are best used where minimal cleansing is desired.

After completing cleansing, the sensitive-skin patient requires moisturization. The moisturizer should create an optimal environment for barrier repair, while not inducing any type of skin reaction. For example, the product should not contain any mild irritants that may present as an acneiform eruption in the sensitive-skin patient due to the presence of follicular irritant contact dermatitis. The best moisturizers are simple oil-in-water emulsions. The most common oil used is white petrolatum, but dimethicone and cylcomethicone are also acceptable oils in the sensitive-skin population for decreasing the greasiness of a simple petrolatum and water formulation. As mentioned previously, the fewer ingredients the better.

Sensitive-skin females also require recommendations on proper cosmetic selection. This can be a challenge for the physician, because cosmetic formulations change rapidly as dictated by the needs of fashion. One possible aid to the female patient who wants general cosmetic selection guidelines is to present the list of recommendations in Table 2. This compilation presents the basis for selecting cosmetics that are less likely to be problematic. Of course, the provocative-use test performed by applying a 2-cm area of product lateral to the eye for five consecutive nights is recommended for any new cosmetic purchased by the patient.

SUMMARY

The treatment of sensitive skin is a medical challenge. Any treatment must address the barrier disruption, immune hyperreactivity, and heightened sensory responsiveness that characterize sensitive skin. If the sensitive skin is due to a visible dermatosis, the treatment can be streamlined, but if the sensitive skin is invisible, a long-treatment algorithm must be followed to further elucidate valuable diagnostic information. Finally, basic skin-care and cosmetic recommendations can be made to the sensitive-skin patient to minimize the chances of encountering a problem.

REFERENCES

1. Draelos ZD. Noxious sensory perceptions in patients with mild to moderate rosacea treated with azelaic acid 15% gel. Cutis 2004; 74:257.
2. Draelos ZD. Cumulative benefit of topical polyhydroxy acids in combination with azelaic acid for the treatment of rosacea. J Cosmet Dermatol. In press.
3. Berardesca E, Distante F, Vignoli GP, Oresajo C, Green B. Alpha hydroxyacids modulate stratum corneum barrier function. Br J Dermatol 1997; 137:934–938.
4. Draelos ZD. Sensitive skin: perceptions, evaluation, and treatment. Contact Dermatitis 1997; 8:67.
5. Joyeux M, Lobstein A, Anton R, Mortier F. Comparative antilipoperoxidant, antinecrotic and scavenging properties of terpenes and biflavones from Ginkgo and some flavonoids. Planta Med 1995; 61:126.
6. Fox C. Technically speaking. Cosmet Toiletries 2001; 116:42.
7. Katiyar SK, Elmets CA. Green tea and skin. Arch Dermatol 2000; 136:989.
8. Katiyar SK, Elmets CA, Agarwal R, et al. Protection against ultraviolet-B radiation-induced local and systemic suppression of contact hypersensitivity and edema responses in C3H/HeN mice by green tea polyphenols. Photochem Photobiol 1995; 62:861.
9. McKeown E. Aloe vera. Cosmet Toiletries 1987; 102:64.
10. Waller T. Aloe vera. Cosmet Toiletries 1992; 107:53.

21

Tests for Sensitive Skin

Manuela Carrera and Enzo Berardesca
San Gallicano Dermatological Institute, Rome, Italy

INTRODUCTION

Sensitive skin is a condition of subjective cutaneous hyperreactivity to environmental factors. Subjects experiencing this condition report exaggerated reactions when their skin is in contact with cosmetics, soaps, and sunscreens, and they often report worsening after exposure to dry and cold climates.

Although no sign of irritation is commonly detected, itching, burning, stinging, and a tight sensation are constantly present. Generally, substances that are not commonly considered irritants are involved in this abnormal response. They include many ingredients of cosmetics such as dimethylsulfoxide (DMSO), benzoyl peroxide preparations, salicylic acid, propylene glycol, amyldimethylaminobenzoic acid, and 2-ethoxyethyl methoxycinnamate (1).

Sensitive skin and subjective irritation are widespread but still far from being completely defined and understood. Burckhardt (2) hypothesized a correlation between sensitive skin and constitutional anomalies and/or other triggering factors such as occupational skin diseases or chronic exposure to irritants. In contrast, Bjornberg (3) supported that no constitutional factors play a role in the pathogenesis of sensitive skin, although the presence of dermatitis demonstrates a general increase in skin reactivity to primary irritants lasting months.

EPIDEMIOLOGIC STUDIES

Recent findings suggest that higher sensitivity can be due to different mechanisms. Hyperreactors may have a thinner stratum corneum (SC) with a reduced corneocyte area causing a higher transcutaneous penetration of water-soluble chemicals (4).

Until 1977, Frosch and Kligman (5), by testing different irritants, showed a 14% incidence of sensitive skin in the normal population, likely correlated with a thin, permeable SC, which makes these subjects more susceptible to chemical irritation. Many epidemiologic studies have been carried out to assess whether a correlation with sex, age, skin type, or race could be found (6).

Contradictory findings have been reported. Some authors (7–9) documented a higher reactivity to irritants mostly in females; others noted that male subjects were directionally or significantly more reactive than female (6). Other experimental studies did not confirm this observation. Bjornberg (10), using six different irritants by patch-test application, found no sex-related differences. Moreover, Lammintausta et al. (11), studying the response to open- and patch-test application of sodium lauryl sulfate (SLS), found mild interindividual variations in transepidermal water loss (TEWL) and dielectric water content values but no sex-related differences in the reaction pattern.

In 1982, Frosch and Wissing (12), using DMSO, demonstrated a correlation between the minimal erythema dose (MED) and the response to irritants: the higher the inflammation, the lower the MED. Subsequently, a correlation between skin reactivity and skin type was reported: stronger reactions were detected in subjects with skin type I (13). However, in a total of 110 subjects covering all six skin types, the SLS dose–response generated by applying the substance under four-hour occlusion demonstrated that there was no significant difference between the groups. Even for type VI skin, the dose–response curve fell within the general pattern (14). In fact, conflicting findings have been reported on the incidence of allergic contact dermatitis in different races (15–18). Although there is a clinical consensus that blacks are less reactive and Asians are more reactive than Caucasians, the data supporting this hypothesis rarely reach statistical significance (19). Conflicting data have also been found on subjective (sensory) irritation. Frosch and Kligman (20) reported that most common "stingers" were light-complexioned persons of Celtic ancestry who sunburned easily and tanned poorly. Grove et al. (21) found no skin-type propensity to stinging; they noted that increased stinging was related mainly to the person's history of sensitivity to soaps, cosmetics, and drugs. Arakami et al. (18), instead, found no significant differences after SLS testing, but significant subjective sensory differences between Japanese and German women. So, they concluded that Japanese women may complain about stronger sensations reflecting a different cultural behavior rather than measurable differences in skin physiology; however, a faster penetration of SLS in Japanese cannot be excluded.

Moreover, in eczema, skin reactivity is enhanced (22). Studies performed on animal models demonstrated that strong irritant reactions in guinea pigs significantly reduced the threshold of skin irritation (23). In contrast, hyporeactive states may be induced by skin treatment. Subclinical dermatitis, after repeated cutaneous irritation by open application, may induce skin hyporeactivity (24). This can also be one of the mechanisms of false-negative patch test.

Skin reactivity seems also to change depending on age. The literature is contradictory. For example, Nilzen and Voss Lagerlund (25) reported higher reactivity patch-test reactions to soaps and detergents in the elderly, whereas Bettley and Donoghue (26) reported a lower reactivity in the same group. Coenraads et al. (27) demonstrated a higher skin reactivity to croton oil in the older patient group, but no differences by testing thimochinone or croton aldehyde. In 1993, Grove (28), by testing croton oil, cationic and anionic surfactants, weak acids, and solvents, reported a lower susceptibility in older subjects in terms of less severe skin reactions. Recently, Robinson (6) confirmed this low reactivity; in fact, in his study, subjects of the oldest age (56–74 years) were directionally or significantly less reactive than younger subjects. Moreover, Wohrl et al. (9) noted that although the rate of positive reactions to nickel and thimerosal decreased with ages, fragrance mix, and metallic mercury stayed at the same level through all ages. The overall sensitization rate was highest in children less than 10 years old and decreased steadily with increasing age, being lowest among patients more than 70 years.

Aged skin seems to have a reduced inflammatory response either to irritants or to irritation induced by ultraviolet light (UV) (29). The UV-B-induced increase in both TEWL and DNA synthesis was significantly diminished, with decreased epidermal hyperplasia evident in intrinsically aged epidermis against that of young mice (30).

In contrast, after irritating the skin, increased TEWL values were recorded in the older subjects when compared with the young. This finding could be related to a deficient "early warning detection system" in the elderly.

The lack of any visible response can lead to a continued exposure to external irritants and to a higher risk of damage to skin barrier function.

CLINICAL PARAMETERS

Sensitive skin can be defined in both subjective and objective terms. Subjective perceptions of sensitive skin are derived from the patient's observations regarding stinging, burning, pruritus, and tightness following various environmental stimuli. Because of the lack of clinical signs, the phenomenon of sensitive skin is difficult to document. Attempts to identify clinical parameters in subjects with subjective irritation indicate that these individuals tend to have a less hydrated, less supple, more erythematous, and more telangiectatic skin when compared with the normal population. In particular, significant differences were found for erythema and hydration/dryness (31).

TESTS FOR SENSITIVE SKIN

Approximately 50% of patients with sensitive skin demonstrate their uncomfortable symptoms without accompanying visible signs of inflammation (32).

For this reason, new methods of sensory testing have been increasingly utilized to provide definite information.

QUANTIZATION OF CUTANEOUS THERMAL SENSATION

The superficial skin layer includes sensory nerve fibers connected to specialized receptors such as corpuscles or naked nerve endings. Three types of fibers are generally recognized in the subclass of sensory fibers.

1. A-β fibers, myelinated (conduction velocity of 2–30 m/sec) and the largest fibers, mediate the touch, vibration, and pressure sensation.
2. A-δ fibers, smaller and myelinated (conduction velocity of >30 m/sec), mediate cold and pain sensation.
3. C-fibers, slowest, smaller, and non-myelinated (conduction velocity of <2 m/sec), mediate warm and itching sensation. C-fibers subserve most of the autonomic peripheral functions.

Quantitative sensory testing (QST) methods have been utilized mainly to study the impairment of somatosensory function in neurological diseases; particularly, in dermatology, thermal sensation testing analysis is becoming the most utilized QST technique (33). It assesses the function in free nerve endings and their associated small myelinated and non-myelinated fibers. Thermal somatosensory testing allows the clinician to test small nerve fibers. In this technique, thresholds for warmth, cold, as well as hot and cold pain are quantitatively measured and then compared with age-matched normal population values. A deviation from the normal range can indicate the existence of peripheral nerve disease. A small device, called a thermode, is attached to the patient's skin. The device is capable of heating or cooling the skin, as needed. Technically, the thermode is based on Peltier elements. It consists of semiconductor junctions that, by the passage of an electric current, produce a temperature gradient between the upper and lower stimulator surfaces produced.

In the center of the thermode, a thermocouple records the temperature. TSA-II® (Medoc Company, Ramat Yshai, Israel) is considered one of the most advanced portable thermal sensory testing devices. It operates between 0 and 54°C.

The TSA-II measures thresholds for four sensory submodalities:

1. Warm sensation, usually at 1 to 2°C above adaptation temperature, mediated by a C-fiber sensation.
2. Cold sensation, at a similar range below adaptation, mediated by A-δ fibers.
3. Heat-induced pain, threshold around 45°C, mediated by C-fiber sensation mostly, with some involvement of A-δ fibers.
4. Cold-induced pain, the most variable and difficult to assess of all previous modalities, at about 10°C, mediated by a combination of both C and A-δ fibers.

Basically, it measures the hot or cold threshold and the suprathreshold pain magnitude. The thermode in contact with the skin produces a stimulus whose intensity increases or decreases until the subject feels the sensation. As the sensation is felt, the subject is asked to press a button. The test is then repeated two more times to get a mean value. Using this method, artifacts can occur because of the lag time the stimulus needs to reach the brain. This inconvenience can be avoided by using relatively slow rates of increasing stimuli.

The stimulus can also be increased stepwise and the subject is asked to say whether the sensation is felt. When a positive answer is given, the stimulus is decreased by one-half the initial step and so on, until no sensation is felt. The subject's response determines the intensity of the next stimulus. The limitation of this second method is that a longer performance time is required.

STINGING TEST

Stinging seems to be a variant of pain that develops rapidly and fades quickly any time the appropriate sensory nerve is stimulated. Although this method lacks objective criteria, it is widely accepted as a marker of sensitivity and has often been utilized in skin irritation studies (5,31). It provides information to establish those subjects experiencing invisible cutaneous irritation.

It is performed by applying hydrosoluble substances such as lactic acid or capsaicin to the skin. This test is usually carried out on the nasolabial fold, a site richly innervated with sensory fibers. This may be performed utilizing two methods (34):

1. Subjects first undergo a facial sauna for 5 to 15 minutes or are conditioned to a state of profuse sweating in an environmental chamber at 110°F and 80% relative humidity, then an aqueous 5% lactic acid solution is applied with a cotton swab on the test site.
2. A 10% aqueous solution of lactic acid at room temperature is rubbed with a cotton swab on the test site.

To have a more reliable response, it is recommended to apply an inert control substance, such as saline solution, to the contralateral test site. After application, within a few minutes, a moderate-to-severe stinging sensation occurs for the "stingers group." These subjects are then asked to describe the intensity of the sensation using a point scale. Hyperreactors, particularly those with a positive dermatologic history, have higher scores. An alternative test involves the application of 2 mL of 90% aqueous DMSO in a small glass cup on the cheek for five minutes. This procedure causes intense burning in stingers and, after application, tender wheal and persistent erythema often occur. In contrast, lactic acid produces no visible changes.

Using this screening procedure, 20% of the subjects exposed to 5% lactic acid in a hot, humid environment were found to develop a stinging response (5). Lammintausta et al. (35) confirmed these observations. In this study, 18%

of subjects were identified as stingers. In addition, stingers were found to develop stronger reactions to materials causing non-immunologic contact urticaria, to have increased values of TEWL, and to have increased blood flow velocimetric values after application of an irritant under patch test.

NICOTINATE TEST AND ERYTHEMA FOLLOWING SLS OCCLUSION TEST

A different approach to identify sensitive skin patients relies on vasodilation of the skin as opposed to cutaneous stinging. Many investigators prefer this approach because objective changes can be visually and biomechanically assessed. These two tests are the nicotinate test (36) and erythema assessment following SLS exposure (37). In the first test, methyl nicotinate, a potent vasodilator, is applied to the upper third of the ventral forearm in concentrations varying between 1.4% and 13.7% for a period of 15 seconds. The vasodilatory effect is assessed by observing the erythema and employed laser Doppler velocimetry (LDV). Similar analysis can be performed following application of various concentrations of SLS to the forearm.

EVALUATION OF ITCHING RESPONSE

Recent studies show that a new class of C-fibers with an exceptionally lower conduction velocity and insensitivity to mechanical stimuli can be likely considered afferent units which mediate the itchy sensation (38).

Indeed, this subjective feeling has been extensively investigated but no explanation of the individual susceptibility to the itching sensation, without any sign of co-existing dermatitis, has been found. Laboratory investigation of the itch response has also been limited.

An itch response can experimentally be induced by topical or intradermal injections of various substances such as proteolytic enzymes, mast cell degranulators, and vasoactive agents.

Histamine injection is one of the more common procedures: histamine dihydrochloride (100 μg in 1 mL of normal saline) is injected intradermally in one forearm. Then, after different time intervals, the subject is asked to indicate the intensity of the sensation using a predetermined scale and the duration of itch is recorded. Information is always gained by the subject's self-assessment.

A correlation between whealing and itching response produced by applying a topical 4% histamine base in a group of healthy young females has been investigated by Grove. The itching response was graded by the subjects using the following scale: none, slight, moderate, and intense. The data showed that although 90% of the wheals were greater than 8 mm in diameter, only 50% of the subjects experienced pruritus; patients with large wheals often had no complaints of itching, suggesting that the dimensions of the wheals do not correlate well with pruritus. Also, itch and sting perception seem to be poorly correlated.

Grove (28) compared the cumulative lactic acid sting scores with the histamine itch scores in 32 young subjects; all the subjects who were stingers were also moderate-to-intense itchers, whereas 50% of the moderate itchers showed little or no stinging response.

Yosipovitch et al. (39), studying the effects of drugs on C-fibers during experimentally induced itch, demonstrated that topically applied aspirin rapidly decreases histamine-induced itch. This result can be attributed to the role that prostaglandins play in pain and itch sensation (40).

Localized itching, burning, and stinging can also be a feature of non-immunologic contact urticaria. This condition, still not completely defined, is characterized by a local wheal and flare after exposure of the skin to certain agents. Different combinations of mediators such as non-antibody-mediated release of histamine, prostaglandins, leukotrienes, substance P, and other inflammatory mediators may likely be involved in the pathogenesis of this disorder (41). The fact that prostaglandins and leukotrienes may play a role in the inflammatory response is supported by the inhibition of the common urticants by both oral acetylsalicylic acid and indomethacin and by topical diclofenac and naproxen gel (1). Several substances such as benzoic acid, cinnamic acid, cinnamic aldehyde, and nicotinic acid esters are capable of producing contact non-immunologic urticaria, eliciting local edema and erythematous reactions in half of the individuals. Provocative tests are usually utilized to identify subjects experiencing this condition: benzoic acid, sorbic acid, or sodium benzoate in open application will reproduce the typical symptoms in subjects suspected of contact non-immunologic urticaria.

WASHING AND EXAGGERATED IMMERSION TESTS

The aim of these tests is to identify a subpopulation with an increased tendency to produce a skin response.

In the washing test (42), subjects are asked to wash their face with a specific soap or detergent. After washing, individual sensation for tightness, burning, itching, and stinging is evaluated using a point scale previously determined.

The exaggerated immersion test is based on soaking the hands and forearms of the subjects in a solution of anionic surfactants (such as 0.35% paraffin sulfonate, 0.05% SLS-2EO) at 40°C for 20 minutes.

After soaking, hands and forearms are rinsed under tap water and patted dry with a paper towel. This procedure is repeated two more times, with a two-hour period between each soaking, for two consecutive days. Prior to the procedure, baseline skin parameters are evaluated. The other evaluations are taken two hours after the third and sixth soakings and 18 hours after the last soaking (recovery assessment). All the skin parameters are performed after the subjects have rested at least 30 minutes at $21 \pm 1°C$.

BIOENGINEERING TESTS

Recently, there has been great interest in the development of non-invasive mechanistic skin assessment allowing presumably more accurate evaluation of small cutaneous changes. Bioengineering tests should be able to measure preclinical disease, without altering the underlying skin condition. So, the physiologic changes indicative of sensitive skin can be detected at low levels prior to clinical disease presentation (43). The most useful tests are TEWL, corneometry, colorimetry, and LDV.

Transepidermal Water Loss

TEWL is used to evaluate water loss that is not attributed to active sweating from the body, through the epidermis, to the environment. It is widely used to characterize the SC barrier function, both in physiological and pathological conditions, to perform predictive irritancy tests and to evaluate the efficacy of therapeutic treatments on diseased skin (44,45). TEWL assessment can be performed using different techniques (closed-chamber method, ventilated-chamber method, and open-chamber method) (46,47). The measurements of TEWL are based on the estimation of water pressure gradient above the skin surface. The evaporative TEWL is approximately proportional to the difference between the vapor pressures measured at two different fixed heights situated perpendicularly above the skin surface and within the zone of diffusion. These open-chamber instruments consist of a detachable measuring probe connected by a cable to a portable main signal-processing unit. The Teflon® capsule of the probe head has a cylindrical measuring chamber, open at both ends where relative humidity sensors (hygrosensors) are paired with temperature sensors (thermistors). From this gradient, the evaporative TEWL value, in $g/m^2/h$, is calculated by the signal-processing units in the probe handle and main unit and digitally displayed. The instrument is extremely sensitive to any disturbances in the microclimate, whether due to environment-, instrument-, or subject-related variables.

By the use of a closed-chamber instrument, the disturbance related to external or body-induced airflows on the measurement can be avoided. The instrument consists of a closed cylindrical chamber with an air volume of 2.0 cm^3 and an open contact area of 1.0 cm^2. The chamber contains sensors for relative humidity and temperature. The humidity sensor is based on a thin-film capacitive sensor with features of rapid response time and insensitive to temperature changes in the chamber between 15 and 40°C. The sensor was directly integrated to a hand-held microprocessor-controlled electronic unit provided with a digital readout for the TEWL value.

Corneometry

Corneometry is a method to measure SC water content (electrical measurement) (48,49). The importance of water to the proper functioning of the SC is well recognized. The reliable quantification of water in the corneum and its interaction with topically applied products are, in fact, essential to understand skin physiology and develop efficient skin-care formulation. This instrument is described as being a "capacitance"-measuring device operating at low frequency (40–75 MHz), which is sensitive to the relative dielectric constant (or permittivity) of material placed in contact with the electrode surface. Because increasing the water content of the SC will, in general, increase its relative permittivity (although by a very complex and variable relationship), the device can estimate in about 20 msec the SC water content in arbitrary (relative) units. However, it should be noted that this result is based on the assumption of ceteris paribus, which may not always be valid. The probe exerts a constant pressure on the skin surface of 3.5 N and covers an area of 49 mm^2. It estimates water content in the epidermis to an approximate depth ranging between 60 and 100 μm. The presence of salts or ions on the surface of the skin tends to affect the readings. The instrument consists of a probe that should be placed normally to a hair-free skin surface with slight pressure just sufficient to start the measurement process. It is advisable to measure at least three times, once at each of three different but nearby sites, and calculate the median, to have more reproducible data (50).

Laser Doppler Velocimetry

A monochromatic light from a helium–neon laser is transmitted through optical fibers to the skin. The light is reflected with Doppler-shifted frequencies from the moving blood cells in the upper dermis at the depth of ~1 mm. The LDV extracts the frequency-shifted signal and derives an output proportional to the flux of erythrocytes in the blood flow. The shift increases with the increasing velocity. In a mechanical model that simulates the microvascular pattern of the skin, a linear relationship between LDV and blood flow was detected for low and moderate flow rates. For higher flow, photo multiple scattering and increased light absorption due to higher erythrocyte volume fraction cause a slight underestimation of the blood flow (51). LDV seems useful to discriminate between negative and positive reactions but fails to quantify strongly positive reactions (52,53). LDV is useful to evaluate the degree of skin irritation (54). The degree of the experimentally induced irritant contact dermatitis usually correlates well with the blood flow detected by LDV; however, dithranol and sodium hydroxide may give discordant results. Although LDV can be used to quantify the strength of allergic and irritant skin reactions, the technique cannot discriminate between these two types of reactions (53). LDV is one of the most important parameters to predict early signs of skin irritation (55).

Colorimetry

Surface color may be quantified using the CIE (Commission Internationale de L'Eclairage) system of tristimulus values. Commercially available devices that utilize high-sensitivity silicon photocells assure good reproducibility and accuracy. The measuring head of these units contains a high-power pulsed-xenon arc lamp, which provides two CIE illuminant standards. The color is expressed in a three-dimensional space. The coordinates of such space are expressed as L (brightness, i.e., integrated reflection of light from the surface), a^* value (color range from green to red), and b^* value (color range between blue and yellow). Natural skin tones can be stored in the colorimeter memory for direct comparison. The colorimeter allows for quantitative comparison of erythema in individuals and between individuals comparable by visual assessment: the a^* value, related to skin erythema, shows an increase in relation to irritation and skin damage (56).

CORNEOSURFAMETRY

This method investigates the interaction of surfactants with the human SC, using the reflectance colorimetry (57). It is performed as follows: cyanoacrylate skin surface stripping is taken from the volar aspect of the forearm and sprayed with the surfactant to be tested. After two hours, the sample is rinsed with tap water and stained with basic fuchsin and toluidine blue dyes for three minutes. After rinsing and drying, the sample is placed on a white reference plate and measured by reflectance colorimetry (Chroma Meter® CR200, Minolta, Osaka, Japan).

The index of redness (colorimetric index of mildness = Luminacy L^* − Chroma C^*) is taken as a parameter of the irritation caused by the surfactant. This index has a value of 68 ± 4 when water alone is sprayed on the sample and decreases when surfactant is tested, with stronger surfactants lowering the values.

Piérard et al. (58), testing different shampoo formulations in volunteers with sensitive skin, demonstrated that corneosurfametry correlates well with in vivo testing. A significant negative correlation ($P < 0.001$) was found between values of colorimetric index of mildness (CIM) and the skin compatibility parameters that include a global evaluation of the colorimetric erythemal index and the TEWL differential, both expressed in the same order of magnitude.

In the same study, corneosurfametry showed less interindividual variability than in vivo testing, allowing a better discrimination among mild products.

An interesting finding showed that sensitive skin is not a single condition. Goffin et al. (59) hypothesized that the response of the SC to an environmental threat might be impaired in different groups of subjects experiencing sensitive skin. Data of the corneosurfametry performed after testing eight different house-cleaning products showed that the overall SC reactivity, as calculated by the average values of the corneosurfametry index and the CIM, is significantly different ($P < 0.01$) between detergent-sensitive skin and both non-sensitive and climate/fabric sensitive skin, as well.

CONCLUSIONS

Sensitive skin represents a widespread condition of susceptibility to exogenous factors. The reason why some subjects react with subjective symptoms such as itching, burning, stinging, prickling, or tingling is unclear. However, a correlation of increased reactivity in subjects with a history of dermatitis and the association of increased reactivity with skin type I has been reported. Non-invasive evaluation of sensitive skin may successfully predict individual susceptibility to cosmetic-related adverse reaction. All the efforts in this direction appear undoubtedly important to improve tolerance to the majority of cosmetic products.

REFERENCES

1. Amin S, Engasser PG, Maibach HI. Side effects and social aspect of cosmetology. In: Baran R, Maibach HI, eds. Textbook of Cosmetic Dermatology. London: Martin Dunitz, 1998:709–746.
2. Burckhardt W. Praktische und theoretische bedeutung der alkalineutralisation und alkaliresistenzproben. Arch Klin Exp Dermatol 1964; 219:600–603.
3. Bjornberg A. Skin reactions to primary irritants in patients with hand eczema. Thesis. Goteborg: Isaccsons, 1968.
4. Berardesca E, Cespa M, Farinelli N, Rabbiosi G, Maibach HI. In vivo transcutaneous penetration of nicotinates and sensitive skin. Contact Dermatitis 1991; 25:35–38.
5. Frosch PJ, Kligman AM. A method for appraising the stinging capacity of topically applied substances. J Soc Cosmet Chemist 1977; 28:197–209.
6. Robinson MK. Population differences in acute skin irritation responses. Contact Dermatitis 2002; 46(2):86–93.
7. Agrup G. Hand eczema and other hand dermatoses in South Sweden. Academic dissertation. Acta Derm Venereol 1969; 49(suppl):161.
8. Fregert S. Occupational dermatitis in 10 years material. Contact Dermatitis 1975; 1:96–107.
9. Wohrl S, Hemmer W, Focke M, et al. Patch testing in children, adults, and the elderly: influence of age and sex on sensitization patterns. Pediatr Dermatol 2003; 20(2):119–123.
10. Bjornberg A. Skin reactions to primary irritants in men and women. Acta Derm Venereol 1975; 55:191–194.
11. Lammintausta K, Maibach HI, Wilson D. Irritant reactivity in males and females. Contact Dermatitis 1987; 17:276–280.
12. Frosch P, Wissing C. Cutaneous sensitivity to ultraviolet light and chemical irritants. Arch Dermatol Res 1982; 272:269–278.
13. Lammintausta K, Maibach HI, Wilson D. Susceptibility to cumulative and acute irritant dermatitis: an experimental approach in human volunteers. Contact Dermatitis 1988; 19:84–90.
14. McFadden JP, Wakelin SH, Basketter DA. Acute irritation thresholds in subjects with type I-type skin. Contact Dermatitis 1998; 38(3):147–149.
15. Berardesca E, Maibach H. Ethnic skin: overview of structure and function. J Am Acad Dermatol 2003; 48:S139–S142.
16. Berardesca E, Maibach HI. Contact dermatitis in Blacks. Dermatol Clin 1998; 6(3):363–368.

17. Robinson MK. Racial differences in acute and cumulative skin irritation responses between Caucasian and Asian populations. Contact Dermatitis 2000; 42(3):134–143.
18. Arakami J, Kawana S, Effendy I, et al. Differences of skin irritation between Japanese and European women. Br J Dermatol 2002; 146(6):1052–1056.
19. Modjtahedi SP, Maibach HI. Ethnicity as a possible endogenous factor in irritant contact dermatitis: comparing the irritant response among Caucasian, Blacks and Asians. Contact Dermatitis 2002; 47(5):272–278.
20. Frosch P, Kligman AM. A method for appraising the stinging capacity of topically applied substances. J Soc Cosmet Chem 1981; 28:197.
21. Grove GL, Soschin DM, Kligman AM. Adverse subjective reactions to topical agents. In: Drill VA, Lazar P, eds. Cutaneous Toxicology. New York: Raven Press, 1984:200–210.
22. Bettley FR. Non-specific irritant reactions in eczematous subjects. Br J Dermatol 1964; 76:116–121.
23. Roper SS, Jones EH. An animal model for altering the irritability threshold of normal skin. Contact Dermatitis 1985; 13:91–97.
24. Lammintausta K, Maibach HI, Wilson D. Human cutaneous irritation: induced hyporeactivity. Contact Dermatitis 1987; 17:193–198.
25. Nilzen A, Voss Lagerlund K. Epicutaneous tests with detergents and a number of other common allergens. Dermatologica 1962; 124:42–52.
26. Bettley FR, Donoghue E. The irritant effect of soap upon the normal skin. Br J Dermatol 1960; 72:67–76.
27. Coenraads PJ, Bleumink E, Nofer JP. Susceptibility to primary irritants: age dependence. Contact Dermatitis 1975; 1:377–381.
28. Grove GL. Age-associated changes in intertegumental reactivity. In: Léveque JL, Agache PG, eds. Aging Skin: Properties and Functional Changes. New York, Basel, Hong Kong: Marcel Dekker, 1993.
29. Haratake A, Uchida Y, Mimura K, et al. Intrinsically aged epidermis displays diminished UVB-induced alterations in barrier function associated with decreased proliferation. J Invest Dermatol 1997; 108(3):319–323.
30. Gilchrest BA, Stoff JS, Soter NA. Chronologic aging alters the response to ultraviolet-induced inflammation in human skin. J Invest Dermatol 1982; 79:11–15.
31. Seidenari S, Francomano M, Mantovani L. Baseline biophysical parameters in subjects with sensitive skin. Contact Dermatitis 1998; 38:311–315.
32. Simion FA, Rau AH. Sensitive skin. Cosmet Toiletries 1994; 109:43–50.
33. Yosipovitch G, Yarnitsky D. Quantitative sensory testing. In: Maibach HI, Marzulli FN, eds. Dermatotoxicology Methods: The Laboratory Worker's Vade Mecum. New York: Taylor & Francis, 1997.
34. Facial Sting Task Group, ASTM Committee; E-18.03.01.
35. Lammintausta K, Maibach HI, Wilson D. Mechanisms of subjective (sensory) irritation: propensity of non-immunologic contact urticaria and objective irritation in stingers. Dermatosen Beruf Umwelt 1988; 36(2):45–49.
36. Guy RH, Maibach HI. Rapid radial transport of methyl nicotinate in the dermis. Arch Dermatol Res 1982; 273:91–95.

37. Agner T, Serup J. Skin reaction to irritants assessed by non-invasive bioengineering methods. Contact Dermatitis 1989; 20:352–359.
38. Schmelz M, Schmidt R, Bickel A, Handwerker HO, Torebjörk HE. Specific C-receptors for itch in human skin. J Neurosci 1997; 17(20):8003–8008.
39. Yosipovitch G, Ademola J, Lui P, Amin S, Maibach HI. Topically applied aspirin rapidly decreases histamine-induced itch. Acta Derm Venereol (Stockh) 1977; 77:46–48.
40. Lovell CR, Burton PA, Duncan EH, Burton JL. Prostaglandins and pruritus. Br J Dermatol 1976; 94:273–275.
41. Lahti A, Maibach HI. Species specificity of nonimmunologic contact urticaria: guinea pig, rat and mouse. J Am Acad 1985; 13:66–69.
42. Hannuksela A, Hannuksela M. Irritant effects of a detergent in wash and chamber tests. Contact Dermatitis 1995; 32:163–166.
43. Andreassi L. Bioengineering in dermatology: general aspects and perspectives. Clin Dermatol 1995; 13(4):289–292.
44. Pinnagoda J, Tupker RA, et al. Guidelines for transepidermal water loss (TEWL) measurement. A report from the Standardization Group of the European Society of Contact Dermatitis. Contact Dermatitis 1990; 22(3):164–178.
45. Berardesca E, Vignoli GP, et al. Effects of water temperature on surfactant-induced skin irritation. Contact Dermatitis 1995; 32(2):83–87.
46. Wilson DR, Maibach H. Transepidermal water loss: a review. In: Lévêque JL, ed. Cutaneous Investigation in Health and Disease: Noninvasive Methods and Instrumentation. New York: Marcel Dekker, 1989:113–133.
47. Lévêque JL. Measurement of transepidermal water loss. In: Lévêque JL, ed. Cutaneous Investigation in Health and Disease: Noninvasive Methods and Instrumentation. New York: Marcel Dekker, 1989:135–153.
48. Fluhr J, Gloor M, Lazzerini S, et al. Comparative study of five instruments measuring stratum corneum hydration (corneometer CM 820 and CM 825, Skicon 200, Nova DPM 9003, DermaLab). Part I. In vitro. Skin Res Technol 1999; 5:161–170.
49. Barel AO, Clarys P. In vitro calibration of the capacitance method (Corneometer CM 825) and conductance method (Skicon-200) for the evaluation of the hydration state of the skin. Skin Res Technol 1997; 3:107–113.
50. Berardesca E. EEMCO guidance for the assessment of the stratum corneum hydration: electrical methods. Skin Res Technol 1997; 3:126–132.
51. Andersen KE, Staberg B. Quantization of contact allergy in guinea pigs by measuring changes in skin blood flow and skin fold thickness. Acta Derm Venereol 1985; 65(1):37–42.
52. Serup J, Staberg B. Quantification of weal reactions with laser Doppler flowmetry: comparative blood flow measurements of the oedematous centre and the perilesional flare of skin-prick histamine weals. Allergy 1985; 40(4):233–237.
53. Staberg B, Serup J. Allergic and irritant skin reactions evaluated by laser Doppler flowmetry. Contact Dermatitis 1988; 18(1):40–45.
54. Bircher A, De Boer EM, et al. Guidelines for measurement of cutaneous blood flow by laser Doppler flowmetry. A report from the Standardization Group of the European Society of Contact Dermatitis. Contact Dermatitis 1994; 30(2):65–72.
55. Zuang VR, Archer G, Berardesca E. Detection of skin irritation potential of cosmetics by non-invasive measurements. Skin Pharmacol Appl Skin Physiol 2000; 13:358–371.

56. Agner T, Serup J. Sodium lauryl sulphate for irritant patch testing: a dose–response study using bioengineering methods for determination of skin irritation. J Invest Dermatol 1990; 95(5):543–547.
57. Piérard GE, Goffin V, Piérard Franchimont C. Corneosulfametry: a predictive assessment of the interaction of personal care cleansing products with human stratum corneum. Dermatology 1994; 189:152–156.
58. Piérard GE, Goffin V, Hermanns-Le T, Arrese JE, Piérard Franchimont C. Surfactant-induced dermatitis: comparison of corneosulfametry with predictive testing on human and reconstructed skin. J Am Acad Dermatol 1995; 33:462–469.
59. Goffin V, Piérard Franchimont C, Piérard GE. Sensitive skin and stratum corneum reactivity to household cleaning products. Contact Dermatitis 1996; 34:81–85.

22

Cosmetic Intolerance Syndrome

Marina Goldovsky, Patricia G. Engasser, and Howard I. Maibach
*Department of Dermatology, University of California,
San Francisco, California, U.S.A.*

Is there a specific trigger to the cosmetic intolerance syndrome? What is the underlying pathophysiology? These are the questions that the clinician caring for these patients must attempt to answer in order to treat these patients successfully.

Cosmetic intolerance syndrome has been described as an adverse skin reaction of individuals who are no longer able to tolerate a wide range of cosmetic products (1). As, frequently, there is a discrepancy between objective signs of disease and patients' perception of symptoms, this syndrome can be particularly challenging to physicians' diagnostic abilities and management options. Such patients often confront dermatologists treating reactions to cosmetics, by complaining of facial burning, itching, or stinging after applying eye shadows, sunscreens, moisturizers, cleansers, and so on. Allergic reactions due to cosmetics occur much less commonly than irritant reactions in these cases.

These patients may manifest objective inflammation of the skin or have only subjective symptoms. Fisher (2) used the term "status cosmeticus" for the condition in which a patient is no longer able to tolerate the use of any cosmetic. Indeed, some of these patients seem to experience irritation (subjective and/or objective) from cosmetics, but during the evolution of this disorder, they become intolerant of many, if not all, topical agents, including drugs. Some patients have occult allergic contact dermatitis (ACD), allergic photocontact dermatitis, or contact urticarial reactions, and the causal agents are documented by careful chemical review and patch testing. Overall, however, patch testing for ACD and photopatch testing for photo-ACD are negative in the majority of these patients.

Lachapelle and Maibach (3) provide details of diagnostic patch, photo-patch, open, and prick tests to rule in or out allergic, photoallergic, and contact urticaria. Wohlrab et al. (4) described six patients with morbus morbihan (MM) in their study to have transient symptoms including reddening, swelling, and itching shortly after the application of cosmetics. Allergologic examination showed the origin of these episodes to be correlated with immunologic contact urticaria (ICU) caused by fragrances and preservatives. In their study of MM, a prolonged inflammatory response with edema and increased blood flow was observed after ICU induction in the area of the affected facial skin and was monitored by ultrasound and laser Doppler flowmetry. Hypothetically, an impaired function of the cutaneous lymphatic vessels might play a crucial role in the development of MM as well as of cosmetic intolerance. Amin et al. (5) details the contact urticaria syndrome.

The etiology and pathophysiology of the cosmetic intolerance syndrome are complex, but they are often secondary to a combination of endogenous and exogenous factors (Table 1). Cosmetic intolerance syndrome is associated with the following endogenous conditions: rosacea, seborrhea, and atopic dermatitis. Patients with a seborrheic/rosacea diathesis with or without inflammation seem to have induced cosmetic intolerance by overusing cleansers, toners, moisturizers, and cosmetics. Both of these conditions may be accompanied by facial erythema or scaling.

Rosacea, atopic dermatitis, and seborrheic dermatitis when present in atypical forms often confuse the clinician. We believe the face (as well as palm, scalp,

Table 1 Facial Intolerance to Cosmetics and Skin-Care Agents: A Profile of Intolerant Skin

Exogenous	
Subjective irritation	Common but difficult for some patients to realize the cause-and-effect relationship
Objective irritation	Common but often difficult morphology to observe on face [i.e., occult (hidden) dermatitis]
ACD	Often not morphologically obvious on the face
Photo-ACD	Rare, discerned by phototesting
Contact urticaria	
Endogenous	
Seborrheic dermatitis	Common with a small percentage having an atypical morphology
Rosacea diathesis	Highly complex biology
Atopic dermatitis	May be only residual of childhood atopic dermatitis
Status eczematous[a] (status cosmeticus)	Some patients may have no other definable endogenous or exogenous factors
Dysmorphobia[a]	Rare, psychologic diagnosis made by exclusion

[a]The patients are the most difficult to treat successfully.
Abbreviations: ACD, allergic contact dermatitis; photo-ACD, photoallergic contact dermatitis.
Source: From Ref. 1.

and scrotum) hides the inflammation. Frequent close examination of the face as well as other anatomic areas helps rule in or out these entities. This assessment is important because some patients with endogenous components or cosmetic intolerance require anti-inflammatory therapy to reverse the condition.

Maibach et al. (6) noted, when studying irritant dermatitis, that workers whose hand dermatitis appeared "healed" after an absence from work for weeks to months may relapse quickly on return to work despite protective measures. Other workers' dermatitis may fail to clear despite a prolonged absence from work. Although the skin appears healed, it is not functionally intact and is even more vulnerable to further irritation.

Freeman and Maibach (7) examined this question by the application of 2% aqueous sodium laurel sulfate (SLS) with occlusive patch testing. The protocol used daily challenges and the recording of visual and palpation grades, as well as instrumental analysis. Transepidermal water loss increased after trauma as expected but healed after the first application. The highest level was immediately after patch removal. By the seventh day, the skin appeared normal on visual examination. However, an additional SLS patch produced an even greater response than initially and a much slower return to normal. This strongly suggests that although the skin can look normal, it is not functioning at a normal level. Thus, there may exist a biological dichotomy between the normal appearing phenotype and the underlying biochemical/pathophysiologic condition. We hypothesize a similar condition exists in the cosmetic intolerance syndrome. These patients have frequently used multiple skin-care products that have left their facial skin vulnerable.

Cosmetic intolerant patients usually present with multiple subjective complaints. Therefore, a thorough and often repeated history is essential. Patch testing (Table 2) to standard allergens as well to all the patient's skin-care products can be useful at times but proves to be negative in the majority of cases. Nevertheless, the physician should recommend the patient to stop the usage of cosmetics.

Table 3 outlines a management strategy. Even if one cannot identify the underlying cause, an intervention of "skin rest" should be implemented. Prolonged compliance with the proposed elimination program aids most patients.

Table 2 Patch, Photopatch, and Open/Prick Tests

Condition	Test
ACD	Patch test (3)
Photo-ACD	Photopatch test (3)
ICU and non-immunologic contact urticaria	Open/prick tests (3)

Abbreviations: ACD, allergic contact dermatitis; photo-ACD, photoallergic contact dermatitis; ICU, immunologic contact urticaria.
Source: From Ref. 3.

Table 3   Patient Management: Intolerant to Cosmetic Usage[a]

Examine every cosmetic and skin-care agent, including semiquantitative chemical
 composition
Patch and photopatch tests to rule out occult ACD and photo-ACD
Careful history and examination of chemical components to rule in or out NICU and ICU
 (see text for details). Open testing, and, if negative, prick testing is indicated to rule in or
 out this diagnosis.
Limit skin to
 Water washing without soap or detergent
 Lip cosmetics, as desired, unless lip symptoms are present
 Eye cosmetics, as desired, if the eyelids are not symptomatic
 Face powder, as desired (rare exceptions only)
 Glycerin and rose water as moisturizer, only if needed
 Three to six months of avoidance of other skin-care agents and cosmetics
Watch for and test, if necessary, depression and other neuropsychiatric aspects

[a]Patients requiring such testing are identified by BSI history (burn, sting, and/or itch) in minutes after
exposure.
Abbreviations: ACD, allergic contact dermatitis; photo-ACD, photo-allergic contact dermatitis;
NICU, non-immunologic contact urticaria; ICU, immunologic contact urticaria.
Source: From Ref. 1.

After three to six months, they are able to gradually return to the use of other
cosmetics. Additions to their regimens of skin care should be made one at a
time—not more frequently than every two to four weeks (Table 3). Physician
supervision and communication remains critical at this juncture. The final
program should be simple and limited in the number of cosmetics and frequency
of usage.

Cotterill (8) reported that some patients who experience continuous facial
burning without objective signs have a disturbed body image, dysmorphobia, and
complain of physical defects without objective evidence. Frequently, these
patients suffer from depression and even suicidal ideation. They require time-
consuming care. It is often difficult for these patients to accept the skilled psychiatric care that some of them need.

The cosmetic intolerance syndrome is not a simple entity but rather a sign
and symptom complex due to multiple contributing factors. There are endogenous and exogenous components involved, and the pathophysiology involves
cytokines and chemokines released in response to irritation. Even though the
skin may appear normal, it is not and requires a lengthy recovery period prior
to slowly reinitiating cosmetic usage. Baron, Barel, and Shai detail related
issues of cosmetic physiology, chemistry, and pathophysiology; Zhai and
Maibach (9) document dermatotoxicologic principles in preventing such
adverse reactions.

REFERENCES

1. Maibach HI, Engasser PG. Dermatitis due to cosmetics. In: Fisher AA, ed. Contact Dermatitis. 3rd ed. Philadelphia: Lea & Febiger, 1986:368–382.
2. Fisher AA. Current contact news (cosmetic actions and reactions: therapeutic, irritant and allergic). Cutis 1980; 26:22.
3. Lachapelle J-M, Maibach HI. Patch Testing and Prick Testing. Berlin: Springer, 2003.
4. Wohlrab J, Lueftl M, Marsch WC. Persistent erythema and edema of the midthird and upper aspect of the face (morbus morbihan): evidence of hidden immunologic contact urticaria and impaired lymphatic drainage. J Am Acad Dermatol 2005; 52:595.
5. Amin S, Lahti A, Maibach HI. Contact Urticaria. Boca Raton: CRC Press, 1997.
6. Maibach HI, et al. Tendency to irritation: sensitive skin. J Am Acad Dermatol 1989; 21:833.
7. Freeman S, Maibach HI. Study of irritant contact dermatitis produced by repeat patch testing with sodium lauryl sulfate and assessed by visual methods, transepidermal water loss and laser Doppler velocimetry. J Am Acad Dermatol 1988; 18:65.
8. Cotterill JG. Dermatological nondisease: a common and potentially fatal disturbance of body image. Br J Dermatol 1981; 104:611.
9. Zhai H, Maibach HI. Dermatotoxicology. 6th ed. Boca Raton: CRC Press, 2004.

Index